P9-AGN-474

SECOND EDITION

Health Behavior Theory
for Public Health

Principles, Foundations, and Applications

Ralph J. DiClemente, PhD

Charles H. Candler Professor
Rollins School of Public Health
Emory University
Atlanta, GA

Laura F. Salazar, PhD

Professor
Institute of Public Health Georgia
State University
Atlanta, GA

Richard A. Crosby, PhD

Good Samaritan Endowed
Professor
Department of Health Behavior
College of Public Health
University of Kentucky
Lexington, KY

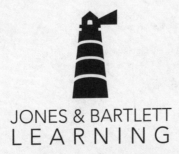

JONES & BARTLETT
LEARNING

World Headquarters
Jones & Bartlett Learning
5 Wall Street
Burlington, MA 01803
978-443-5000
info@jblearning.com
www.jblearning.com

Jones & Bartlett Learning books and products are available through most bookstores and online booksellers. To contact Jones & Bartlett Learning directly, call 800-832-0034, fax 978-443-8000, or visit our website, www.jblearning.com.

Substantial discounts on bulk quantities of Jones & Bartlett Learning publications are available to corporations, professional associations, and other qualified organizations. For details and specific discount information, contact the special sales department at Jones & Bartlett Learning via the above contact information or send an email to specialsales@jblearning.com.

Copyright © 2019 by Jones & Bartlett Learning, LLC, an Ascend Learning Company

All rights reserved. No part of the material protected by this copyright may be reproduced or utilized in any form, electronic or mechanical, including photocopying, recording, or by any information storage and retrieval system, without written permission from the copyright owner.

The content, statements, views, and opinions herein are the sole expression of the respective authors and not that of Jones & Bartlett Learning, LLC. Reference herein to any specific commercial product, process, or service by trade name, trademark, manufacturer, or otherwise does not constitute or imply its endorsement or recommendation by Jones & Bartlett Learning, LLC and such reference shall not be used for advertising or product endorsement purposes. All trademarks displayed are the trademarks of the parties noted herein. *Health Behavior Theory for Public Health: Principles, Foundations, and Applications, Second Edition* is an independent publication and has not been authorized, sponsored, or otherwise approved by the owners of the trademarks or service marks referenced in this product.

There may be images in this book that feature models; these models do not necessarily endorse, represent, or participate in the activities represented in the images. Any screenshots in this product are for educational and instructive purposes only. Any individuals and scenarios featured in the case studies throughout this product may be real or fictitious, but are used for instructional purposes only.

This publication is designed to provide accurate and authoritative information in regard to the Subject Matter covered. It is sold with the understanding that the publisher is not engaged in rendering legal, accounting, or other professional service. If legal advice or other expert assistance is required, the service of a competent professional person should be sought.

Production Credits

VP, Product Management: David D. Cella
Director of Product Management: Michael Brown
Product Specialist: Carter McAlister
Production Manager: Carolyn Rogers Pershouse
Vendor Manager: Molly Hogue
Senior Marketing Manager: Sophie Fleck Teague
Manufacturing and Inventory Control Supervisor:
    Amy Bacus
Composition: codeMantra U.S. LLC

Project Management: codeMantra U.S. LLC
Cover Design: Michael O'Donnell
Rights & Media Specialist: Merideth Tumasz
Media Development Editor: Shannon Sheehan
Cover Image (Part Opener, Chapter Opener):
    © lzf/Shutterstock, Henrik Sorensen/Getty Images,
    MeskPhotography/Shutterstock, Hero Images/Getty Images
Printing and Binding: Edwards Brothers Malloy
Cover Printing: Edwards Brothers Malloy

Library of Congress Cataloging-in-Publication Data
Names: DiClemente, Ralph J., author. | Salazar, Laura Francisca, 1960-
   author. | Crosby, Richard A., 1959- author.
Title: Health behavior theory for public health / Ralph DiClemente, Laura
   Salazar, Richard Crosby.
Description: 2nd. | Burlington, Massachusetts: Jones & Bartlett Learning,
   [2019] | Includes bibliographical references and index.
Identifiers: LCCN 2018008730 | ISBN 9781284129885 (paperback: alk. paper)
Subjects: | MESH: Public Health | Health Behavior | Health Promotion |
   Models, Theoretical
Classification: LCC RA776.9 | NLM WA 100 | DDC 614.4—dc23
LC record available at https://lccn.loc.gov/2018008730

6048

Printed in the United States of America
22 21 20 19 18   10 9 8 7 6 5 4 3 2 1

Dedications:

To my three girls, Gina, Sahara, and Sianna. You are my Love, my Joy, my Passion, my Hope, and my Life. RJD

To my wonderful and inspiring co-authors whose friendship, support, and mentorship mean the world to me and whose dedication and contribution to public health are an inspiration to all. LFS

This book is dedicated to the next generation of public health professionals – the future of this profession, and the people it serves, are in your hands. RAC

Special Dedication:

James W. Curran, MD, MPH

Dean, Rollins School of Public Health, Emory University

To a friend, colleague, and public health leader. You have made an indelible footprint on the landscape of public health. Your leadership, passion, and scholarship are widely respected and an inspiration for all of us fortunate to serve with you in your effort to champion a public health of consequence.

Contents

Foreword

John S. Santelli, MD, MPH

Dr. Santelli is a Professor in the Department of Population and Family Health and Pediatrics in the Mailman School of Public Health at Columbia University.

Theory is essential in understanding health behaviors and is critical in guiding health research. Theory helps us organize and understand information; it focuses attention on key issues; and it helps us select constructs for questionnaires. Theory is fundamental in designing, implementing, and evaluating interventions and in constructing policies to improve health and prevent disease. Thus, theory is essential to the work of public health.

Health behaviors are influenced by factors related to the individual but are also shaped by the myriad of social and structural influences. For example, to understand adolescent contraceptive use, drug use, smoking, and drinking patterns, one needs to understand the origins of these behaviors and the social and environmental forces supporting them. Physicians who work in public health and address human behavior are well aware of this importance; while medicine is principally guided by a variety of biological theories, physicians rapidly come to understand that effective pharmacologic interventions often fail unless they address the behaviors of patients. Public health professionals intuitively grasp the importance of behavior change in influencing behaviors across the lifespan—from adolescent pregnancy prevention, to injury prevention and prevention of chronic disease, to promoting healthy aging.

The "new public health" focuses on health promotion and the factors that enable individuals and communities to attain optimal health (Awofeso, 2004). In this new era, social education, and economic actions are provided to support attitudinal, behavioral, and social change. For example, health behavior theory has been highly influential in human immunodeficiency virus (HIV) prevention and treatment over the past 30 years, although the focus of interventions and the specifics of health behavior theory have shifted over time. In the early years of the HIV pandemic, behavioral risk reduction—coupled with latex condoms and clean needles—was the only public health tool for prevention of new HIV infection (Lyles et al., 2007). With the advent of highly effective pharmacologic treatments, the new behavioral challenge became encouraging adherence to drug regiments. And when we discovered that effective pharmacologic treatment could be an effective HIV prevention strategy (so-called "treatment as prevention" approach, Cohen, McCauley, & Gamble, 2012), we realized again that behavioral change was essential to the success of this new biomedical strategy.

In my field, adolescent health, understanding the origins of and influences on health risk behaviors is critical to effective health promotion. A recent *Lancet* Commission report outlined the triple dividend of investing in adolescent health: improving the health adolescents today, across the lifespan, and for the next generation (Patton et al., 2016). These investments need to address the social and structural factors (Viner et al., 2012) that influence adolescent risk behaviors. Behavioral theory is essential to understanding these social forces and promoting adolescent health and well-being.

Health Behavior Theory for Public Health, Second Edition addresses the need to provide students with a highly accessible (easy to understand) collection of basic "tools" needed to design, implement, and evaluate health promotion programs. The most essential of these tools is an accurate understanding of the tenets and constructs comprising commonly used behavioral and social science theories. The selection of theories is carefully balanced to provide students with the diverse skill sets that are needed to design effective health promotion programs.

In this new edition, all chapters have been updated and refined to improve the student learning experience—and new chapters added. All chapters also now contain pull quotes to highlight key points relevant to the chapter objectives. Chapter 9 on ecological strategies has been greatly augmented by adding two key theories commonly used to help resolve social inequalities: minority stress theory and intersectionality theory. The authors have updated applied examples, with one featuring the highly successful structural-level of intervention of Citibike in New York City and a second illustrating an ecological intervention in a campus-based violence prevention program. A new chapter (Chapter 13) teaches students the value of combining multiple theories to better understand—and thus better resolve—social inequalities in preventing disease. Using Intervention Mapping as the framework, this chapter provides an efficient set of practices that can be vital to public health professionals who are faced with challenges not easily addressed by the use of one theory in isolation.

Finally, the three authors of this revised text (Ralph, Rick, and Laura) are among the "best of the best", superb social and behavioral scientists who have devoted years to improving health via theory-driven, innovative public health interventions. Their life's work has been dedicated to health promotion. Their thinking in this new edition is very much aligned with modern thinking about ecological influences. Moreover, because it is an authored text, there is strong integration of the chapters. Visuals, margin quotes, learning objectives, practice questions, make the text a unified learning experience. With this second edition, they have created a "one-stop shop" to prepare the next generation of public health professionals to carry on the important work of behavior change.

▶ References

Awofeso, N. (2004). What's new about the "new public health"? *American Journal of Public Health, 94*(5), 705–709.

Cohen, M. S., McCauley, M., & Gamble, T. R. (2012). HIV treatment as prevention and HPTN 052. *Current Opinion in HIV and AIDS, 7*(2), 99.

Lyles, C. M., Kay, L. S., Crepaz, N., Herbst, J. H., Passin, W. F., Kim, A. S., … Mullins, M. M. (2007). Best-evidence interventions: Findings from a systematic review of HIV behavioral interventions for US populations at high risk, 2000–2004. *American Journal of Public Health, 97*(1), 133–143.

Patton, G.C., Sawyer, S. M., Santelli, J. S., Ross, D. A., Afifi, R., Allen, N. B., … Viner, R. M. (2016). Our future: A *Lancet* commission on adolescent health and wellbeing. *The Lancet, 387*(10036), 2423–2478.

Viner, R. M., Ozer, E. M., Denny, S., Marmot, M., Resnick, M., Fatusi, A., & Currie, C. (2012). Adolescence and the social determinants of health. *The Lancet, 379*(9826), 1641–1652.

Prologue

Health promotion is a cornerstone of public health practice. In turn, the primary task of health promotion involves leveraging and sustaining long-term health-protective behaviors across diverse populations. Meeting the very difficult challenges inherent in fostering health-protective behaviors requires the wise and parsimonious use of behavioral and social science theories. These theories can best be viewed as the tools of the trade, and this text is designed to help you master those all-so-important tools. Before you begin this learning process, it is crucial that you understand a basic principle: learning about the full array of currently used theories in health promotion practice is essential to the ultimate success of any public health program you may design and implement. In many ways, your work in health promotion is similar to that of a highly skilled craftsperson. You will be crafting interventions and it is unlikely that any two programs will be "built" in the same way. This is true because even if you plan to change the same behavior in a subsequent program, the population served by that program is bound to be markedly different than the population originally served by the same program. So, think of yourself as a craftsperson who can effectively assess the needs of any population relative to their long-term adoption of health-protective behaviors. Your theory "toolbox" will facilitate this assessment and it will also allow you to develop an effective intervention approach.

Another important preliminary lesson is that each of the theories in your toolbox may, at first blush, appear to be distinctively different. As you read this text, rest assured that the theories you learn about each have a unique role in changing health behavior. Learning about and using only a few of the many theories is unlikely to lead to successful health promotion programs. Similarly, learning about theory in the absence of learning about core practices such as measurement, evaluation, and planning will not be adequate if your goal is to truly have an impact on population health. As such, the second edition of *Health Behavior Theory for Public Health* will provide you with a balanced professional education—one that teaches you about the essential spectrum of theoretical tools as well as the core practices.

This text will open by providing you with a firm foundation (Section I) for developing expertise in public health theory and related core practices. Please pay special attention to the concepts and terminology, as this added effort will certainly pay great dividends in your career. Section I is focused on health, public health, health behavior, and health promotion planning, rather than theory per se. Indeed, you will learn in this section that there is much more to understanding and changing health behavior than simply being well-versed in theory.

Section II provides you with the ability to gain a command of the theories and approaches most commonly applied in public health research and programs. We have taken great strides to present this material in a very straightforward manner and within the context of current relevant challenges in the field. As you finish this section you will see how theory "fits" into the larger scope of public health research and practice as described in Section I.

The text will close by providing you with a diverse set of application "tools" (Section III). These fairly advanced chapters were designed to bring all that you have learned in Section I and Section II into a more practical light. Here, you will learn about the essential tasks of translation, learning to combine theories, measurement, and program evaluation. Again, we emphasize the point that understanding and changing health behavior is challenging and requires multiple skills beyond the ability to apply theory.

Finally, we invite you to use an evaluative eye as you read this text. By using this phrase, we are suggesting that you should avoid the academic trap of looking at ideas as being correct or incorrect. Instead, think of each new idea as an opportunity to indulge in critical thinking. When learning about various theories or core practices, you may want to ask yourself questions such as "Is this approach logical and can it be reasonably translated into practice?" Learn to think in terms that transcend the universal terms of correct or

incorrect and challenge yourself to think about questions such as, "When would this approach work best and when would it work poorly, or not at all?"

Our goal for the next generation of public health professionals is for them to develop effective programs designed to avoid premature morbidity and mortality. We recognize that this work is as important as the work of traditional medical professionals and that effective public health programs can make a difference that transcends the limitation of a medical paradigm. This text will provide you a broad acumen of knowledge and skills that will ultimately serve your needs in the work you do to advance health promotion practice. We trust that your dedication to preventing disease will become greater than ever as you gain the ability to truly have an impact on the lives of others.

Acknowledgment

We wish to thank Mike Brown of Jones & Bartlett Learning for believing in this text and encouraging us to write this second edition. His collegiality, great humor, and dedication to quality are all greatly appreciated traits. We look forward to working with him in the future.

Contributors

John Acker, BA
Department of Psychology
University of Georgia

Michael T. Amlung, MS
Department of Psychology
University of Georgia

James G. Emshoff, PhD
EMSTAR Research, Inc.

James MacKillop, PhD
Department of Psychology
University of Georgia
Center for Alcohol and Addiction Studies
Brown University

Cara M. Murphy, BS
Department of Psychology
University of Georgia

Seth M. Noar, PhD
Associate Professor
School of Journalism and Mass Communication
Lineberger Comprehensive Cancer Center
University of North Carolina at Chapel Hill

Rita K. Noonan, PhD
Behavioral Scientist
Centers for Disease Control & Prevention

Lara Ray, PhD
Department of Psychology
University of California, Los Angeles

Colleen A. Redding, PhD
Research Professor
Cancer Prevention Research Center
University of Rhode Island

James H. Walker, BA, BS
Rollins School of Public Health
Emory University

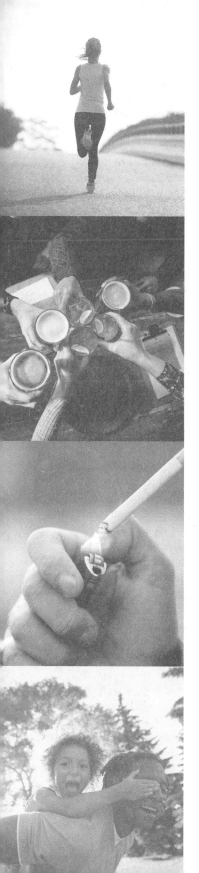

SECTION I
Overview

▶ Introduction

Above all else in life, the maintenance of health may be the one universal value. Being healthy means being free of disease and having the resources to take active measures to fortify the body against the onset of both chronic and infectious diseases—this level of prevention also provides people with a vitality that leads to productive and satisfying lives. Unfortunately, many societies (including the United States) broadly support recovery from chronic and infectious diseases at the expense of the more complicated task of preventing these problems in the first place. The ethic of placing prevention on the "pedestal of medicine" is a largely unrealized vision. A more practical vision is known as "upstream thinking," which implies that preventing the onset of disease or injury is the greatest priority in public health. The concept of upstream thinking implies that nations should prioritize prevention over treatment. Given the overarching influence of social determinants on health, this concept also implies that social equity must become a frontline effort of health-promotion programs.

Health equity is the obtainment of the highest level of health for all members of a population. Health inequities then are differences in health that are avoidable and therefore unjust. To achieve health equity, we need to foster efforts pertaining to eliminating those avoidable health inequities and their corresponding outcomes (i.e., health disparities). Health equities pertain to health, whereas social equities pertain to equal opportunities for all people, regardless of race, ethnicity, gender, sexual orientation, or religious beliefs. Social equity guarantees health equity because it promotes unfettered access (and comparable access) to the advantages of a society that protect health and prevent disease. Achieving social equity, however, implies that some members of a population will need more support/access than others to bring them to the same level of opportunity. Stated differently, social disadvantages create an initial unequal starting point for some people—these people cannot be said to have social equity until those deficits are made up. This means that some people will have more support/access needs than others, and thus, a need exists for disproportionate distribution of resources before true social equity.

Upstream thinking is not always an easy paradigm. It demands an understanding of why people place themselves at risk of disease and why they adopt health-protective behaviors. It also demands an understanding of how people manage to successfully adopt health-protective behaviors, especially those behaviors requiring daily repetition. Most importantly, it demands a thorough understanding of the social determinants of health and a corresponding commitment to achieving equity on the distribution of these determinants. Fortunately, a vast range of theories can be used to traverse these multiple challenges of upstream thinking. Modern theory spans a range from those that locate the behavior and change efforts strictly at the individual level to ecological theories, suggesting that behavior is a product of multiple and often interlocking environmental influences.

All theories are ultimately useful in the larger process of changing health-risk behaviors. This process, however, is far more involved than one might first imagine. A central starting point is to empirically identify the determinants of health-risk and health-protective behaviors. Determinants that are potentially modifiable can then be conceived as hypothesized mediators of behavior change. Theory can be used to define specific objectives meant to alter these hypothesized mediators in a way that leads to effective behavior change for large numbers of people, even entire populations The wise selection of theory is, of course, vital, because the process just described is one that can easily go wrong if program objectives are ill-conceived because of a theory that poorly matches the identified health-promotion challenge at hand.

In the first two chapters, you will learn much more about the concept of upstream thinking, particularly with respect to the concepts of primary prevention and universal care. Some of what you learn may challenge current beliefs you hold regarding health and medical care, and may even challenge the concept that apparently simple health behaviors may be influenced by a complex web of ecological factors. We suggest that any challenges to your current belief systems be embraced, as this is the first and most critical stage of your growth as a health-promotion professional. Further, we suggest that you diligently learn the basic vocabulary of health promotion as shown by the bolded terms in these two chapters. You will soon become proficient at using

terms such as *construct, proximal influence, distal influence,* and *multilevel intervention.*

We also implore you to study Chapter 3 quite carefully. This chapter provides you with a widely used framework that is useful for conceptualizing the entire process of planning a health-promotion program. As you study Chapter 3, please bear in mind that theory application and program planning are not synonymous. Think of theory application as a subset of program planning. Program planning is a larger concept simply because it includes elements related to problem assessment, goal setting, and evaluation. Chapter 3 introduces a long-standing and highly practical approach known as the PRECEDE–PROCEED model. For several decades, this planning model has served public health effectively through its ability to achieve targeted and judicious use of resources and health-promotion efforts.

An important caveat is warranted before you begin reading these three chapters: public health practice is an activity rather than a specific discipline. This statement reflects the growing tendency of public health practice to implicate a spectrum of likely intervention points for any given health behavior. Thus, public health efforts span a continuum ranging from media-based health communication programs to making products easily accessible (e.g., condoms, low-fat foods, bicycle helmets, exercise facilities). The continuum spans further to include changes to public policy and laws. It will become apparent that people from numerous professional backgrounds are needed to promote conditions favoring widespread and long-term adoption of health-protective behaviors.

The question you may then ask is, "What holds all of these various professionals together in a unified effort to promote health in an upstream thinking paradigm?" To this question, we respectfully suggest that the concepts you will learn about in the entire text represent a type of shared wisdom that indeed defines the work of health promotion. Your dedication to these chapters will have an important influence on your ability to protect the health of the public through prevention of disease and conditions that would otherwise limit the quality and longevity of people's lives.

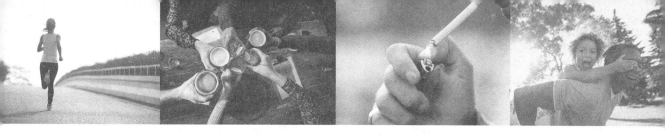

CHAPTER 1

Health Behavior in the Context of the "New" Public Health

Laura F. Salazar, Richard A. Crosby, and Ralph J. DiClemente

The health of the people is really the foundation upon which all their happiness and all their powers as a state depend.

—**Benjamin Disraeli**, British Politician (1804–1881)

PREVIEW

Unhealthy behaviors contribute to the leading causes of early mortality. As such, if health-promotion efforts can prevent people from engaging in many of these behaviors, then health-promotion can make a significant impact on the rates of early mortality and morbidity. Using a wide range of theories in its endeavors, health promotion seeks to change environments, settings, policies, regulations, and individuals so that optimal health can be achieved.

OBJECTIVES

1. Compare and contrast the three levels of prevention.
2. Understand the different types of health behaviors.
3. Define health promotion and understand the multidisciplinary nature of health promotion.
4. Understand the importance of multiple theories in health-promotion efforts.
5. Understand that health behavior is highly influenced by the physical, economic, legal, and social environments that define people's daily existence; thus, a broad range of theoretical approaches provides increased assurance of leveraging change.

▶ Introduction

Without question, health should be the most valuable thing in a person's life. An old Arabic proverb states, "He who has health, has hope; and he who has hope, has everything." But what, exactly, is health? Some would argue that health is simply the absence of disease. According to the World Health Organization (WHO), health is not merely the absence of disease or infirmity; rather, **health** should encompass a state of complete physical, mental, and social well-being. Expanding on this definition at a seminal conference in Ottawa, Ontario, Canada, the WHO reconceptualized health, in that it should be defined from an ecological perspective to encompass the "extent to which an individual or group is able, on the one hand, to realize aspirations and satisfy needs; and, on the other hand, to change or cope with the environment. Health is, therefore, seen as a resource for everyday life, not the objective of living; it is a positive concept emphasizing social and personal resources, as well as physical capacities" (World Health Organization, 1986). Using these definitions, health would seem to transcend an individual's state of physical being at any given moment to also include his or her *ability* to optimize his or her health and the availability of environmental resources that enable him or her to maintain his or her health over time. Thus, to embrace these definitions of health requires perhaps a paradigm shift in terms of conceptualizing what health is, what the determinants of health are, and most importantly how to promote health. A basic premise of *Health Behavior Theory for Public Health: Principles, Foundations, and Applications* is that, as Benjamin Disraeli so succinctly stated, an important goal for any nation is the health of its people, but we advocate that the means to this end lie in adopting strategies that modify environments, settings, and policies/regulations while also targeting the many individual factors that influence health.

> *Health is not merely the absence of disease or infirmity; rather, **health** should encompass a state of complete physical, mental, and social well-being.*

A key principle in health promotion involves understanding the nature of the diseases that are most likely to occur in a population. At the turn of the 20th century (see **FIGURE 1-1**), the top three causes of death were attributed to infectious disease agents that caused pneumonia, tuberculosis, diarrhea, and enteritis (Centers for Disease Control and Prevention [CDC], 1999). Early public health efforts were very successful in implementing important new biomedical advances (e.g., vaccinations and antibiotics) and developing public health programs that remedied many types of infectious diseases (e.g., water sanitation to reduce cholera), eradicated some diseases (e.g., smallpox), and mitigated many afflictions. However, as the incidence of these diseases decreased, chronic diseases (e.g., cardiovascular disease, diabetes, and cancer) flourished.

Toward the end of the 21st century, individual lifestyle **behaviors**, such as smoking, poor diet and exercise, alcohol consumption, and the use of illicit drugs, were primary contributors to the six leading causes of death (Mokdad, Marks, Stroup, & Gerberding, 2004). These behaviors are deemed "lifestyle behaviors" because they take place within the context of individuals' everyday lives. These specific lifestyle behaviors have been cited as **actual causes** of death because they have been linked directly to the top five chronic diseases: heart disease, cancer, cerebrovascular disease, respiratory disease, and diabetes (McGinnis & Foege, 1993; Mokdad et al., 2004).

Clearly, a person who contracts an infectious disease such as cholera, pneumonia, or tuberculosis would most likely hold the perception that they were not healthy; however, it may not be as clear to people who smoke, eat high-fat foods, do not exercise, consume too much alcohol, or use illicit drugs that they are *unhealthy*. They may hold an inaccurate perception of their health, which is most likely due to the *hidden* contribution of engaging in unhealthy lifestyle behaviors to the development of **chronic diseases**, rather than the more noticeable **infectious** or **communicable diseases**.

Chronic diseases manifest over time, are not always apparent, and may be long-lasting or recurring. In **TABLE 1-1**, we list various chronic diseases that may result from engaging in several unhealthy lifestyle behaviors and are linked to the leading

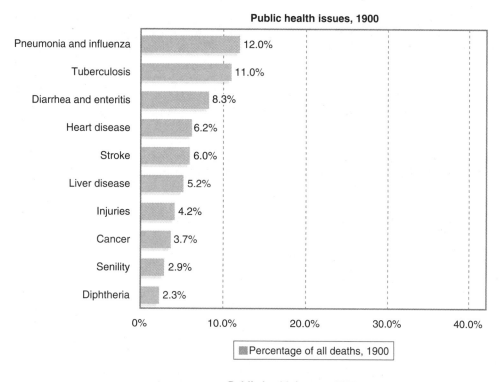

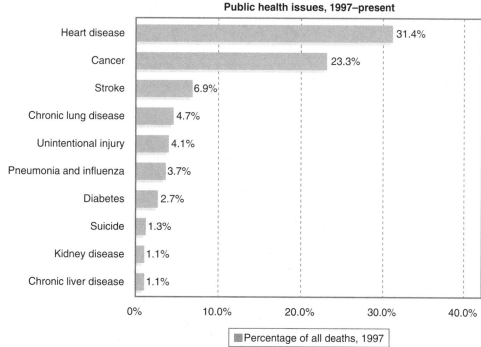

FIGURE 1-1 The 10 leading causes of death, as a percentage of all deaths—the United States, 1900, 1997

Centers for Disease Control and Prevention, National Center for Health Statistics. (1999). Achievements in Public Health, 1900–1999: Control of infectious diseases, 1900–1999. *Morbidity & Mortality Weekly Report, 48,* 621–629.

TABLE 1-1 Chronic Diseases Associated with Unhealthy Lifestyle Behaviors

SMOKING: Acute myeloid leukemia; cancers of the cervix, kidney, bladder, esophagus, larynx, lung, mouth, pancreas, and stomach; abdominal aortic aneurysms; cataracts; periodontitis; pneumonia; chronic lung disease; chronic heart and cardiovascular diseases; osteoporosis; peptic ulcers; reproductive problems

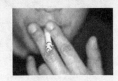

HIGH-FAT DIET: Coronary heart disease, type 2 diabetes, cancers (endometrial, breast, and colon), hypertension (high blood pressure), dyslipidemia (e.g., high total cholesterol or high levels of triglycerides), stroke, liver and gallbladder disease, sleep apnea and respiratory problems, osteoarthritis (a degeneration of cartilage and its underlying bone within a joint), gynecological problems (abnormal menses, infertility)

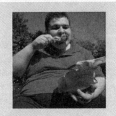

ALCOHOL: Cardiovascular disease; liver disease; chronic pancreatitis; pancreatic, breast, liver, oral, colon, and throat cancers

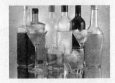

ILLICIT DRUGS: Suicide, homicide, motor vehicle injury, HIV infection, pneumonia, violence, mental illness, hepatitis

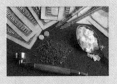

Photos from top to bottom, © Photos.com, © Digital Vision/Photodisc/Thinkstock, © SunnyS/Shutterstock © Vladimir V. Georgievskly/Shutterstock

causes of death in the United States. In viewing the associated disease outcomes, you may surmise that many people are unaware that these diseases are significantly linked to these unhealthy behaviors. Although there is no definitive answer as to exactly how many years of unhealthy lifestyle behavior it takes to develop some of these chronic diseases, it is generally agreed that the time is best thought of in terms of years. Thus, it is understandable why so many people engaging in these lifestyle behaviors may not perceive themselves at risk for disease in the same way as a person who was recently exposed to someone coughing on an airplane or who may have worked in an environment that was harmful (e.g., manufacturing of asbestos textiles).

If the consummate goal is to ensure the health of the people, then individual perceptions of health or what constitutes "unhealthy" may exert some influence on whether appropriate action is taken by society or by the individual. This text emphasizes that public health initiatives to combat both chronic and infectious diseases and improve the health of the public should be multidimensional—that is, health-promotion efforts should target systems and political structures to affect the underlying social determinants of health and their corresponding health behaviors. This emphasis on the significant role of environmental influences in shaping individual behavior and affecting health is the driving force behind the "new public health." An expedient summary of the new public health is provided by the director of the Centers for Disease Control and Prevention, under the Obama administration. **FIGURE 1-2** illustrates the relative strength

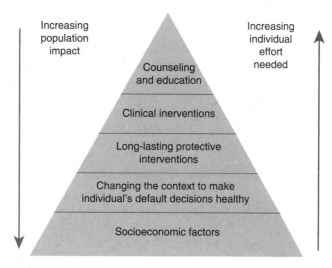

FIGURE 1-2 Frieden pyramid

Reproduced from Frieden, Thomas. A Framework for Public Health Action: The Health Impact Pyramid. American Journal of Public Health. 2010 April; 100(4): 590–595.

of five factors influencing public health, with the largest (i.e., strongest) contribution coming from socioeconomic status. This is precisely why the new public health has an emphasis on social equity. Beyond socioeconomic status, in order of strength, the remaining four factors involve making ecological changes that enable the "easy" adoption of health-protective behaviors, the use of planned intervention programs shown to have long-lasting effects on health behavior, clinical interventions, and counseling/education-based programs. Noteworthy in this pyramid is that clinical interventions occupy a relatively small fraction of the overall influence on the health of a population.

Public health initiatives to combat both chronic and infectious diseases and improve the health of the public should be multidimensional—that is, health-promotion efforts should target systems and political structures to affect the underlying social determinants of health and their corresponding health behaviors.

This chapter provides an overview of the importance of health behavior (i.e., reducing unhealthy behaviors while also promoting healthy ones) in achieving optimal health. We describe how the best approach emphasizes prevention and targets settings where behavior takes place. You have most likely heard the famous adage attributed to Benjamin Franklin: "An ounce of prevention is worth a pound of cure." He believed that it is wiser and more cost-effective to try and prevent a disease from manifesting rather than to treat it. Public health, in general, embraces this adage; its mission is **prophylaxis**, or prevention, of early **mortality**, **morbidity**, and associated negative health outcomes. Changing or modifying health behaviors that are associated with morbidity and early mortality is considered one aspect of a prevention approach. Because health behaviors can contribute significantly to early mortality and morbidity, understanding and changing health behaviors and the surrounding conditions that influence behavior are critical to achieving public health's mission.

We also provide an overview of public health and describe the rationale for public health approaches that target whole populations rather than only those individuals at heightened risk. We articulate the role of health promotion in the context of public health and the basic principles and strategies used. We express that the field of public health is multidisciplinary and involves a process, rather than being a unified field, like physics or chemistry. Finally, we highlight the role of theory in public health research and practice and the importance of choosing the proper framework.

▶ Key Concepts

Why the Emphasis on Prevention?

Once one is afflicted with a disease, medical approaches must be used for treatment. Treatment can be very costly, not everyone has access to treatment, and furthermore, treatment is not always a panacea; treatment cannot "fix" many health issues (e.g., dead heart muscle tissue). In 2015, the United

States spent $3.2 trillion (representing 17.8% of the gross domestic product) on health care or $9,990 per person (Centers for Medicaid and Medicare Services [CMS], 2015). As shown in **FIGURE 1-3**, the United States spends more on health care, both as a proportion of gross domestic product and on a per capita basis, than any other country in the world (WHO, 2009). Given the enormous price tag associated with U.S. healthcare costs, you would imagine that the United States should be getting what they pay for in terms of much lower early mortality and morbidity rates. Unfortunately, statistics do not support this assertion. In fact, the United States ranks 47th in terms of life expectancy, 9th in terms of cancer death rates, 13th in heart disease death rates, and 1st in obesity rates (http://www.NationMaster.com). Despite its drastically smaller population size (approximately 300 million), the United States ranks with India (approximately 1.1 billion people) and China (approximately

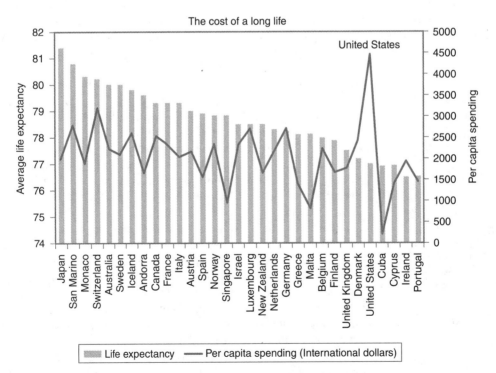

FIGURE 1-3 Per capita healthcare costs and life expectancy around the world

Reproduced from UC Atlas of Global Inequality, http://ucatlas.ucsc.edu/spend.php, Health care spending.

1.3 billion people) in terms of the number of estimated cases of diabetes.

Diabetes is an excellent example of a prime opportunity for improved population-based prevention. Type 2 diabetes is the most common form of diabetes and has been linked to obesity, inactivity, and genetic factors. Ignoring the genetic component (as this is largely not amenable to change), obesity is considered a **modifiable** risk factor as it can be changed. If the rates of obesity and inactivity among the population were somehow reduced significantly, a reduction in the prevalence of type 2 diabetes should be experienced as well, thereby reducing the associated mortality rate. Now consider that one out of every five U.S. federal healthcare dollars is spent *treating people with diabetes* (American Diabetes Association, 2008). If treating people with diabetes represents 20% of healthcare dollars spent, then a better approach may be to *prevent* diabetes rather than *treat* diabetes. Unfortunately, according to former U.S. Surgeon General Dr. David Satcher, of the total dollars spent on national health care in the year 1999, only 1% went to population-based prevention.

Some estimates suggest that the U.S. government spends $1390 per person to treat disease, while spending only $1.21 per person on prevention. Although this represents an enormous imbalance in the amount of money spent on treatment versus prevention, the United States does make a concerted effort. To combat many of the lifestyle diseases afflicting its populace in the later part of the 20th century and to enhance the health of its people, the United States created a national prevention agenda. The 1979 Surgeon General's Report on health promotion and disease prevention, *Healthy People*, outlined the tremendous gains made in combating infectious diseases in the earlier part of the 20th century, stating that "the health of the American people has never been better." However, he also stated that further improvements could be achieved through a "renewed national commitment to efforts designed to prevent disease and to promote health" (U.S. Department of Health, Education & Welfare, 1979, p. 3). *Healthy People* laid the foundation for a national prevention agenda that spanned a wide range of health goals focused

on reducing early mortality and morbidity, such as a reduction in smoking, an increase in physical activity, and a reduction in injuries. Most important is that *Healthy People* as a policy signified that the United States must take responsibility for the health of its people. The agenda has since been updated and goals reexamined every 10 years. The 1980 *Promoting Health/Preventing Disease: Objectives for the Nation and Healthy People 2000: National Health Promotion and Disease Prevention Objectives* both established national health objectives and served as the basis for the development of state and community plans. Presently, *Healthy People 2020* has built on the work of the past three decades and has implemented a 10-year health-promotion program with four overarching goals:

1. Attain high-quality, longer lives free of preventable disease, disability, injury, and premature death.
2. Achieve health equity, eliminate disparities, and improve the health of all groups.
3. Create social and physical environments that promote good health for all.
4. Promote quality of life, healthy development, and healthy behaviors across all life stages.

The focus is on different health areas (e.g., sexually transmitted diseases, substance abuse, tobacco use, diabetes, cancer, HIV), accompanied by 600 public health objectives and leading health indicators to measure the progress toward meeting its goals. The question remains, however, as to whether the U.S. government will balance the scales and devote enough funds toward prevention so that it can meet these goals. Passage of the Affordable Care Act in 2010 created historic strides toward shifting funds to the prevention of disease. Whether these strides continue in the future will be crucial to the health of U.S. citizens.

Health Behavior Is Complex

The central question, irrespective of funding, is: how do we work toward achieving these prevention goals? Focusing on type 2 diabetes, specifically, how do we prevent people from becoming obese? How can we motivate and enable people to adopt better dietary habits, lose weight, and exercise more? What systems-level changes or policy/regulations changes can be made to promote consistent exercise behaviors and improved dietary habits among persons most at risk of diabetes? What social inequities must be addressed and rectified to optimally prevent diabetes? We may think that all we need to do is tell people that they are at risk and that making people aware of their risks will result in them changing their dietary and exercise behaviors. Unfortunately, changing behavior is not as simple as it seems. Persuading a person to change his or her habits is a major challenge indeed, especially when the behavior is viewed as enjoyable (e.g., eating a juicy hamburger) or when they may not have complete control (e.g., a child whose parent makes the decisions about food or a person who can only afford high-calorie foods of low nutritional value such as fast-food "bargains"). The reality is that human behavior is complex and influenced by many factors; therefore, changing it requires a thorough understanding of the range of influences. For example, changing dietary habits such that whole foods (i.e., foods that are unrefined and unprocessed) compose the majority of the daily caloric intake implies understanding (1) why people prefer processed foods; (2) what people do not like about whole foods; (3) the benefits that people perceive from consuming less processed foods; (4) the physical, economic, political, cultural, and social barriers that people perceive relative to the consumption of whole foods; (5) the barriers to stocking produce and other whole foods among grocery stores; and (6) the national and local policies that translate to the cost-prohibitiveness of providing whole foods. In essence, reducing the obesity epidemic will involve health-promotion efforts that address all six of these questions, with an emphasis on the latter three.

Before we can change health behavior,

> *Before we can change health behavior, we must understand the **determinants** of the behavior, the nature of the behavior, and the motivation for the behavior.*

we must understand the **determinants** of the behavior, the nature of the behavior, and the motivation for the behavior. Influencers (also referred to as "drivers") of behavior can theoretically be infinitesimal and can include a range of factors, such as biological characteristics, personality characteristics, family, peers, the community, society, and the built environment. Moreover, the nature of health behaviors can vary along many dimensions. For example, some health behaviors may occur once in a lifetime (e.g., polio vaccine), some on a daily basis (e.g., diet, exercise), and some are conditional to the context (e.g., using a condom). Furthermore, motivation for engaging in a health behavior or to stop engaging in an unhealthy behavior will also be affected by numerous individual, environmental, and policy/regulatory factors.

So, how do we begin to make a dent in achieving the prevention goals of *Healthy People 2020* and eventually *Healthy People 2030*? First, understanding what factors contribute, cause, precede, influence, and motivate health behaviors, and then how to effectively modify those factors so that behavior change is achieved is the basic premise of health promotion. Health promotion is an integral part of the "new public health" approach and involves two aspects: research and practice. Indeed, public health professionals are increasingly recognizing that the mainstays of epidemiology and healthcare service administration lack the ability to change population-level indicators of health. The realization is that changing behaviors in a population and creating environments conducive to healthy behaviors are possibly the ultimate solutions to the long-standing question of how best to improve the health of the public. Health-promotion research is at the forefront of understanding the underlying individual, environmental, and policy/regulatory factors that influence health behavior. Conversely, health-promotion practice is at the forefront of designing and implementing interventions to modify those factors and to ultimately change behavior. Thus, health promotion can be viewed as a process for which many public health, medical, and education professionals, whether on the research side or the practice side, have a responsibility and play an integral role in promoting health. The tool used for health-promotion research and practice is theory.

A theory is a set of testable propositions that is used to explain a group of facts or phenomena. In health promotion, theory enables researchers to better understand health behavior and make predictions about how to change behavior. Just as there are a multitude of health behaviors, there are many theories that attempt to explain these health behaviors. Unfortunately, in this text, we cannot cover all of them; however, we do describe many of the theories widely used today in health promotion research and practice. Before we proceed to the description of these theories, it may be helpful to provide a foundation of health behavior in the context of public health.

Prevention and the Public Health Approach

In broad terms, public health seeks to promote health, prevent early mortality and morbidity, and enhance or ensure quality of life. Prevention is the basic principle underlying the public health approach. In fact, the leading public health agency in the United States—the Centers for Disease Control and Prevention (CDC)—has the following mission statement: "To promote health and quality of life by preventing and controlling disease, injury, and disability." The CDC motto of "Saving Lives, Protecting People" is very much a reflection of a prevention-based orientation. From a public health perspective, the essence of

prevention is creating healthy populations, meaning that the incidence of chronic disease, infectious disease, and injury decline dramatically. In our experience, the implications of a prevention-oriented approach to public health are often difficult for students to fully comprehend without first "divorcing" themselves from a medical orientation to public health. **FIGURE 1-4** provides a visual depiction, suggesting that the prevention of disease entails far more than averting clinically observable illness.

As shown in Figure 1-4, clinically observable illness can be viewed as the midpoint of a continuum ranging from optimal wellness to extreme illness. Coronary vascular disease serves as a good example to illustrate this division. Clinically observable early warning signs of a heart attack, for example, can be diagnosed through a treadmill stress test. Proxy measures of pending blockages in coronary arteries include high serum cholesterol levels, high blood pressure, and high body mass index (BMI). From a medical orientation, the prevention of a heart attack is about defining a threshold for high blood serum cholesterol, high blood pressure, and a risky level of BMI. Once these thresholds are established, any person who exceeds any one threshold can be "treated" under the prevailing medical paradigm. Failure to do so will presumably result in increased coronary occlusion followed by the eventual blockage of the blood supply to the heart, possibly inducing death.

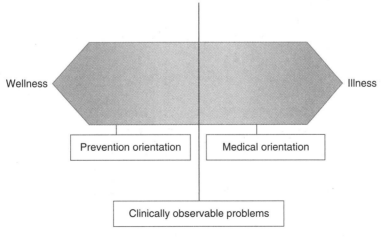

FIGURE 1-4 Wellness–illness continuum

The problem with the "prevention ← medical" orientation is that it begins with a diagnosis and is reactive, thereby restricting the arena of the doctor–patient relationship and defining prevention in medical terms. This limits the public health approach to changing people literally one at a time. Conversely, the "prevention → medical" orientation (left part of Figure 1-4) lends itself to a population-level approach because it is not predicated on an individual medical diagnosis. Instead, this orientation acknowledges that defining what levels constitute *high* cholesterol, *high* blood pressure, and *high* body mass is problematic and that everyone in a population can benefit from lower cholesterol, lower blood pressure, and less body fat. In this orientation, prevention activities are most often implemented *before* clinically defined levels of risk are reached by people. The intent is to figuratively "pull" people further to the left of the continuum (as far away from illness as possible). Unlike the medical approach, this orientation does lend itself to intervening with entire populations, rather than taking a one-at-a-time approach to public health. Unfortunately, the one-at-a-time approach to prevention has been frequently applied without success to the task of changing health behaviors, as well as changing risk factors (such as high cholesterol) through medication. This individual-level approach to behavior change is not necessarily relegated to the right side of the wellness–illness continuum shown in Figure 1-4. Thus, at this juncture, a second figure may be quite useful.

The public health orientation, in contrast, is perhaps best embodied by the motto of the Bloomberg School of Public Health at Johns Hopkins University: Protecting Health, Saving Lives—Millions at a Time. This extension of the CDC motto clearly defines health at the population level. In his book titled *The Strategy of Preventive Medicine*, Geoffrey Rose, a British physician, developed the skewed distribution curve shown in **FIGURE 1-5**, also known as the Rose curve (Rose, 1992) that guides thinking about population-level intervention.

This drawing is quite useful because it gives a visual image of those considered "at risk" because of their diet and the associated negative health outcomes as composing the right-end tail of the distribution; those not at risk would fall under the rest of the area under the curve. Think of the tail in this curve as being the portion of a population located on the right side of the wellness–illness continuum. It follows, then, that the remaining area under the curve represents that portion of a population somewhere to the left of the center point in the wellness–illness continuum. The medical orientation can be

> *The inherent problem of intervening only at the tail is that even when success occurs and these people join the masses near the mean, more people will continue to move into the tail.*

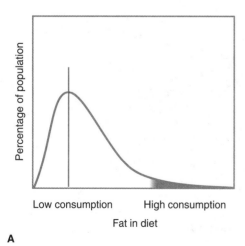

A

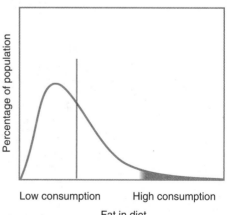

B

FIGURE 1-5 Example of a Rose curve

viewed as a type of intervention that only happens with people located in the tail of the curve. The inherent problem of intervening only at the tail is that even when success occurs and these people join the masses near the mean, more people will continue to move into the tail. This occurs because the social inequities, system influences, and policy/ regulatory influences do not change. Thus, the task of intervening with people who are already ill becomes never ending. Think of Sisyphus rolling his boulder up the hill for all of eternity! The following reference to the Multiple Risk Factor Intervention Trial (MRFIT) depicts this concept:

> [E]very time we helped a man in [MRFIT] to stop smoking, on that day, probably one to two children in a schoolyard somewhere were taking their first tentative puffs on a cigarette . . . So, even when we do help high-risk people to lower their risk, we do nothing to change the distribution of disease in the population because, in one-to-one programs . . . we do nothing to influence forces in society that caused the problem in the first place
>
> (Syme, 1996, p. 463)

As a result of the limitations that accompany the at-risk paradigm, public health strategies have increasingly been directed at the goal of moving the population mean to the left of the curve shown in Figure 1-5. By shifting the mean to the left, everyone in the distribution benefits and ultimately the population as a whole experiences an increase in health behavior, and perhaps a decrease in eventual morbidity and mortality (Syme, 1996). The concept of moving the population mean to the left of the Rose curve corresponds quite nicely with a prevention-orientation goal—the goal is to lower everyone's level of risk rather than targeting only those at greatest risk or those who have manifested the disease. This goal allows intervention to transcend a one-at-a-time approach, thereby allowing for change strategies that can be applied to entire populations. This involvement at the level of entire populations is the essence of public health.

A popular analogy to illustrate the concept of population-based prevention versus individual treatment is the "upstream allegory." In this story, fishermen fishing downstream observe streams of people coming down the river struggling not to drown. The fishermen must spend all their time pulling these individuals out of the river to save them. After exhausting their efforts, they finally decide to move upstream to see why so many people have fallen into the river. They quickly ascertain that there is no protective barrier at the edge of the riverbank; thus, when people are drawn to the riverbank, it is quite easy for them to fall into the raging waters. Consequently, community leaders decide to put up a railing at the edge of the riverbank, which results in significantly fewer people falling into the water. Not only does this benefit the people who would have fallen in, but it also benefits the fishermen, as they do not have to spend their time and resources rescuing people. This "intervention," in turn, benefits the entire community: the community has reduced rates of early mortality; they have more fish to eat; and they sell what is left over to the neighboring community, generating economic revenue. Thus, everyone's quality of life has improved in many ways.

From this story, it is easy to see why the medical approach is considered a downstream approach (treating individuals on a case-by-case basis after falling in), whereas public health is considered an upstream approach (instituting changes to prevent large numbers of people from ever falling in). The upstream approach equates with **primary prevention**, which is one of three levels of prevention identified by epidemiologists Hugh Leavell and Guerney Clark (1960), with **secondary** prevention and **tertiary** prevention being the other two levels. Using our analogy, secondary prevention equates with saving people who perhaps have just fallen in, but well before they have been caught up in the current and are drowning. Tertiary prevention in public health targets people who can treat the disease and/or people who have the disease with the goal of mitigating the disease's effects; thus, tertiary prevention would equate with targeting the fishermen and teaching them how to more effectively save drowning people or targeting the drowning people and teaching them to tread water to buy them more time so that they can be saved. These different levels of prevention equate with the three stages of the

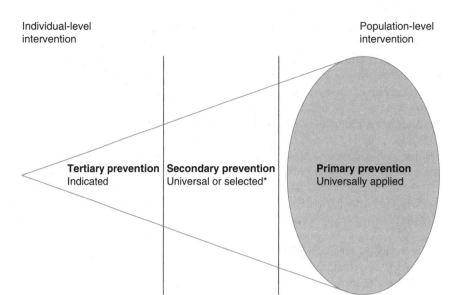

Individual-level intervention

Population-level intervention

Tertiary prevention | **Secondary prevention** | **Primary prevention**
Indicated | Universal or selected* | Universally applied

*Depending on the disease/condition in question.

FIGURE 1-6 Three levels of prevention

disease, injury, or behavioral process, where each stage may require a different prevention strategy. A graphic depiction is provided in **FIGURE 1-6**.

The public health approach is predicated on primary prevention. In primary prevention, efforts are made to intercept the onset or occurrence of disease, injury, or behavior. Primary prevention examples include vaccination programs, water fluoridation, abstinence programs, motorcycle helmet laws, bicycle helmet laws for children, mandatory seatbelt and child safety seat laws, mandatory minimum smoking/drinking age requirements, and antismoking media campaigns. These are just a few examples, and many of these initiatives have been very effective in reducing associated morbidity and early mortality. For example, increasing price may be the most effective way to prevent teens from becoming daily smokers. A joint study from the University of Illinois at Chicago and the University of Michigan Institute for Social Research conducted an analysis where they matched price hikes of cigarettes with teen smoking rates over a period of 6 years. They found that a 10% price increase would decrease the number of children who started to smoke between 3% and 10%, depending on their stage of smoking (Chaloupka & Warner, 2000).

Moreover, analyses indicate that in addition to preventing disease, pain, suffering, disability, death, or loss of function, many prevention programs are also cost-effective. Primary prevention involves intervening before disease onset. In the context of public health, it must be broad in scope and aimed at large portions of the population. This is defined as adopting a **universal approach**, and it corresponds with the notion of intervening at the "bell" rather than the tail in the Rose curve shown in Figure 1-5. A universal approach is when an entire population (e.g., a nationwide crime-prevention media campaign) or subgroups of the population (e.g., children 16 years of age and under to enforce bicycle helmet use) are targeted regardless of whether individuals in the group have specific risk factors. Because whole populations are targeted, a large number of individuals are reached and the economic benefits of prevention become substantial. Moreover, if the focus of the preventive effort (e.g., diabetes,

In primary prevention, efforts are made to intercept the onset or occurrence of disease, injury, or behavior.

obesity, motor vehicle injury, alcohol abuse) corresponds to a high rate within the population, then the universal approach is extremely cost-effective. However, it is important to note that if the rate is infrequent, then an ounce of prevention *may not* equate with a pound of cure (see Cohen, Neumann, and Weinstein (2008) for detailed analyses on this subject).

In some situations, instead of taking a universal approach, primary prevention efforts target those in the population who are at heightened risk. This type of approach is called a **selective approach**. Typically, those individuals are targeted on the basis of biological, psychological, social, or environmental risk factors known to be associated with the disease or condition. For example, as mentioned previously, obesity is a risk factor for type 2 diabetes. A selective primary intervention to combat type 2 diabetes would target those individuals whose BMI is above 25, but who have not yet developed type 2 diabetes. Thus, although the focus is on those who are at increased risk, this approach is still considered primary prevention. Indeed, this approach was used by Knowler et al. (2002) in their randomized controlled trial of a primary prevention educational intervention (curriculum to affect diet and exercise behaviors) in preventing type 2 diabetes. They targeted clinic patients who had a BMI above 24 and whose glucose levels were elevated but not diagnostic of diabetes. At the 2-year follow-up, they found the educational intervention was nearly twice as effective as pharmaceutical treatment (metformin) in preventing the onset of diabetes.

Secondary and tertiary are the other two levels of prevention identified by Leavell and Clark. Secondary prevention occurs when a disease process is diagnosed in an early stage of progression, thereby enhancing the odds of treatment success. The focus of secondary prevention is to minimize consequences through early detection and intervention. Screening programs for sexually transmitted diseases, cancer, or diabetes and smoking cessation programs are examples of secondary prevention. A good example is the use of mammography to diagnose localized tumors of the breast before these tumors progress. A tumor may indeed form, but with mammography the early diagnosis may lead to a simple lumpectomy as opposed to what may have become a radical mastectomy. Pap testing and colonoscopy are also common forms of secondary prevention because they screen for cervical dysplasia and polyps, respectively.

The focus of secondary prevention is to minimize consequences through early detection and intervention.

Tertiary prevention occurs when a disease state is diagnosed in time to apply treatment that may prevent further organic damage or death. Thus, the difference between secondary and tertiary prevention can essentially be thought of as the difference between early and late diagnosis. Tertiary prevention involves mitigating the consequences of disease or an injury after the fact.

Tertiary prevention involves mitigating the consequences of disease or an injury after the fact.

The goal of tertiary prevention is to provide treatment and rehabilitation so that negative impact is reduced and function can be restored. An **indicated approach** is used in tertiary prevention. Examples of tertiary prevention would include providing patients who have type 2 diabetes with educational pamphlets to help them better manage their disease, providing mental health counseling for rape victims, and instituting outreach programs to monitor people with mental disorders who live in the community to ensure they are adhering to their medication regimens. In many ways, tertiary prevention in the public health model is similar to treatment in the medical model.

Primary, secondary, and tertiary prevention can be integrated with the concepts of universal, selective, and indicated approaches. Figure 1-6 provides a visual depiction of this integration. As shown by the wide angle of this cone, the vast majority of health-promotion practice is primary prevention applied on a universal basis. This application can and should occur at the population level. Conversely, the least prevalent form of health promotion occurs with the indicated application of tertiary prevention—this application occurs at the individual level. This bipolar continuum therefore leaves secondary prevention in the middle of the cone, suggesting that it is practiced less often than primary prevention but more often than tertiary prevention. Consistent with our description of a selective approach, secondary prevention may be universally applied to an entire population or selectively applied to a defined subset of a population.

Prioritizing and Conceptualizing Health Behaviors

To fulfill the public health mission of prevention, public health professionals must first have a clear understanding of which diseases and types of injuries are having the greatest impact, so that efforts are correctly positioned. Epidemiologists conduct surveillance studies and analyze records to determine the rates of diseases and the leading causes of death. Consequently, the causes and contributing

risk factors have been well established. Although in the 21st century chronic diseases are at the top of the list, there are many other public health concerns. Injury from firearms and motor vehicle crashes are on the list, while infectious diseases such as influenza, HIV/AIDS, tuberculosis, chlamydia, human papillomavirus (HPV), Ebola, and methicillin-resistant *Staphylococcus aureus* (MRSA), to name a few, are also responsible for substantial morbidity and early mortality. From a global perspective, infectious diseases still remain a significant source of morbidity and early mortality. Six infectious diseases—pneumonia, HIV/AIDS, diarrhea, tuberculosis, malaria, and measles—account for half of the premature deaths globally. The top causes of death worldwide are listed in **TABLE 1-2**.

Although the etiology is quite different for chronic and infectious diseases, as well as for sustaining injury, all can be prevented to some degree. At a minimum, onset can be delayed and the risk

TABLE 1-2 Top Causes of Death Worldwide, 2004		
Cause of Death	**Number of Deaths in Millions**	**Deaths (%)**
Coronary heart disease	7.20	12.2
Stroke and other cerebrovascular diseases	5.71	9.7
Lower respiratory infections	4.18	7.1
Chronic obstructive pulmonary disease	3.02	5.1
Diarrheal diseases	2.16	3.7
HIV/AIDS	2.04	3.5
Tuberculosis	1.46	2.5
Road traffic accidents	1.27	2.2
Prematurity and low birth weight	1.18	2.0

Reproduced from World Health Organization. (2008). The 10 leading causes of death by broad income group (2004). Retrieved from http://www.who.int /mediacentre/factsheets/fs310/en/index.html

of death mitigated. Many of these 21st-century "scourges" have underlying health behaviors, and public health efforts that target these health behaviors are integral to a comprehensive preventive effort. For example, one in four child deaths from malaria could be prevented if children at risk slept under bed nets at night to avoid mosquito bites (WHO, 1999). In the United States, motor vehicle injuries are the leading cause of death for children aged 4–11 years (CDC, 2008). For children aged 4–7 years, the use of belt-positioning booster seats reduces this risk by 59%, compared with the use of seat belts alone (Durbin et al., 2003).

"Using a bed net" and "using a booster seat" are merely two types of health behaviors that can be affected or modified to prevent the acquisition of malaria or the risk of auto accident injury, respectively; however, there are other health behaviors that could be changed to prevent malaria and injuries. When conceptualizing health behavior, many people may not perceive that "using a bed net" or "buying a booster seat" should be classified as health behaviors. Generally speaking, when people think of health behavior, they think of things like exercising or taking vitamins. They might not consider that their decision to get a mammogram or to get a flu shot is a health behavior. Furthermore, they might not categorize testing their home for the presence of radon as a health behavior.

Regardless of the general public's perceptions of what constitutes a health behavior, it should be defined so that health-promotion research can be used to gain a better understanding of health behavior, and subsequently, health-promotion practice can be used to alter it. **Behavior** in the broadest sense is the manner in which something acts, functions, responds, or reacts. This definition can apply not only to individual people but also more broadly to collectives and systems. Along these lines, **health behavior** can be defined as the actions, responses, or reactions of an individual, group, or system that prevent illness, promote health, and maintain quality of life. Examples of individual health behaviors would be using a condom, buckling up the seat belt, or getting vaccinated. Collective health behaviors could be a neighborhood association making changes to the built environment to encourage physical activity (e.g., putting in sidewalks, installing better lighting), initiating a safety patrol, or starting a local co-op farmer's market. Sociopolitical system behaviors could involve instituting a citywide smoking ban, implementing community-wide condom accessibility/availability programs, or banning trans fats in restaurants. Again, we emphasize the importance of using a multilevel approach to promote health in a population; a focus on only one of these levels is unlikely to be productive. We also emphasize that any approach taken must be made with the goal of social equity in mind. This implies that intervention resources and efforts will be intensified for marginalized populations, most at risk of morbidity and early mortality. Often, with extreme social inequities, intervention efforts as simple as food provision are tremendously helpful (see **FIGURE 1-7**).

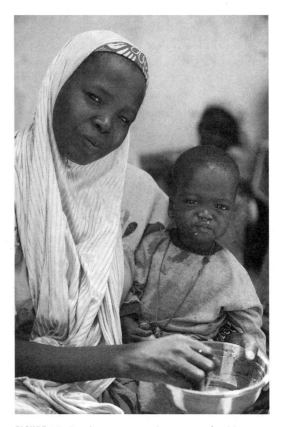

FIGURE 1-7 Food provision is a basic part of public health practice

Courtesy of WFP/Rein Skullerud

Health behavior can be defined as the actions, responses, or reactions of an individual, group, or system that prevent illness, promote health, and maintain quality of life.

Just as there are different levels to prevention, health behaviors can be similarly qualified according to the nature of the health behavior. Most health behaviors can be classified into three categories: **preventive**, **illness**, or **sick role** (Gochman, 1988; Kasl & Cobb, 1966). These categories are presented in **TABLE 1-3**. Generally, the health-related behaviors of healthy people and those who try to maintain their health are considered preventive behaviors and are strongly tied to primary prevention. The previous examples of different health behaviors can be viewed as preventive health behaviors. Illness behavior is defined as any behavior undertaken by individuals who *perceive* themselves to be ill and who seek relief or definition of the illness. Illness behaviors are linked closely to secondary prevention as the goal is the early intervention and control of a disease. Some examples of illness behaviors would be seeking care from a healthcare provider to obtain a diagnosis, turning to self-help strategies to lose weight if overweight or to reduce anxiety, or seeking help for a drinking problem by going to a 12-step program. Illness behavior stems from the perception that something may

be wrong physically and/or psychologically and is therefore subject to an individual's interpretation of the situation or symptoms. Furthermore, even if people perceive that they may be sick, they may not seek care due to lack of health insurance or other resources.

A logical extension of illness behavior is sick-role behavior. Once an individual is diagnosed with a disease, the treatment plan constitutes the sick-role behavior. Sick-role behavior is denoted as any behavior undertaken to get well. Thus, sick-role behavior is typical of patients in clinical settings and is related to tertiary prevention. One example of sick-role behavior would be adherence to a medically prescribed regimen such as antiretroviral therapy (ART) for patients diagnosed with HIV or switching to a low-carbohydrate/high-fiber diet and exercise regimen for patients diagnosed with type 2 diabetes or cardiovascular disease. Given that patient adherence with medication regimens may be exceedingly poor, sick-role behavior is increasingly being viewed as necessitating individual and environmental intervention and is fast becoming a public health issue. Numerous behavioral, social, economic, medical, and policy-related factors contribute to poor adherence and must be addressed if rates are to improve. For instance, as few as of one of every six people living with HIV receive, and become adherent to, the life-saving advantages of ARTs (Gardner, McLees, Steiner, Del Rio, & Burman, 2011). Adherence issues include lack of

TABLE 1-3 Categories of Health Behaviors and Link to Prevention Level

Type of Health Behavior	State of Person	Behavior	Prevention Level
Preventive	Healthy	Exercise, high-fiber diet, colonoscopy at 50 wear bicycle helmet	Primary
Illness	Perceives health problem	Doctor visit, alternative medicine therapies, join Weight Watchers®, mammogram at 40	Secondary
Sick role	Receives diagnosis	Adherence to treatment regimen (medication, exercise, diet, etc.)	Tertiary

awareness among clinicians about basic adherence management principles, poor communication between patients and clinicians, operational aspects of pharmacy and medical practice, and professional barriers, all of which compromise the effectiveness of therapy. Given all these issues, it is no wonder that adherence to drugs that decrease hypertension and lower cholesterol, for example, is problematic even among people recovering from a heart attack (Ho, Bryson, & Rumsfeld, 2009). As C. Everett Koop, former surgeon general of the United States, stated succinctly, "Drugs don't work in patients who don't take them."

Health Promotion: Definition and Background

Public health seeks to create healthful living conditions. In the 19th century, the focus was on creating safe and healthy environmental infrastructures to reduce the spread of infectious diseases. Early in the 20th century, the focus shifted to the individual with large-scale immunization programs. Beginning in the late 20th century and continuing into the 21st century, a new public health movement emerged where both ends of the spectrum were and are continuing to be addressed. Public health initiatives became multidimensional by targeting individuals, systems, and political structures to affect health behaviors. More importantly, a shift occurred that emphasized the significant role of environmental influences in shaping individual behavior and affecting health; the said influences included but were not limited to culture, public policy, areas of technology, work, energy production, and urbanization. Also, along the same lines as the old public health, the new public health considered the influence of not only built environments but also the natural environment, and thus, conservation of natural resources became a primary goal. This shift in theoretical perspective and scope has been deemed the "new public health" (Macdonald & Bunton, 1992). Although in some ways the new public health has come full circle from the early beginnings of the old public health (i.e., focusing on environmental structures to affect health outcomes), the new public health also includes an emphasis on how those relevant environmental structures and influences affect individual health behavior, which in turn is linked to health outcomes. The new public health embraces the role of individuals in changing their health behavior while also emphasizing the relevant environmental and structural elements within their context to facilitate the adoption of health-promoting behaviors.

The new public health embraces the role of individuals in changing their health behavior while also emphasizing the relevant environmental and structural elements within their context to facilitate the adoption of health-promoting behaviors.

Health promotion emerged as a field against this backdrop of the new public health; it arose out of necessity in part from the insufficiency and costliness of biomedical approaches in improving the public's health, but also from the inability of medical professionals to understand fully how to affect health behavior. In simple terms, health promotion can be viewed as a *process* of enabling people to increase control over, and to improve, their health and the conditions that affect their health (WHO, 1986). Thus, health promotion is concerned not only with empowering people to remain free from illness but also with enhancing their ability to avoid, resist, or overcome illness—moving them to the left side of the wellness–illness continuum shown in Figure 1-4. By enabling people to recognize health threats and creating conditions that facilitate protective action, health promotion can be viewed as a "behavioral" inoculation in the same way that a traditional vaccine inoculates against infectious agents (Ewart, 1991).

Although there are many other definitions of health promotion, we provide one that is more comprehensive and also "official" in the sense that it was used as part of legislation introduced

Health promotion is defined as the art and science of motivating people to enhance their lifestyle to achieve complete health, not just the absence of disease. Complete health involves a balance of physical, mental, and social health.

in the U.S. Senate in 2004. Health promotion is defined as the art and science of motivating people to enhance their lifestyle to achieve complete health, not just the absence of disease. Complete health involves a balance of physical, mental, and social health. As a first impression, this definition of health promotion indicates that health-promotion's objectives are diverse, broad, and complex, and that it embraces a multifaceted and integrated approach in achieving those objectives (e.g., "facilitate behavior change" and "develop supportive environments"). But the unanswered question is: how does health promotion accomplish such lofty and wide-ranging goals?

Health-Promotion Strategies

In **FIGURE 1-8**, we depict the different strategies that health promotion uses to achieve goals. As you can see, the strategies are general and are not limited to any one specific health problem or to a specific set of behaviors. Each strategy can be applied to a range of settings, risk factors, population groups, diseases, or negative health outcomes. Moreover, these strategies are not typically applied in isolation, but overlap and are integral to achieving health-promotion objectives. For example, research is at the forefront of any health-promotion endeavor, and it also informs all of the other strategies shown in the figure. Research can reveal the **epidemiology** (i.e., the scope, causes, and risk factors of disease) of the health issue, the underlying environmental and individual determinants, and the negative outcomes, as well as provide insight into targeted, at-risk populations and their environments. Furthermore, research provides a valid and reliable way to understand the health issue from multiple theoretical perspectives and to

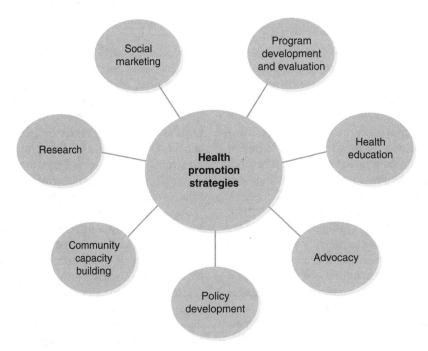

FIGURE 1-8 Health-promotion strategies

inform health-promotion activities, whether they are part of a health education program, a social marketing program, or activities involved in policy development.

Research is also critical in determining whether the health-promotion initiative was effective in reaching its goals, and, if so, research can also show *how* the goals were achieved. This type of research is critical in supporting evidence-based health-promotion practice so as to improve the quality and cost-effectiveness of health-promotion interventions. Against this research backdrop, advocacy represents an important and related strategy. Advocacy is necessary to gain the political commitment, policy support, social acceptance, and systems support for a particular health program. Advocacy may be carried out through lobbying, social marketing, a health education program, or community organizing. Finally, building community capacity is a key strategy for sustaining health-promotion efforts. Community capacity represents the community's ability to do things that promote and sustain its well-being. A number of factors have been proposed as contributing to capacity building, such as leadership, resources, knowledge, skills, and collaboration (Provan, Nakama, Veazie, Teufel-Shone, & Huddleston, 2003). Achieving community capacity by affecting all of these factors may not be feasible, yet many of these factors are modifiable through the use of other health-promotion strategies. For example, health education can be used to convey information and knowledge and impart skills to community members and service organizations; social marketing can also be used in tandem with health education efforts to raise awareness of health information or to inform community members about resources; and research can be used to create an inventory of social organizations, agencies, and other stakeholders within the community so that a network of resources can be constructed. Thus, in reviewing these strategies used in health promotion, you can appreciate why health promotion is considered a process that employs multiple strategies in partnership to achieve its goals of optimal health.

Theory in Health-Promotion Research and Practice

What is missing from Figure 1-8, however, is the inclusion of another circle that would convey that the cornerstone of all health-promotion strategies is theory. Health-promotion researchers, policymakers, and practitioners use theory to guide many of their health-promotion strategies. Theory informs what variables to measure, how to measure them, and how they are interrelated. Within the context of health promotion, theory is viewed as a tool for enhancing our understanding of complex situations versus something that offers universal explanations or predictions (Green, 2000). This more practical perspective is grounded in praxis and acknowledges that theory should be relative to the context in which it is used. *Health Behavior Theory for Public Health* describes many of the more relevant theories used in health promotion. We acknowledge that, like any tool, theory must be used correctly and with fidelity, but even when it is, different results could be observed depending on the context.

Because health promotion involves a *process* that seeks to change both environments and individuals in order to facilitate behavior change and achieve health, it may not be perceived as a specific field of study in its own right. Rather, health promotion has defined itself more in terms of its goals and strategies rather than the subject of its inquiries. Therefore, it has had to borrow from other disciplines to create its body of knowledge. Significant contributions from clinical and social psychology, child development, sociology, and education have shaped the discipline of health promotion by providing

Significant contributions from clinical and social psychology, child development, sociology, and education have shaped the discipline of health promotion by providing a wide range of theoretical perspectives to utilize in its inquiries and to guide its strategies.

a wide range of theoretical perspectives to utilize in its inquiries and to guide its strategies. These theoretical perspectives are the driving force behind health-promotion research and practice and provide the framework for implementing health-promotion strategies in achieving its behavioral, social, environmental, political, and economic goals. Other fields such as philosophy, social policy, and marketing have also made significant theoretical contributions, but not to the same degree (Macdonald & Bunton, 1992).

Health Behavior Theory for Public Health aims to educate students, researchers, and practitioners in many of these theories and in their applications to the various health behaviors described in this chapter. Furthermore, we maintain throughout this text that an ecological approach to health promotion involves using multiple theories that help to identify and understand the relationships among the social causes of health within and across multiple levels. The intervention strategies should also be guided by multiple theories. Although perhaps a daunting task, the end result is the creation of a new body of knowledge that expands the current theoretical boundaries and informs evidence-based practice (see **FIGURE 1-9**).

We maintain that one theory alone cannot begin to adequately address the complexities involved in attempting to fully understand the behavior and to change it; thus, we emphasize that when reviewing and learning about the various theories presented in this text, it is important to keep in mind that multiple theories are required for both understanding the problem and providing more complex and effective solutions.

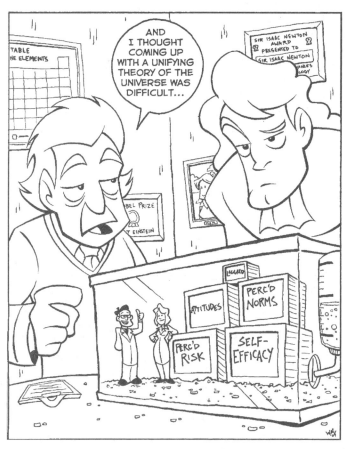

FIGURE 1-9 Great minds struggle to develop a "theory of the solution"

Copyright 2011 by Justin Wagner; with permission

> # Take Home Messages

- Health is not only a state of physical, mental, and social well-being, but also includes the opportunity and available resources that enable people's ability to achieve optimal health.

- The new public health of the 21st century deals with the prevention of both infectious and chronic diseases that contribute greatly to the rates of early mortality and morbidity. The emphasis is on population-based health conditions where personal health behavior is but one "condition." Thus, for public health to be achieved, changes to relevant environmental factors must also be emphasized.

- The new public health utilizes and embraces strategies from earlier times, but also includes an emphasis on the importance of understanding behavior within the context of our natural and built environments.

- Surveillance initiatives into the prevalence of disease, as well as research into the determinants and mediators, combine to promote healthful behavior.

- Health promotion is a process involving many health and education professions, disciplines, and practices for altering health behavior and conditions that affect health behavior.

- Theory is at the core of effective public health approaches that seek to make changes to the environment, which ultimately will enhance health behavior and achieve the health of the people.

> # References

American Diabetes Association. (2008). Economic costs of diabetes in the U.S. in 2007. *Diabetes Care, 31*(3), 596–615.

Centers for Disease Control and Prevention. (1999). Achievements in public health, 1900–1999: Control of infectious diseases, 1900–1999. *Morbidity & Mortality Weekly Report, 48*, 621–629.

Centers for Disease Control and Prevention. (2008). CDC Childhood Injury Report. Retrieved from http://www.cdc.gov/safechild/images/CDC=childhoodinjury.pdf

Centers for Medicare & Medicaid Services. (2015). National health expenditure data. Retrieved from https://www.cms.gov/research-statistics-data-and-systems/statistics-trends-and-reports/nationalhealthexpenddata/nationalhealthaccountshistorical.html

Chaloupka, F. J., & Warner, K. E. (2000). The economics of smoking. In A. J. Culyer & J. P. Newhouse (Eds.), *Handbook of health economics: Vol. 1* (1st ed., pp. 1539–1627). Amsterdam, The Netherlands: Elsevier.

Cohen, J. T., Neumann, P. J., & Weinstein, M. C. (2008). Does preventive care save money? *The New England Journal of Medicine, 358*, 661–663.

Durbin, D. R., Elliott, M. R., & Winston, F. K. (2003). Belt-positioning booster seats and reduction in risk of injury among children in vehicle crashes. *Journal of the American Medical Association, 289*(21), 2835–2840.

Ewart, C. K. (1991). How integrative behavioral theory can improve health promotion and disease prevention. In R. G. Frank, A. Baum, & J. L. Wallander (Eds.), *Handbook of clinical health psychology: Models and perspectives in health psychology* (Vol. 3, pp. 249–289). Washington, DC: American Psychological Association.

Gardner, E. M., McLees, M. P., Steiner, J. F., Del Rio, C., & Burman, W. J. (2011). The spectrum of engagement in HIV care and its relevance to test-and-treat strategies for prevention of HIV infection. *Clinical Infectious Disease, 52*, 793–800.

Gochman, D. (1988). Health behavior: Plural perspectives. In D. Gochman (Ed.), *Health behavior: Emerging research perspectives* (pp. 3–18). New York, NY: Plenum Press.

Green, J. (2000). The role of theory in evidence-based health promotion practice. *Health Education Research, 15*, 125–129.

Ho, P. M., Bryson, C. L., & Rumsfeld, J. S. (2009). Medication adherence: Its importance in cardiovascular outcomes. *Circulation, 119*, 3028–3035.

Kasl, S., & Cobb, S. (1966). Health behavior, illness behavior, and sick role behavior. *Archives of Environmental Health, 12*, 246–266.

Knowler, W. C., Barrett-Connor, E., Fowler, S. E., Hamman, R. F., Lachin, J. M., Walker, E. A., ... Diabetes Prevention Program Research Group. (2002). Reduction in the incidence of type 2 diabetes with lifestyle intervention or metformin. *The New England Journal of Medicine, 346*, 393–403.

Leavell, H. D., & Clark, E. G. (1960). *Preventive medicine for the doctor in his community: An epidemiologic approach.* New York, NY: McGraw-Hill.

Macdonald, G., & Bunton, R. (1992). Health promotion: Discipline or disciplines? In R. Bunton & G. MacDonald (Eds.), *Health promotion: Disciplines and diversity* (pp. 6–19). London, England: Routledge Press.

McGinnis, J. M., & Foege, W. H. (1993). Actual causes of death in the United States. *Journal of the American Medical Association, 270*(18), 2207–2212.

Mokdad, A. S., Marks, J. S., Stroup, D. F., & Gerberding, J. L. (2004). Actual causes of death in the United States, 2000. *Journal of the American Medical Association, 291*, 1238–1245.

Provan, K. G., Nakama, L., Veazie, M. A., Teufel-Shone, N. I., & Huddleston, C. (2003). Building community capacity around chronic disease services through a collaborative interorganizational network. *Health Education & Behavior, 30,* 646–662.

Rose, G. (1992). *The strategy of preventive medicine.* New York, NY: Oxford Press.

Syme, S. L. (1996). To prevent disease: The need for a new approach. In D. Blane, E. Brunner, & R. Wilkinson (Eds.), *Health and social organization: Toward a healthy policy for the twenty-first century.* London, England: Routledge Press.

U.S. Department of Health, Education & Welfare. (1979). Healthy people: The Surgeon General's report on health promotion and disease prevention. Retrieved from http://www.eric.ed.gov/PDFS/ED186357.pdf

World Health Organization. (1986). The Ottawa charter for health promotion. Retrieved from http://www.who.int/hpr/NPH/docs/ottawa_charter_hp.pdf

World Health Organization. (1999). Report on infectious diseases: Removing obstacles to healthy development. Retrieved from http://www.who.int/infectious-disease-report/indexrpt99.html

World Health Organization. (2009). Health systems performance assessment. Retrieved from http://who.int/bulletin/volumes/87/1/08=061945/en/

Section Opener: © lzf/Shutterstock; © Henrik Sorensen/Getty Images; © MeskPhotography/Shutterstock; © Hero Images/Getty Images
Chapter Opener: © lzf/Shutterstock; © Henrik Sorensen/Getty Images; © MeskPhotography/Shutterstock; © Hero Images/Getty Images

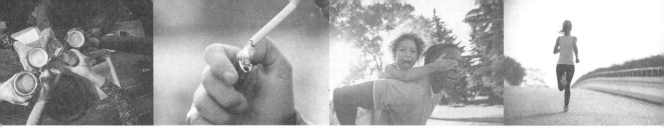

CHAPTER 2

How Theory Informs Health Promotion and Public Health Practice

Richard A. Crosby, Laura F. Salazar, and Ralph J. DiClemente

If vegetables tasted as good as bacon we would have an outbreak of good health.

—**Gary Larson**

PREVIEW

Health behaviors are diverse and sometimes complex, therefore fostering their adoption is a challenging process. The challenge often begins by understanding the multiple influences on any given health behavior. This understanding is facilitated by the use of theory, thus making theory an indispensable tool in public health and health promotion.

OBJECTIVES

1. Understand that health behaviors are diverse.
2. Understand proximal and distal influences on health behavior.
3. Describe the importance of theory in health promotion and understand how theory informs health-promotion practice and research.
4. Describe how challenges in health-promotion practice can be understood through the use of theory.
5. Understand and appreciate the use of theory in multilevel prevention approaches.

▶ Introduction

In the past few decades, behavioral and social science theories have been used to advance our ability to achieve the public health objectives of the nation. Theory has become an indispensable tool for the development, implementation, and evaluation of public health initiatives because it enables researchers to better understand and change health behavior. Key documents, such as *Healthy People 2020*, inform health-promotion efforts in the United States and globally advocate for the application of theory. Theory can be used in diverse ways to achieve meaningful changes in behavior that translate into reduced morbidity and mortality at the population level. This chapter provides the contextual background needed to understand how public health—and specifically, health promotion—programs can be designed to change a broad range of health behaviors. Next, the chapter provides a framework for understanding how theory can most effectively be used to inform and guide interventions designed to reduce health risk behaviors associated with morbidity and mortality. Of note, in our experience, students learning about the use of theory in public health practice often feel "stuck" in a sea of terminology, but terms are simply a way to represent concepts. Thus, we suggest that the best way to feel confident about terminology is to have a firm grasp of the concepts behind the terms. Approach this chapter with great care as it prepares you for much of what follows in the rest of the text.

Theory has become an indispensable tool for the development, implementation, and evaluation of public health initiatives because it enables researchers to better understand and change health behavior.

▶ Key Concepts

Health Behaviors Are Diverse

Based on what you learned in Chapter 1, you now understand that health behaviors are extremely complex and diverse. This diversity necessitates that an equally diverse range of theories be available for application in health-promotion practice and research. Indeed, students learning about theories used in health promotion typically ask, "Why do we need so many different theories?" The answer to this question becomes apparent upon considering the broad spectrum of differences among health behaviors. To represent this spectrum, we have identified three dimensions to health behavior: complexity, frequency, and volitionality. These three dimensions can be applied to illustrate the variation in health behaviors.

The first dimension is **complexity**. Behaviors may be highly complex, meaning they involve higher levels of knowledge, skill, or resources to perform than simple behaviors. Consider, for example, eating a low-sodium diet. Sodium is in many foods and at varying levels, so one challenge is to become educated on which foods are high in sodium and should be avoided. Another challenge to think about is how to know which foods are low in sodium and also good-tasting. Another example of a complex health behavior is using male condoms. The correct use of male condoms involves at least 10 steps. Multiple studies indicate that very few people perform all 10 steps correctly.

Not all behaviors are complex; some, such as getting vaccinated against influenza, brushing teeth, or wearing sunscreen, are less complex. The key lies in understanding that these behaviors are relatively easy to perform and may be viewed as less demanding in terms of necessary knowledge, skills, or resources.

A critical point here is that the dimension of complexity is not always inherent in the behavior, which may be counterintuitive. Complexity is also a function of the environment. For example, boiling drinking water is not a complex behavior in a nation like the United States; however, in a resource-poor nation, boiling water could be considered complex given an absence of a reliable heat source or pots. Similarly, getting the flu vaccine may not be complex for a middle-class American, whereas the same behavior may be cost-prohibitive and logistically problematic for a person living in isolated, rural poverty. To make this picture complete, it is also vital to understand that complexity may vary as a function of the population. For example, the complexity of having a first mammogram for a woman who just turned 50 years of age is likely to be quite different compared to a woman having "just another mammogram" at age 65. Further, one 50-year-old woman may have ready access to preventive health care, while another may have no such access, thereby greatly magnifying the complexity level of this first mammogram.

In addition to the dimension of complexity, there is the second dimension of **frequency**. Health behaviors can be frequent and repetitive (diet and exercise), one time only (screening for radon), or periodic (obtaining a mammogram or having a flu shot). As you can observe, this second dimension greatly complicates things as a health behavior may be highly complex but require only infrequent repetition (being screened for colorectal cancer), or a behavior could be highly complex and require daily repetition (consuming a low-fat diet).

The concept of **volitionality** is yet another important dimension that can be used to differentiate between various health behaviors. Volitionality represents the degree of personal control over the behavior; specifically, a highly volitional behavior is one in which the person has complete control in performing the behavior—the behavior does not require external resources, assistance, or support. Conversely, behaviors that are low in volitionality require (to some extent) a reliance on external resources, assistance, or support. It is easy to imagine that many health behaviors fall into the latter category. An example of low volitionality may be consuming fresh fruits and vegetables, because performing this behavior requires having access to fresh fruit and vegetables, which are not always affordable or even available. Examples of highly volitional behaviors include flossing, using seat belts, and performing moderate indoor exercises.

Like the dimension of complexity, volitionality is very much tied to the environment. For example, the use of contraceptives for women can vary in terms of volitionality depending on the environment. In many cultures, the use of contraception may not be highly volitional for women because it is their male partners who have control over sexual behaviors and contraceptive-related decisions.

FIGURE 2-1 displays the three dimensions (complexity, frequency, and volitionality) with specific examples of behaviors that vary across these dimensions. In viewing this figure, it becomes clear that health behaviors are quite diverse. Thus, theories applied to the process of understanding and changing health behavior must also be equally diverse. The next section highlights the various dimensions to theory.

Theory Is Relevant at Multiple Levels

Much like health behaviors, theories are also diverse. Although a vast number of theories relevant to health behavior exist, each is somewhat unique in its approach to understanding and changing health behavior. An important paradigm for understanding this range of potential theories is based on the concept that theories can be applied at several "levels" within the environment. Environmental levels represent different influences on individual behavior. The concept of environmental levels is drawn from a classic model of an ecological approach to health promotion as popularized by Bronfenbrenner (1979). **FIGURE 2-2** displays this model.

The model suggests that outer levels influence inner levels all the way down to the individual ("I" in the innermost circle). Although the "I" is often construed as the "target" of all intervention efforts, it is important to note that making changes at any of the levels can

Much like health behaviors, theories are also diverse.

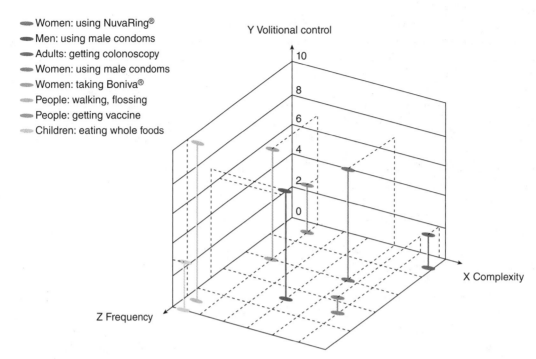

Women: using NuvaRing®
Men: using male condoms
Adults: getting colonoscopy
Women: using male condoms
Women: taking Boniva®
People: walking, flossing
People: getting vaccine
Children: eating whole foods

FIGURE 2-1 Three dimensions of health behavior

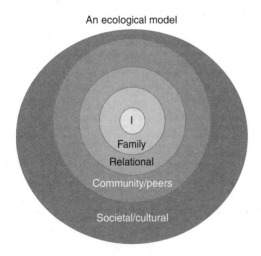

An ecological model

FIGURE 2-2 Socioecological model

influence individual health behavior. In essence, the model suggests that the outermost level influences all other levels and that the next outermost level influences all remaining levels, and so forth. The ultimate implication of this model is that interventions targeting multiple levels represent an ecological approach. Ecological approaches

are widely believed to be more effective compared to single-level approaches and are representative of the new public health. A synonymous term is "multi-level approach," meaning that two or more levels of ecological influence are the targets of the planned health-promotion program.

An applied example will illustrate the principle of an ecological approach to understanding and changing health behavior. Consider the long-standing public health challenge of childhood obesity. Gittelsohon and colleagues (2014) designed and implemented an ecological (i.e., multi-level approach) intervention designed to prevent childhood obesity in the city of Baltimore, MD (USA). The intervention used four levels of influence: individual, household, institutional, and city policy. At the individual-level the targets of the intervention included knowledge, motivation, and skill relative to food selection. At the household-level the intervention sought to teach parents food preparation skills, and portion control measures, that would lead to healthier eating for their children. At the institutional-level targets included a variety of food outlets, including large and small grocery stores, carryout food outlets, recreation centers that serve food, and even wholesale food distributors. Intensive efforts were made at the policy-level to create regulations designed to make healthy food options accessible and affordable.

This is an interesting study in that it provides a clear example of how a health behavior (food consumption) can be understood at multiple levels of causation. From an individual perspective, the behavior is highly resistant to long-term change; however, this multi-level perspective provides ample support structures that optimize the odds of changing the eating behaviors of children over time, and across large populations thereby providing a strong potential for actually lowering the prevalence of childhood obesity. Indeed, the dominant paradigm in health promotion is the use of as many levels as is feasible within a multi-level framework. Thus, theory selection is predicated upon the composition of the applicable levels that best describe a given health behavior.

Proximal Versus Distal Influences on Health Behavior

Many theories exist to understand and change factors found in the inner levels of Bronfenbrenner's ecological model that influence health behavior, whereas a markedly smaller number of theories exist to understand and change those factors located in the outer levels. Inner-level factors are called **proximal influences** because these influences are in close proximity to the individual ("I" level). Conversely, factors located in the outer levels are called **distal influences** because these influences do not always directly or immediately affect the individual due to their location in the model. For example, taxes on cigarettes and tobacco smoking regulations, as well as marketing regulations, are considered distal influences on the behavior of tobacco use. These influences have a broad impact that ultimately can affect tobacco use at the individual level.

The concept of outer levels influencing the inner levels is a key point here. For instance, taxes on tobacco (distal influence) may work through other variables, such as affecting a person's evaluation of the desirability of cigarettes. When a person begins to perceive that the cost of purchasing cigarettes

outweighs the benefits, then he or she may decide to reduce smoking or even quit entirely. The distal influence may have led to the opinion that the "cost of cigarettes is too high." Because proximal influences demonstrate an immediate influence on the health behavior, the perception that the "cost is too high" would be considered a proximal influence on smoking reduction. Please note, however, that this proximal influence was the result of the distal influence of a tax increase. **BOX 2-1** displays several other examples that will help you gain a better understanding of the difference between proximal and distal influences on health behaviors.

To streamline health-promotion efforts, programs need to be designed so that the critical constructs (proximal and distal) are identified and the corresponding intervention methods and strategies for modifying these constructs can be implemented. This process can be overwhelming without the availability of a guide; therefore, the concept of theory-derived intervention activities has been widely embraced in health promotion. Theory keeps us from randomly attempting to change behavior. Indeed, theory helps us to develop an organized, systematic, and efficient approach to investigating health behaviors. Once these investigations produce satisfactory results and are replicated the findings can be used to inform the design of theory-based intervention programs.

Getting Started: An Inductive Approach to Defining the Problem

An inductive approach to defining the problem comprises three informal steps. The first is your own hunch about the nature of the health behavior in question and its underlying causes. The second is to think about the health behavior from a theoretical perspective. The third is to conduct an empirical evaluation (often relying on published literature) that suggests underlying causes of risk behavior

> *Theory helps us to develop an organized, systematic, and efficient approach to investigating health behaviors.*

BOX 2-1 Examples of Distal and Proximal Influences

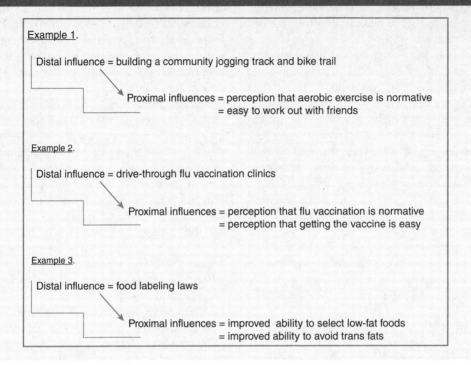

Example 1.

Distal influence = building a community jogging track and bike trail

Proximal influences = perception that aerobic exercise is normative
= easy to work out with friends

Example 2.

Distal influence = drive-through flu vaccination clinics

Proximal influences = perception that flu vaccination is normative
= perception that getting the vaccine is easy

Example 3.

Distal influence = food labeling laws

Proximal influences = improved ability to select low-fat foods
= improved ability to avoid trans fats

and potential antecedents to the adoption of health-protective behaviors. Collectively, the three steps serve the central and initial goal: to identify the determinants of the specific health behavior. Simply stated, **determinants** influence the health behavior; they are the levels of influence shown in Bronfenbrenner's ecological model. Therefore, the identification of determinants can greatly enhance our understanding of those factors that influence health behavior. Determinants should be targeted to affect behavior change; thus, it is the determinants that programs seek to change, not the behavior, per se. Although fostering health behavior change is the ultimate goal, that goal is achieved through planned strategies designed to change multiple determinants. By changing multiple determinants, the goal of lasting behavior change may indeed become a reality. As you will learn when reading Chapter 13 (a chapter that introduces the concept of intervention mapping), theory guides the process of identifying the determinants most likely to alter and support the long-term adoption of health-protective behaviors.

Determinants can be identified through an exercise that is best described by the phrase "determining the theory of the problem." Please note that the word "theory" is used in the generic sense here. Three methods constitute a theory-of-the-problem analysis: (1) literature reviews relevant to the behavior and the population, (2) formal needs assessments, including assessments at the community level and policy level, and (3) empirical investigations using theory as a guide. The last method is the crux of defining and understanding any given health behavior. Stated differently, an initial step is to understand the health behavior from the perspective of the target population and within the context of the relevant environmental factors. Many different theories can facilitate the identification of determinants of behavior. For example, the health belief model hypothesizes that perceived susceptibility to a health-related outcome (e.g., influenza) is one potential determinant of the health-related behavior (e.g., getting vaccinated). Theories of health behavior that identify determinants of risk or protective behaviors that are

An initial step is to understand the health behavior from the perspective of the target population and within the context of the relevant environmental factors.

amenable to change can be very useful in providing program planners with a starting point for producing behavior change.

Determinants of health behavior may range from individual characteristics, such as knowledge, attitudes, and beliefs, to environmental factors such as family, friends, community, culture, and society. As such, an important question becomes, "Where do you start in finding those factors that are related to the health behavior?" A fundamental starting point in any health-promotion effort is to identify the relevant determinants by revealing the answers to questions such as:

- Do people perceive their current behavior as being risky or problematic and, if so, what are their perceptions?
- Are people sufficiently convinced that taking the recommended protective actions will truly be effective?
- What are the reinforcements for engaging in the current risk behaviors?
- What aspects of the immediate social, economic, physical, and legal environments detract from the ability to adopt protective behaviors?
- What aspects of the immediate social, economic, physical, and legal environments support the adoption of protective behaviors?
- What forms of self-confidence (self-efficacy) and actual skill are needed to attempt to perform the behavior in question?

Fortunately, the process of finding answers to these questions is streamlined by the use of theory. If, for example, preliminary investigations suggest that teen pregnancy often results from deliberate attempts to conceive rather than failed attempts at contraception, then a theory should be selected to help enrich this understanding. For instance, a rather popular theory known as social cognitive theory (SCT, see Chapter 8) has often been applied to the prevention of teen pregnancy.

As applied to guiding an investigation of the preceding questions, SCT would dictate that a theoretical construct known as **self-efficacy** be examined. In this example, self-efficacy can be viewed as perceptions that teens hold about their ability to successfully manage pregnancy, childbearing, and parenthood in the context of modern society. Self-efficacy can also be investigated to advance our understanding relative to teens' acquisition and use of contraceptives, condoms, or even their self-control to abstain from sex. Further, an SCT-guided investigation would assess other factors (e.g., response efficacy, the expectation that condoms confer protection against pregnancy and sexually transmitted diseases, peer norms surrounding condom use) that reinforce both risk and protective behaviors among the target population of teens. Environmental factors such as access to contraception and condoms would also be assessed. In essence, the theory would direct the questions asked as part of the research process, and thus indirectly influence the identification of determinants. A word of caution, however, is warranted at this juncture in that the concept of "personal agency" that is implicit is the vast majority of theories used in health behavior may have very limited applicability in societies and cultures characterized by collectivism rather than individualism (DiClemente, Crosby, & Kegler, 2009).

Program Planning

A useful way for developing effective programs with theory is to consider several questions. These questions are characterized by a simple string of statements involving what, who, how, why, and when (see **TABLE 2-1**). Please be aware that Table 2-1 is only a starting point in the learning process.

Once the health behavior in question has been thoroughly analyzed regarding its cause, the next and final step is analyze how it can be changed to promote health. In this process the practitioner determines what has worked in the past to change identified determinants and identifies possible approaches or specific theories that could be applied in the pending program. As previously noted, mastery of multiple theories available in health promotion will optimize your ability

TABLE 2-1 Core Questions Addressed When Theory Is Used to Identify Program Objectives

Elements	Core Question and Meaning
What?	What are the most important socioecological changes that must occur to optimize the odds of program success? The use of any ecological approach requires that supportive structural changes be implemented as part of the planned program.
Who?	Who will be in direct contact with the target population? In essence, this element addresses the heart of the intervention—the actual change agent is the key to success and various theories posit differing agents.
How?	How will community support be gained and maintained? Various theories, models, and approaches exist to achieve the goal of initial and ongoing participation from key people (often referred to as "stakeholders").
Why?	Why might the program fail? The reality is that multiple factors may be immutable to short-term change and thus limit the odds of program success. This is particularly true with social capital, as well as economic and legal factors.
When?	When can the first and subsequent signs of program success be observed? Program planning theories and models provide insight regarding structured milestones that lead to the eventual achievement of a final goal. These milestones are connected to that maintenance of community support.

to affect meaningful behavior change. In essence, your task is to become well-versed in the application of the many "tools" that can be applied to your trade. Like any skilled craftsperson, a quality health-promotion program is built through the use of multiple and diverse tools. Thus, possessing a large repertoire of theory tools is imperative to effective practice. For example, a program may screen injection drug users for hepatitis C and then provide prevention case management to people testing positive. The theory-based needs of such a program may be quite modest compared to a health-promotion effort designed to reduce tobacco consumption. In the former scenario, the challenge is to prevent someone from transmitting the hepatitis C virus to others; this goal will most likely be achieved by conveying to the person a norm of safety relative to protecting others and providing him/her with a set of skills and resources designed to foster harm-reduction practices. Conversely, the latter scenario necessitates not only changing people, but also changing their environment; for example, increases in tobacco tax have been demonstrated to lower tobacco consumption and smoke-free ordinances have been shown to foster smoking cessation. In sum, the application of theory may be as discreet as individual counseling (as in the hepatitis C example) or as broad-based as changing policy and laws (as in the tobacco example). That theory exists across this broad spectrum is a vital point to remember in health-promotion practice.

Because health-promotion practice is vital to public health, the use of theory at multiple levels (see Chapter 13) is a task well-worth the time and resources. As a rule, an ecological approach (see Figure 2-2) should always be considered when program planning occurs. The concept of using the multiple levels within an ecological model

That theory exists across this broad spectrum is a vital point to remember in health-promotion practice.

implies the constant use of the individual level and varying degrees of other levels such as families, peer groups, entire communities, and even social structures such as culture and law. At this juncture, it may suddenly become very easy to get lost in a quagmire of seemingly similar terms such as multilevel, individual level, or environmental level. The picture becomes a bit more complicated by the common use of the term "ecological approach"; as such, please take a moment to carefully think about what you have learned so far by slowly reviewing the following text, as well as examining how the term "ecological approach" can now be fitted into this larger vision of health promotion. The term "multilevel" implies that at least two of the following levels of causation have been examined: individual, familial, relational, peer, community, societal, or policy/legal. When each of these levels is explored, relative to a single health behavior, a more complete understanding of the behavior is obtained. Furthermore, when interactions between the levels are examined, an even greater understanding of the health behavior occurs, thereby magnifying the odds that program planning and subsequent implementation of interventions will be successful. This concept of exploring all applicable levels and their interrelationships constitutes a true ecological approach to understanding health behavior. It is useful, if possible, to intervene at every level of the ecological model. For example, altering policy/legal (e.g., safety belt or child protective seat laws) may facilitate behavior change, although additional educational, persuasion, enforcement, and other actions may be needed to achieve optimal levels of change. Typically, policy/legal, built environments, and related actions can lead to significant changes in the environmental context of a given behavior and, as such, they are sometimes referred to as structural or environmental. Notably then, structural or environmental actions need to be fully explored and undertaken when feasible, as part of an ecological approach.

> *Theories provide program planners with a range of theory-derived hypothesized mediators that will become the targets of intervention efforts.*

Hypothesized Mediators

The use of theory to identify determinants of health behaviors is critical to the success of a program. Stated more formally, theories provide program planners with a range of theory-derived hypothesized mediators that will become the targets of intervention efforts. The term "**mediator**" in this context represents the determinant targeted by the intervention and its association with the health behavior. If the determinant is theory-derived, it is correctly referred to as a **hypothesized mediator**. The hypothesized mediator "comes between" the intervention and the behavioral outcome. In essence, a change in health behavior is achieved by changing the hypothesized mediator associated with that specific behavior. **FIGURE 2-3** provides an example of this point.

After examining Figure 2-3, imagine that you next determine that perceived barriers to influenza vaccination are also important in determining vaccination. Thus, a second hypothesized mediator would be perceived barriers to vaccination. Out-of-pocket cost, for example, may be a common perceived barrier, with the program implication being that making the vaccine available at

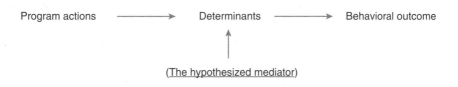

FIGURE 2-3　A simplified planning model for influencing vaccine acceptance

little or no cost to the person may be an effective strategy in enhancing the likelihood of vaccination. Other barriers may include access to vaccination sites. Program implications then become centered on enhancing access to vaccination by perhaps providing highly visible and convenient locations where people may receive vaccination (e.g., banks, supermarkets, public parks). These multiple actions would all be designed to reduce the number and magnitude of perceived barriers to influenza vaccination among people in the target community. Again, the expected behavioral action that would stem from a positive change in this hypothesized mediator would be greater likelihood of influenza vaccination among community members. Common hypothesized mediators in health-promotion practice include:

- Belief that the behaviors will produce the desired results
- The resources and ability to perform the behavior, possibly on a daily basis
- Social norms that provide reinforcement for the behavior
- The presence of structural factors that promote access needed to preform behaviors

Moving from Hypothesized Mediators to Objectives

Once the hypothesized mediators are identified, how are they used as a starting point for changing health behaviors? These hypothesized mediators are the platform for developing intervention objectives. An **objective** is a quantifiable action that, when achieved, will contribute to achieving behavior change. For example, consider the health behavior (especially important in developing countries) of breastfeeding. Suppose that a key hypothesized mediator of breastfeeding among first-time mothers is having the social support of women who have successfully breastfed their infants. The goal is to increase breastfeeding; thus, the intervention objective of enhancing the level of social support for this practice, especially among first-time mothers, becomes the guide to intervention planning. In this case, the objective would be to provide first-time mothers with social support

(in various forms) and education in the process of breastfeeding their newborn infants. Some hypothesized mediators can be quite challenging to change, particularly if they involve health policy or laws. Yet even in these instances, guidance may be available based on insights from theory.

A second question then becomes, "Does theory also apply to this process?" The answer is yes. Theory is used very often in health promotion to guide the process of identifying and developing methods for changing hypothesized mediators. For instance, one theory that may be useful for creating a social support network is the Natural Helper model as described by Eng and Parker (2002). This model provides guidance in the process of using natural helpers (an informal network of people who already serve in this capacity and who are uniquely qualified to work with a specific population) to achieve a defined objective. In this example, the objective would be to increase social support, which theoretically would lead to the behavior change (e.g., adopting the practice of breastfeeding). Utilizing natural helpers would be the intervention to achieve the objective.

A second example to consider is the control of waterborne illness. In this case, one important health-protective behavior might be drinking bottled water rather than tap water. A likely hypothesized mediator might be the theoretical construct of **social norms**. Normative influences have a profound influence on all types of behavior, not just health behavior. In some places in the United States, the norm is to drink from the tap (faucet) and in other places drinking filtered or bottled water is the norm (although bottled water is falling out of favor because of the impact of plastic bottles on the environment). So, what if an outbreak of waterborne illness such as cryptosporidiosis or cholera (see **BOX 2-2**) necessitated that community residents accustomed to drinking tap water had to give up this practice or risk infection? The public health challenge would be to foster the use of filters, boiling water, or bottled water for drinking, cooking, and even brushing teeth. Although large segments of any given population may be receptive to this change, other segments may not be. Simply stated, the alternative may be contrary to the norms of their

BOX 2-2 *Cryptosporidium* and Cholera

Cryptosporidiosis is a gastrointestinal illness caused by parasitic protozoa of the genus *Cryptosporidium* and can produce watery diarrhea lasting 1–3 weeks; one or two cases per 100,000 population are reported annually in the United States. Fecal–oral transmission of *Cryptosporidium* oocysts occurs through ingestion of contaminated drinking or recreational water, consumption of contaminated food, and contact with infected persons or animals (e.g., cattle or sheep). Unlike bacterial pathogens, *Cryptosporidium* oocysts are resistant to chlorine disinfection and can survive for days in treated recreational water venues (e.g., public and residential swimming pools and community and commercial water parks). In 2006, a total of 18 cryptosporidiosis outbreaks were reported to the CDC.

Centers for Disease Control and Prevention. (2006). Cryptosporidiosis outbreaks associated with recreational water use—Five states, 2006. *Morbidity and Mortality Weekly Report, 56,* 729–732.

The cholera epidemic in Africa has lasted more than 30 years. In areas with inadequate sanitation, a cholera epidemic cannot be stopped immediately, and, although far fewer cases have been reported from Latin America and Asia in recent years, there are no signs that the global cholera pandemic will end soon. Major improvements in sewage and water treatment systems are needed in many countries to prevent future epidemic cholera.

The risk for cholera is very low for U.S. travelers visiting areas with epidemic cholera. When simple precautions are observed, contracting the disease is unlikely. All travelers to areas where cholera has occurred should observe the following recommendations:

- Drink only water that you have boiled or treated with chlorine or iodine. Other safe beverages include tea and coffee made with boiled water and carbonated, bottled beverages with no ice.
- Eat only foods that have been thoroughly cooked and are still hot, or fruit that you have peeled yourself.
- Avoid undercooked or raw fish or shellfish, including ceviche.
- Make sure all vegetables are cooked; avoid salads.
- Avoid foods and beverages from street vendors.
- Do not bring perishable seafood back to the United States.

    A simple rule of thumb is "Boil it, cook it, peel it, or forget it."

Centers for Disease Control and Prevention. (2005). Cholera. Retrieved from http://www.cdc.gov/ncidod/dbmd/.cdc.gov/ncidod/dbmd/diseaseinfo/cholera_g.htm

community, network, group, or family, or not within their economic means.

At this point it is vital to understand that theory guides the identification of objectives that, if achieved, will lead to changes in the behavior. In this example, one theory-derived objective might be to foster the adoption of drinking bottled water among highly respected and visible community members who will model the new behaviors for others. This modeling effect may, in turn, foster a new social norm, consequently changing the behavior through the hypothesized mediator.

> *Theory guides the identification of objectives that, if achieved, will lead to changes in the behavior.*

Thus, theory gives direction to channel intervention efforts toward change in hypothesized mediators. **FIGURE 2-4** illustrates this point.

Once the program objectives are firmly in place, the intervention activities that will compose the health-promotion program can be created. Intervention activities may be classified as:

- Strategies
- Methods
- Tactics
- Technology-based tactics

These types of activities will be described in more detail in Chapter 13. For now, the critical concept is to understand that selecting and applying intervention activities is an art rather than a science. Wise use of intervention methods and

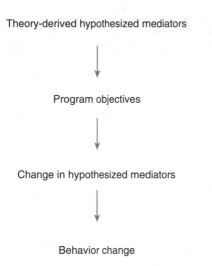

Theory-derived hypothesized mediators

Program objectives

Change in hypothesized mediators

Behavior change

FIGURE 2-4 Sequence of events leading to behavior change

> *The ultimate success of a health-promotion program is in the hands of the practitioner, with the researcher playing a far less prominent role.*

strategies is based on a thorough understanding of the target population and a learned sense of how to effectively communicate with members of that population. In essence, the ultimate success of a health-promotion program is in the hands of the practitioner, with the researcher playing a far less prominent role.

Key questions that may be answered through the use of theory, pertaining to the wise use of intervention activities, are:

- Who will actually conduct the intervention with members of the target population? Will these interveners be paid employees or volunteers?
- What structural-level supports should exist to optimize the odds that members of the target population will adopt the desired protective behaviors? What plans exist for sustaining these changes, and who is ultimately responsible for gaining the political and community support needed to make these changes?

- How will "buy in" from key community stakeholders be achieved and maintained throughout the intervention period? How will the program be institutionalized so that it evolves and continues within the target community after initial resources have been depleted?
- What are the short-term goals, intermediate goals, and long-term goals of the program, and how will progress toward these endpoints be monitored and achieved?
- What assets and liabilities exist, within the community, that are relevant to the overall success of the program as well as its short-term and intermediate goals?

Theories Have Differences and Similarities to Each Other

Any one theory described in this text can be said to possess unique properties that make it distinct from other theories. Various theories share common goals, but they typically employ differing approaches and use different constructs. Thus, theories are indeed as diverse as the range of potential challenges to changing health behavior. All too often students and professionals in public health become confused about theory, and their subsequent response is to learn one or two theories well and only apply these theories, irrespective of the health behaviors targeted or the hypothesized mediators identified, throughout their career. This is unfortunate because learning about theory need not be a complicated process at all. At their core, theories that identify hypothesized mediators of health behavior may share relatively similar constructs—understanding the similarities and differences form the basis for a much more efficient understanding and effective use of theories.

TABLE 2-2 provides a list of common theoretical constructs found in many of the theories often used to identify hypothesized mediators of health behavior. For example, many of these theories posit that people adopt a given health behavior, in part, based on a feeling of perceived threat. Threat is generally viewed by most theories to lead people to a contemplative stage that may involve a

TABLE 2-2 Common Theoretical Constructs	
Elements	**Meaning**
Perceived threat*	This is the theoretical basis for all voluntary behavior change. When people can freely choose to reject unhealthy behaviors and adopt healthy behaviors, this shift must be motivated by some internal (cognitive) sense of impending trouble.
Self-efficacy	Adapted from social cognitive theory, this element simply represents a person's perceived ability to perform a health-protective behavior and/or to avoid a given risk behavior. This is not a generic trait of people; instead, self-efficacy is specific to the behavior under consideration.
Outcome expectations	Also adapted from social cognitive theory, the concept is simply described as the perceptions that people hold regarding personal gain if a given health-protective behavior is adopted or a given risk behavior is avoided. Gains can be physical, emotional, relational, social, or economic. Gains can also be short-term or longer-term.
Barriers to change	This concept of "cost" represents any and all disadvantages to adopting a health-protective behavior or avoiding a risk behavior. In the former scenario, these costs may be physical, emotional, relational, social, or economic; in the latter scenario, these costs typically comprise the perceived loss of a feeling or social connection that is highly valued.
Facilitators of change	These are the structural supports that enable change. They may involve access issues, social support, time, practical constraints, economic constraints, and even legal issues that preclude change.
Support to maintain change	These structural supports are specific to the ongoing practice of health-protective behaviors. For behaviors that require repetition, a host of social, economic, and legal supports are necessary to prevent relapse.

*Generally speaking, perceived threat is considered to be a combination of perceived severity (e.g., how bad is the disease or condition?) and perceived susceptibility (e.g., can "it" happen to me?).

personal assessment of self-efficacy to adopt the advocated health behavior(s). This contemplation is also hypothesized to involve a personal estimation of whether the anticipated positive outcomes of the recommended health behavior are likely to occur. The adoption of health behaviors becomes complex when several barriers that may preclude the behavior are identified. Although the barriers may be personal (e.g., lack of requisite skills), they are also quite likely to be structural (e.g., issues related to access, support, and economics). We urge you, however, to bear in mind that Table 2-2 is merely a starting point in the learning process—it provides a basis for an expanded understanding of theory that will result when considering the specific definitions, propositions, and application potentials of the theories described in this text.

Moving Toward an Ecological Approach

The primary function of an ecological approach is the use of every available means that has a reasonably strong potential to ultimately contribute to lasting behavior change. Although intervening with individuals, families, and even entire communities may seem to be standard-fare in health promotion practice, the concept of changing key aspects of the environment is increasingly valuable paradigm. In many cases, changes to the environment can become powerful influences on health behavior; as such, one increasingly important role taken on by the health-promotion practitioner is to become an advocate for changes in policy, regulation, and legislation that enhance people's long-term adoption of health-protective behaviors. Past examples of policy-level changes that greatly influenced public health include the widespread fortification of table salt with iodine to prevent goiter (a thyroid disorder) or the addition of fluoride to water supplies to prevent tooth decay. Note that in each case the concept of changing a hypothesized mediator is moot because the behavior is not chosen (i.e., people do not consume salt with the intent to avoid goiter and they do not drink water with the intent to prevent tooth decay).

Ecological approaches may be most appropriate to the health behaviors that are complex, require frequent repetition, and require external resources, such as the challenging scenario of changing lifestyle behaviors such as those leading to obesity and diabetes. Consider the case of over eating. While identifying hypothesized mediators such as depression that may lead to overeating is an important individual-level strategy, other determinants may relate to poverty and access to healthy foods. The question, however, becomes whether these determinants can truly be classified as hypothesized mediators given that they may not be immediately amenable to change. This juncture is exactly where an ecological approach (including changes at the environmental-level) comes into play. Although it is beyond the scope of public health to eliminate poverty, it may well be possible to subsidize the cost of healthy (low-calorie) foods such as vegetables, and to advocate for policy that helps assure widespread access to these foods. The determinants may then be appropriately conceived of as hypothesized mediators.

The mediators, however, are not changed through the traditional route of individual-level intervention. Instead, the mediators are changed

through means such as coalition-based advocacy. Thus, intervention activities that target the environment (broadly defined) may be quite useful. Some intervention activities may limit access to empty-calorie foods as has been the case in many school systems throughout the United States (Molnar & Garcia, 2006; Suarez-Balcazar et al., 2007; Wojcicki & Heyman, 2006). Another intervention activity may be providing extra taxes on "junk foods," thereby limiting access. Other approaches to averting the twin epidemics of diabetes and obesity involve promoting exercise behaviors. Various communities have recognized the value of an ecological approach to promote exercise and have invested substantial resources, both fiscal and human, in changing the physical environment to promote walking as part of daily life (Ashe et al., 2007; French, Story, & Jeffery, 2001; Lopez-Zetina, Lee, & Friis, 2006), use of stairs rather than elevators (Eves & Webb, 2006; Hultquist, Albright, & Thompson, 2005; Lang & Froelicher, 2005), and vigorous physical activity through the provisions of public tracks and recreation facilities. Again, the environmental change should be viewed as one aspect of a larger approach designed to encourage exercise on a daily basis.

Just as individuals are constrained by their economic reality, so too are public health professionals. Unfortunately, some of the most powerful approaches to health promotion may be far too expensive for use by public health professionals. Advertising, for example, may be tremendously efficacious in promoting high-calorie foods such as cheeseburgers (indeed, advertising may be directly responsible for making cheeseburgers a part of American culture). Clearly, media promotion of low-calorie food and drink is equally plausible, but funding for such a campaign would be meager in contrast to the money spent by the fast food industry to promote their high-calorie products. Other examples include policy changes such as federal subsidies for grocery stores to make fresh vegetables easily available to consumers (Kuchler, Abebayehu, & Harris, 2005; Seymour, 2004) and laws that regulate the physical location of fast food restaurants (Ashe, Jernigan, Kline, & Galaz, 2003; Hayne, Moran, & Ford, 2004).

A rapidly emerging solution to the public health issues that are ultimately caused by poverty and the corresponding inequities is the use of micro-finance programs. Globally, microfinance programs are being used to provide impoverished women with an economic starting point to open small businesses, thereby helping them to find a long-term solution to inequities. Because these inequities may be mediators of risky behaviors such as engaging in commercial sex work, the environmental-level solution of microfinancing provides a potentially powerful form of intervention.

In sum, theory is clearly a vital tool in health-promotion practice and research. Theory selection and use is best thought of as one essential part of program planning that guides intervention development. Theory should be thought of being objective-specific. In essence, "one size" (i.e., one theory) does not fit all needs. Because program objectives are inherently different from one another, a diverse selection of theories may be quite useful. Indeed, theory selection and application may become the backbone of the planning process.

▶ Take Home Messages

- Health behavior is complex and three-dimensional.
- Because theory is always a tool and never an end product, health-promotion programs should begin with the essential question, "What theories are most likely to be most valuable in guiding the promotion effort?"
- The selected theories can be used in the process of mediator identification and then to guide efforts to change the identified mediators.
- Theory can be used to develop programs designed to promote relatively complex health behaviors that entail frequent repetition or, at the other extreme, those behaviors that are relatively infrequent.
- In addition, theory can be used to identify, and expand upon, opportunities where simple but meaningful changes can result in a favorable impact on health behavior.

▶ References

Ashe, M., Feldstein, L. M., Graff, S., Kline, R., Pinkas, D., & Zellers, L. (2007). Local venues for change: Legal strategies for health environments. *Journal of Law, Medicine, and Ethics, 35*, 138–147.

Ashe, M., Jernigan, D., Kline, R., & Galaz, R. (2003). Land use planning and the control of alcohol, tobacco, firearms, and fast food restaurants. *American Journal of Public Health, 93*, 1404–1408.

Bronfenbrenner, U. (1979). *The ecology of human development.* Cambridge, MA: Harvard University Press.

Centers for Disease Control and Prevention. (2006). Cryptosporidiosis outbreaks associated with recreational water use—Five states, 2006. *Morbidity and Mortality Weekly Report, 56*, 729–732.

DiClemente, R. J., Crosby, R. A., & Kegler, M. (2009). Is theory applicable cross culturally? The adaptation of western theory for global interventions. In R. J. DiClemente, R. A. Crosby, & M. Kegler (Eds.), *Emerging theories in health promotion practice and research* (2nd ed, pp. 551–558). San Francisco, CA: Jossey-Bass Wiley.

Eng, E., & Parker, E. (2002). Natural helper models to enhance a community's health and competence. In R. J. DiClemente, R. A. Crosby, & M. Kegler (Eds.), *Emerging theories in health promotion practice and research* (pp. 126–156). San Francisco, CA: Jossey-Bass.

Eves, F. F., & Webb, O. J. (2006). Worksite interventions to increase stair climbing; reasons for caution. *Preventive Medicine, 43*, 4–7.

French, S. A., Story, M., & Jeffery, R. W. (2001). Environmental influences on eating and physical activity. *Annual Review of Public Health, 22*, 309.

Gittelsohon, J., Steeves, E. A., Mui, Y., Kharmats, A. Y., Hopkins, L. C., & Dennis, D. (2014). Communities for kids: Design of a multi-level intervention for obesity prevention for low-income African American children. *BMS Public Health, 14*, 942–949.

Hayne, C., Moran, P. A., & Ford, M. M. (2004). Regulating environments to reduce obesity. *Journal of Public Health Policy, 25*, 391–407.

Hultquist, C. N., Albright, C., & Thompson, D. (2005). Comparison of walking recommendations in previously inactive women. *Medicine and Science in Sports and Exercise, 37*, 676–683.

Kuchler, F., Abebayehu, T., & Harris, J. M. (2005). Taxing snack foods: Manipulating diet quality or financing information programs? *Review of Agricultural Economics, 27*, 4–17.

Lang, A., & Froelicher, E. S. (2005). Management of overweight and obesity in adults: Behavioral intervention for long-term weight loss and maintenance. *European Journal of Cardiovascular Nursing, 5*, 102–114.

Lopez-Zetina, J., Lee, H., & Friis, R. (2006). The link between obesity and the built environment: Evidence from an ecological analysis of obesity and vehicle miles of travel in California. *Health and Place, 12*, 656–664.

Molnar, A., & Garcia, D. (2006). The battle over commercialized schools. *Educational Leadership, 63*, 78–82.

Nexoe, J., Kragstone, J., & Sogaard, J. (1999). Decisions on influenza vaccination among the elderly: A questionnaire study based on the health belief model and multidimensional locus of control theory. *Scandinavian Journal of Primary Health Care, 17*, 105–110.

Seymour, J. D. (2004). Fruit and vegetable environment, policy, and pricing workshop: Introduction to the conference proceedings. *Preventive Medicine, 39*, 71–74.

Suarez-Balcazar, Y., Redmond, L., Kouba, J., Hellwig, M., Davis, R., Martinez, L. I., & Jones, L. (2007). Introducing systems change in the schools: The case of school luncheons and vending machines. *American Journal of Community Psychology, 39*, 335–345.

Wojcicki, J. M., & Heyman, M. B. (2006). Healthier choices and increased participation in a middle school lunch program: Effects of nutrition policy changes in San Francisco. *American Journal of Public Health, 96*, 1542–1547.

Chapter Opener: © Henrik Sorensen/Getty Images; © MeskPhotography/Shutterstock; © Hero Images/Getty Images; © lzf/Shutterstock

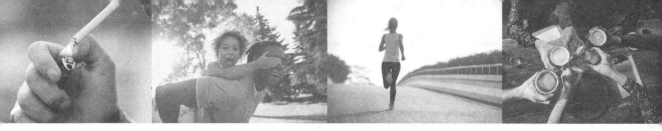

CHAPTER 3

The PRECEDE–PROCEED Planning Model

Richard A. Crosby, Ralph J. DiClemente, and Laura F. Salazar

Strategic planning is worthless—unless there is first a strategic vision.

—**John Naisbitt**, American Author

PREVIEW

As a public health professional, your foremost goal is always the same: to protect the health of the public. This ongoing challenge is best met through strategic planning. This chapter provides you with a framework to streamline the planning process, to select appropriate theories of health behavior, and to utilize diverse methods of achieving improved health outcomes.

OBJECTIVES

1. Understand the value of the PRECEDE–PROCEED model (PPM) in program planning and evaluation.
2. Describe the importance of community involvement and the initial planning phase of social diagnosis.
3. Distinguish between an epidemiological diagnosis, a behavioral diagnosis, and an environmental diagnosis.
4. Understand how and when theory can be applied when using the PPM framework.
5. Describe the utility of the PPM for making policy decisions.
6. Explain how the PPM framework can guide program evaluation efforts.

▶ Introduction

Understanding health behavior requires intimate knowledge of the community and environmental context in which a particular behavior occurs. Context is the ecology that enables, controls, and limits human behavior. Behavior, in essence, occurs as part of a larger system, and once that system is understood, it may be manipulated to encourage health-protective action. These "systems," however, are not divorced from the people who live within them. Indeed, it is artificial to separate systems (i.e., the environment) from people (Green, Richard, & Potvin, 1996). With this basic principle in mind, it then becomes important to adopt a unified approach to health promotion—one that accounts for the reciprocal actions that occur between people and the systems within which they live.

Before we begin describing the various theories used in public health-promotion programs, we feel that it is essential for you to first see the larger and more important picture; specifically, please know that theory is only a tool that is applied in the critical process of program planning. As the planning process unfolds (a process described in this chapter), the specific needs for health behavior theory will become apparent, and the process will dictate the need for theory. It is categorically incorrect to decide upon a theory and then engage in program planning. This distinction may initially sound trivial, but it is not at all minor. After all, the goal is to protect the health of the public; thus, the use of theory "A" or theory "B" is purely an academic question. The PRECEDE–PROCEED model (PPM) is the most widely used planning model in health promotion. It has been described in great detail in online resources such as the Community Toolbox, and it has dominated the field of health-promotion planning for decades. (Workgroup for Community Health and Development, 2017). As such, this model is the next "stop" in your journey to learning more about effective methods of changing health behavior.

FIGURE 3-1 displays the PRECEDE–PROCEED model. The PPM embodies an ecological approach to changing health behavior, and it does so with full recognition that systems/environments enable, control, and limit health behavior. As a public health professional, you will most likely be called upon to solve rather complex issues related to health behavior, and you are quite likely to find that your planning process becomes quickly mired in complexity as you enumerate all of the possible systems' influences on even one health behavior. You may find yourself looking for a method of organizing your thinking and, ultimately, a method to organize your actions. A standard framework would be useful. One useful way to think about a framework is to equate it with a logic model. A logic model is much like a blueprint in that it is a graphical representation of an intervention program, which shows the flow of activities that will lead to successful completion of the objectives. The logic model is somewhat of a master plan that guides each and every action. Ultimately, your actions may require you to employ health behavior theory, but your first and foremost goal is always simply to protect the health of the public.

To begin, it is vital to understand that the PPM is a planning framework, not a theory. Having said this, however, it is equally vital to note that as a planning framework, the model can be used to strategically select one or more theories that can best be applied to the goals of the health-promotion program. The selection and use of theory, however, is driven by the phases in a logic model, meaning that the planning process dictates the use of theory—this puts theory into a different perspective as it is used as needed, rather than as a predetermined action. The PPM has been used in health promotion since the publication of *Health Program Planning: An Educational and Ecological Approach*, initially published in 1980 by Drs. Larry Green and Marshall Kreuter. More detailed descriptions and sample applications of the model can be found in their fourth edition (Green & Kreuter, 2005) and in bibliography of more than 1000 scholarly citations compiled by Dr. Green (Green, 2017).

To begin, it is useful to understand the two acronyms that comprise the model. PRECEDE stands for **P**redisposing, **R**einforcing, and **E**nabling **C**onstructs in **E**ducational/environmental **D**iagnosis and **E**valuation. Generally speaking, the

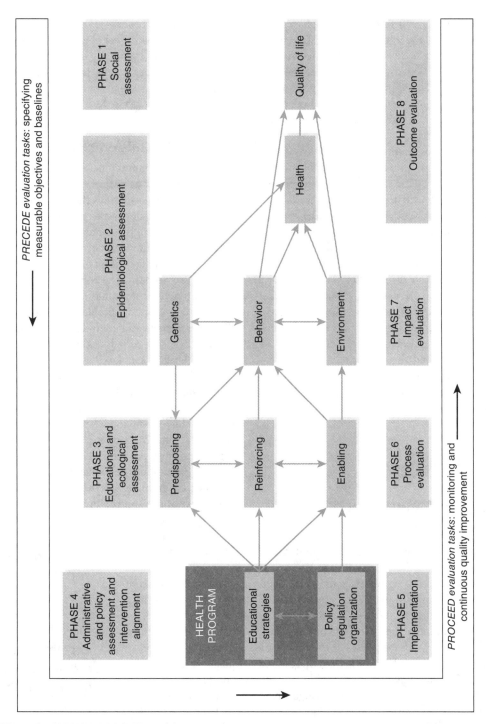

FIGURE 3-1 The PRECEDE–PROCEED model

Reproduced from Green, L.W., & Kreuter, M.W. (2005). *Health program planning: An educational and ecological approach* (4th ed.). New York, NY: McGraw-Hill. With permission.

PRECEDE phases correspond with phases one through four of the model. PROCEED, on the other hand, stands for **P**olicy, **R**egulatory, and **O**rganizational **C**onstructs in **E**ducational and **E**nvironmental **D**evelopment. This aspect of the model begins with the administrative and policy assessment. We will provide an overview of the model in its entirety.

The basic assumption of the PPM is that behaviors are complex and have multidimensional etiologies. This assumption is, of course, quite consistent with the principles you learned in Chapter 2. In essence, then, the model requires program planning to occur with an eye on each and every relevant level of potential intervention across the spectrum of domains or levels articulated in the ecological model shown in Chapter 2 (see Figure 2-2). In particular, planning under this model is directed at distal as well as proximal hypothesized mediators of health behaviors. Moreover, the model includes an intervention pathway specifying that changes to the environment can have a direct influence on health, thus bypassing direct intervention with an individual to modify behavior.

▶ Key Concepts

An Overview of the Planning Phases

The model is actually quite simple to understand once you first realize that it embodies two key aspects of intervention: planning and evaluation. The planning phases begin with the largest goal (improved quality of life) and culminate in an administrative and policy assessment. Because the planning begins with the end in mind, the phases of the model are numbered sequentially beginning from this desired endpoint. The planning process should begin with phase 1 and continue sequentially through phase 4. The arrows you see in Figure 3-1 illustrate the logic model within the PPM. In essence, the arrows show you causal pathways between the phases as the programs and policies from phase 4 are implemented. So, the planning begins at phase 1 and

continues through phase 4; the arrows show how phase 4 actions will affect phase 3 objectives, phase 2 objectives, and eventually the phase 1 objective. The evaluation part of the model is generally far more intuitive to students; it begins at phase 5 and continues through phase 8.

Phase 1: Social Assessment

An important assumption of the PPM is that all actions occurring as part of the health-promotion planning process, as well as the subsequent implementation and evaluation of the program, must be firmly grounded in the context of community participation and relevance. Stated differently, the PPM is predicated on the concept of community involvement at every phase. The concepts of community capacity and community-based participatory research are quite applicable here. In this paradigm, researchers and community members come together to work side-by-side in their efforts to solve the health issues faced by the community (see Jones & Wells, 2007 for a more detailed description of this approach). Health issues may be identified by the community, the researcher, or public health entities. This assumption is valuable simply because community involvement and ownership may yield highly effective programs (Feinberg, Greenberg, Osgood, Sartarious, & Bontempo, 2007). **BOX 3-1** provides an example of a health-promotion program that was planned, implemented, and sustained by a group of highly motivated community members.

Given the prominent role of community involvement in the PPM, the first phase in the planning process is to work in partnership with the community to assess quality-of-life issues that are particularly relevant to the members of that community. An imperative in this phase is to

All actions occurring as part of the health-promotion planning process, as well as the subsequent implementation and evaluation of the program, must be firmly grounded in the context of community participation and relevance.

BOX 3-1 An Example of a Health-Promotion Program Based on Community Coalitions and Community Participation

Feinberg et al. (2007) demonstrated population-level effects of a comprehensive health-promotion program designed by community coalitions and delivered to thousands of adolescents. Known as Communities That Care (CTC), the ethic of the approach was to provide community coalitions with a well-defined set of guidelines for selecting, implementing, and evaluating evidenced-based interventions. The CTC model is designed for flexibility so that it can be used by townships, school districts, defined communities, or entire counties. Evaluating 15 risk factors and 6 health outcomes among Pennsylvania secondary school students, Feinberg and colleagues found evidence suggesting the students in CTC communities had significantly less risk and more favorable outcomes compared to those in communities without CTC programs.

identify and recruit community stakeholders who truly represent the community. To ensure social equity, it is vital to recognize the community as a heterogeneous collection of diverse factions, organization, and agencies. The Interactive Domain model may be very helpful at this juncture given its emphasis on social equity (Kahn, Grouix, & Wong, 2009). This social assessment stage is also the ideal time to begin the process of building community coalitions that will guide the planning, implementation, and evaluation of the health-promotion program. Working within this context, the health-promotion planner can use the social assessment as the basis for the epidemiological assessment (phase 2).

Phase 2: Epidemiological Assessment

In essence, many of the needs identified by the community can most likely be translated into measurable objectives pertaining to health promotion. These health objectives should be written carefully to specify the exact degree of desired improvement in a quantifiable health indicator and to include a definite time frame for reaching the objective. For example, consider this objective: "By the year 2015, the number of people living in the community who are classified as obese will be reduced by 50%." The objective must be measurable, but it must also be realistic. Setting "pie in the sky" objectives (as is often done) may discourage the efforts of community stakeholders (and yourself) when the goals are not met, so as a rule, it is preferable to set realistic objectives. The original objective then might best be rewritten as follows: "By the year 2015, the number of people living in the community who are classified as obese will be reduced by at least 10%." Preferably, the outcomes should be measured in biological terms, for example, mean A1c levels, mean diastolic blood pressure, mean lipids levels in a community. Once constructed, the objectives compose the primary working objectives for all that follows, including various forms of evaluation.

A careful look at Figure 3-1 informs you that the second phase actually comprises two parts. The logic here is simply that meeting the stated health objectives requires changes in behavior and the environment. Of course, the powerful role of genetics and gene–environment interactions must also be considered. The next step in phase 2 is an exercise that forces the planner (with intensive assistance and involvement from community members) to identify environmental and behavioral influences that have strong connections to the health objective. This work is critical because the identified environmental and behavioral factors will become the subobjectives that direct the remainder of the planning and intervention activities. For example, one important environmental factor leading to a reduced prevalence of obesity may be the widespread availability of freely accessible and attractive exercise facilities throughout the community. Of course, simply changing this aspect of the environment will not magically lead to reduced obesity rates, but it may trigger behavior change (i.e., exercising) that, in turn, may lead to reductions in obesity. So, the pathway for this effect

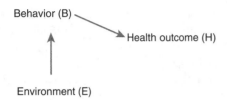

FIGURE 3-2 Simple depiction of environmental and behavioral pathways to health

would be diagrammatically shown as "E" to "B" followed by "B" to "H" as depicted in **FIGURE 3-2**.

As you can imagine, various combinations of the "E" to "B" to "H" pathway could be applied to the reduction of obesity rates in any given community. For example, changing social norms of the community relative to the consumption of high-calorie foods (E) may prompt behavior change (reduced calorie consumption), which, in turn, may lead to reduced obesity.

Direct pathways between "B" and "H" and between "E" and "H" should also be considered. Education programs, for example, may have a direct effect and may be viewed as more proximal mediators (see Chapter 2), thereby changing behavior in the absence of environmental change. This may be true for eating behaviors or exercising behaviors, both of which constitute the energy balance that applies to obesity reduction. Moreover, a direct pathway between "E" and "H" may not exist for the primary objective of obesity reduction; however, it is possible this direct pathway could exist for the primary objectives of injury prevention and reduced tobacco use. For instance, with injury prevention, the mandatory installation of driver air bags prevents injury and death of vehicle operators regardless of behavior. Regarding tobacco, laws prohibiting indoor smoking lead smokers to consume fewer cigarettes in the workplace and other indoor areas—the issue of voluntary behavior change becomes moot because workplace regulations and city ordinances dictate what "must" be done rather than what "should" be done. It is quite possible that employees in workplaces that have bans on tobacco use may be more prone to quit than those working in places without a ban (if all other circumstances are equal). Of course, reductions in tobacco use become more dramatic when the "B" to "H" pathway is used in conjunction with the "E" to "H" pathway. If, for example, mass media campaigns are used to persuade teens not to begin smoking, their abstinence from tobacco may persist into adulthood, thereby reducing community prevalence of tobacco use. The dual action of these two pathways relevant to tobacco-use reduction is portrayed in **FIGURE 3-3**.

> *Meeting the stated health objectives requires changes in behavior and the environment.*

Phase 3: Educational and Ecological Assessment

This phase of the model is by far the most complex, as it requires a type of analysis for each of the behavioral and environmental subobjectives identified in phase 2. The analysis necessitates identification (in partnership with community members) of **predisposing**, **reinforcing**, and **enabling factors** that apply to the subobjectives. Each of these factors is briefly defined in the following list.

- Predisposing factors, such as knowledge, attitudes, beliefs, values, or confidence, facilitate or hinder motivation toward change. Examples include attitude toward the protective behavior (is the benefit greater than the cost?), perceptions of threat (is the consequence of inaction severe?), and personal assessment of skill (can I perform the protective behavior?). One good way to conceptualize predisposing factors is to note that these factors are cognitive, in that they exist "between the ears" of a person.
- Reinforcing factors are rewards (social, personal, or financial) for performing the protective behavior, and these rewards may be internal or external to the person. In essence, people often want to experience a clear and somewhat immediate benefit that derives from the protective behavior. Like predisposing factors, these are also cognitive factors, but they differ in that they are anticipated rewards of performing a given behavior.

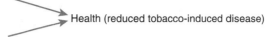

Behavior (teen abstinence from smoking)

Health (reduced tobacco-induced disease)

Environment (regulations and laws against indoor smoking)

FIGURE 3-3 Tobacco-related environmental and behavioral pathways

From a health-promotion planning viewpoint, it is vital to bear in mind that these rewards can indeed be social, meaning that the direct benefit to health need not be the "promised reward." This is, of course, quite important when a health behavior leads only to distant health benefits, as in the case of eating a diet low in saturated fats, avoiding carcinogens, or maintaining a low-sodium diet to prevent the onset of hypertension.

■ Enabling factors allow people to translate their desire to perform a given health-protective behavior into actual behavior. Skill acquisition is a common enabling factor; however, changes to the environment may also be vital (e.g., making cancer-screening services more accessible and affordable). With the exception of actual skill acquisition, enabling factors are external to the person; they facilitate or inhibit the adoption of the behavior and are found in the ecology of a person's environment. Health-promotion programs that make provision for the applicable enabling factors are therefore quite consistent with the concept of an ecological approach. Policy development is often applicable in the process of providing enabling factors to a community.

Returning to the example of obesity reduction, let's assume that one subobjective is to influence the "B" to "H" pathway (see Figure 3-2) by promoting the consumption of vegetables as a replacement for high-fat meats. This third phase of the PRECEDE–PROCEED model demands that you identify (with community involvement) all possible predisposing factors, all possible

With the exception of actual skill acquisition, enabling factors are external to the person.

reinforcing factors, and all possible enabling factors that could be instrumental in changing the behavior. This is naturally a labor-intensive process, but the results of this work are vital because the identified factors become the target of the intervention activities; in more formal language, the identified factors become the hypothesized mediators (see Chapter 2).

The wise selection, and subsequent targeting, of predisposing, reinforcing, and enabling factors is the core of the "PRECEDE" part of the PRECEDE–PROCEED model. Indeed, PRECEDE has been used as stand-alone method of leveraging long-term behavior change. **BOX 3-2** provides an example of using PRECEDE to improve A1c

---

BOX 3-2 An Example of PRECEDE Applied to Population-Level Behavior Change

Salinero-Fort and colleagues (Salinero-Fort et al., 2011) conducted a community-level effectiveness trial of PRCEDE in Madrid, Spain. The goal was to promote behaviors that would lead to the control of Type II Diabetes and the prevention of heart disease. In this study design, nurses/clinicians were randomly assigned to use (or not use) a PRECEDE framework in counseling their patients (*N* = 600). Those randomized to use this framework were trained in the assessment of patients' most relevant predisposing, reinforcing, and enabling factors. They used this information gained from their patients to guide their counseling efforts, thereby creating a PRECEDE-generated intervention program. Compared to patients assigned to control nurses/clinicians, those receiving this PRECEDE-based counseling were significantly more likely to be compliant with behavioral recommendations, and they had significantly lower A1c and systolic blood pressure levels over a 2-year period of observation.

levels and systolic blood pressures, at a population level, in Spain.

At this juncture, a common question raised by students is, "How can I best identify the predisposing, reinforcing, and enabling factors?" The answer goes back to theory! For instance, the theory of reasoned action (see Chapter 4) would suggest that attitudes toward vegetable consumption and subjective norms pertaining to vegetable consumption may each be cognitive factors that are linked with the actual consumption of vegetable in place of high-fat meats. **TABLE 3-1** presents some general examples of predisposing, reinforcing, and enabling factors.

The theory would indeed posit that increasing the community prevalence of favorable attitudes and normative perceptions would create a corresponding increase in vegetable consumption in the community. Thus, two predisposing factors can be identified using the theory of reasoned action as a guide. The theory would also suggest that inhibiting and facilitating factors are important—these correspond to the construct of enabling factors in the PPM. Examples might include easy access to fresh vegetables, price reduction of vegetables, and teaching people how to cook vegetables so

they taste good and therefore satisfy the pleasure needs often associated with eating. Unfortunately, the theory of planned behavior would not be instructive relative to reinforcing factors; however, social cognitive theory (see Chapter 7) might be extremely useful in this regard.

Once all of the possible predisposing, reinforcing, and enabling factors relative to the first subobjective have been identified, the next step is to prioritize these factors according to their relative **importance** as hypothesized mediators and their degree of **changeability**. The most important factors that also rank high in their potential for being changed through intervention then become the top priorities relevant to the first subobjective. The next set of required actions is to repeat the entire analysis as applied to the second subobjective. The second subobjective, for example, might be another "B" to "H" pathway, such as exercising to burn excess calories. Clearly, the entire process of identifying predisposing, reinforcing, and enabling factors must then be repeated from the beginning, as the resulting factors will be quite different from those identified for the previous subobjective. The process may require further repetition for other subobjectives. You can see how the term "labor intensive" applies to this fourth phase of the model. Throughout this process, it is important to bear in mind that subobjectives can exist in three forms: (1) the "B" to "H" pathway, (2) the "E" to "H" pathway, and (3) the "E" to "B" to "H" pathway. A maxim here is that the more pathways you account for in the planning process, the greater the likelihood of achieving your primary objective.

Once you have performed all of the possible analyses relevant to phase 3, you are ready to focus on the administrative aspects and policy.

TABLE 3-1 Predisposing, Enabling, and Reinforcing Factors of Health Behavior	
Factors Affecting Behavior	**Examples**
Predisposing factors	Knowledge, attitudes, cultural beliefs, subjective norms, and readiness to change
Enabling factors	Available resources, supportive policies, assistance, and services
Reinforcing factors	Social support, praise, reassurance, and symptom relief

Phase 4: Administrative and Policy Assessment and Intervention Alignment

In many ways, this is the most challenging and most critical phase of the entire planning process. Your first step is to assess the capacity and resources available to implement programs and change policies in accordance with the needs identified in phase 3. Stated differently, you will need to determine what you may be lacking in resources and capacity so you can begin to identify any additional resources that will be needed to achieve your subobjectives, your larger objectives, and eventually your overall goal. Once this assessment process is complete, you are ready consider intervention alignment.

Intervention alignment is the point where your formative work (PRECEDE) ends and your action (PROCEED) begins. In this part of phase 4, the goals can be divided into two categories: health education and the larger, more encompassing, category of changing policy, regulation, and organizational structures.

> *Intervention alignment is the point where your formative work (PRECEDE) ends and your action (PROCEED) begins.*

Health education remains the front-line method of changing predisposing factors in public health. Whether the identified mediating factors are attitudes, beliefs, or perceptions of risk, health education can be applied at the individual or community-level to favorably alter each factor. Health education may also be an important method of instilling the intrinsic reinforcement designed to promote repetition of health-protective behaviors. Ultimately, however, the mere existence of health education programs is a function of policy, regulation, and organizational structure. The ultimate driving force behind the actions that will be implemented to achieve the primary objectives comes from the lower left-hand corner of the model (the PRO—policy, regulation, and organization—of PROCEED).

Changing policy, regulation, and organizational structure is challenging, but the benefits can be extremely productive, especially with respect to addressing the enabling factors identified as part of phase 3. Other than the enabling factor of skill, which is addressed through health education, the identified enabling factors will be changed through policy, regulation, and organizational structures. These enabling factors typically involve one or more of the following four categories, also known as the four A's (see **FIGURE 3-4**).

- Accessibility (can people easily locate the service or product needed?)
- Affordability (can people afford the service or product needed?)
- Availability (are the services available during convenient hours?)
- Acceptability (is the service or product offered in way that is compatible with the cultural values of the people?)

In each case, the "A" represent targets of change for policy, regulation, and organizational structures. Consider, for example, the public health challenges associated with cancer screening (e.g., mammography, Pap testing, colonoscopy). Although health education programs can predispose people to be screened for cancer, whether their intention is translated into action is likely to be a function of the facilitating and inhibiting factors that apply to the screening procedure. If, for example, Pap testing services are offered from only 9:00 A.M. to 5:00 P.M. on weekdays, the

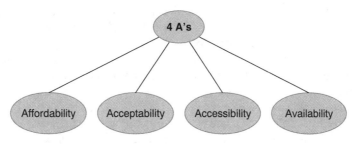

FIGURE 3-4 The four A's

Modified from Singla, Ankush. Dialing for the bottom of the pyramid. Retrieved from http://zalgnis.blogspot.com/2009/12/dialingfor-bottom-of-pyramid.html

screening procedure is not available to women who must work during those hours. In rural areas, if the closest clinic offering Pap testing services is too far away, then the service is not accessible. If the provider of the service is male, then many women may not be comfortable having the test. Finally, if the out-of-pocket costs of Pap testing are too expensive for some women, then the service will not be utilized. In each example, the PRO implications are quite clear: make changes in existing structures that will remedy the **structural barriers** to Pap testing. Indeed, this approach to health promotion is ecological in nature, as it fully recognizes and utilizes the spectrum of potential intervention points that may ultimately culminate in population-level change, thereby leading to declines in morbidity and early mortality (see Chapters 1 and 2).

Phase 4 is the point at which theory selection and application becomes a critical task of the program planner. Theory selection will always be a function of the subobjectives identified in phases 2 and 3, though this is a point that is too often lost on students and even practicing professionals. For example, if the objective for a practitioner is to reduce obesity rates among adolescents by 10% in his or her community, then a subobjective might be to enhance exercise. One way to do this would be to implement an exercise buddy program. Using social cognitive theory (described in detail in Chapter 7) as a framework, you decide that it is important to provide positive reinforcement for exercise and the buddy program will achieve this through enhanced social interaction. In the next section of this textbook, in addition to social cognitive theory, you will learn about many of the theories used in health-promotion practice to change health behavior.

At this juncture, it is worth noting that ultimately, the PPM guides interventions' actions by directing efforts to very specific subobjectives. As you can imagine, literally dozens of subobjectives can be formulated during the planning process. The collective achievement of the identified subobjectives will result in meeting the primary behavioral and environmental objectives that were developed in phase 3 of the process. Achieving these larger objectives

will, in turn, lead to obtaining the goals diagnosed in phase 2 (the epidemiological assessment) and phase 1 (the social assessment). The entire process (see **BOX 3-3**) is firmly embedded in the concept of community-based participatory research and is an ecological paradigm.

> *The collective achievement of the identified subobjectives will result in meeting the primary behavioral and environmental objectives that were developed in phase 3 of the process.*

Phases 5 Through 8: Implementation and Evaluation

Implementation (phase 5) is included in the model to signal the initiation of the program. During this phase, how and when the intervention strategy will be implemented is equally as important as the nature of the intervention to be implemented. Issues surrounding which resources are available for implementation and how policy regulations may affect implementation should be thoroughly considered. Again, reliance on well-informed community members may be an asset at this stage, as they will most likely be aware of these issues. During this phase, additional details regarding the evaluation of the program must be delineated.

Evaluation is a critical phase in the PROCEED process; however, it must be planned *a priori*. Once implementation of the program occurs, the last three phases refer to different pieces of information that should be gleaned about the program. Evaluation is the thread that holds any health-promotion program together—it is not simply an activity that occurs once a program is terminated. For instance, process evaluation (phase 6), which determines whether the program was implemented as intended and reached the targeted population, is designed to establish quality assurance. This assurance is critical to the success of the program simply because even the best laid plans can go awry. The key word here is **fidelity**. In essence, staff may or not faithfully follow protocols

BOX 3-3 A Phase-by-Phase Summary of the Planning Process in the PRECEDE–PROCEED Model

Specific Planning Phases

PRECEDE:

- **SOCIAL ASSESSMENT** (phase 1) brings the planning process to the people. The primary goal is to identify important quality-of-life issues in the community. This step may necessitate performing a community-needs assessment.
- Alternatively, an **EPIDEMIOLOGICAL, BEHAVIORAL, AND ENVIRONMENTAL ASSESSMENT** (phase 2) involves identification of several specific health problems that may contribute to quality-of-life issues.
- Epidemiologic assessments may be based on primary or secondary analyses of data.
- Epidemiologic assessments should always culminate in the creation of measurable objectives related to health outcomes (such as those listed in *Healthy People 2020*—e.g., reduce the incidence of low birth weight by 75%).
- Behavioral assessments seek to identify behaviors that have an important influence on the health outcome(s) under consideration—those that are most important and amenable to change become targets of the intervention (subobjectives are developed).
- Similarly, environmental assessments seek to identify aspects of the physical, social, cultural, political, or family environment that have an important influence on the health outcome(s) under consideration—those that are most important and amenable to change become targets of the intervention (subobjectives are developed).
- **EDUCATIONAL AND ECOLOGICAL ASSESSMENTS** (phase 3) seek to identify hypothesized mediators of the behaviors identified. These are divided into three categories: (1) predisposing factors, (2) reinforcing factors, and (3) enabling factors (subobjectives are developed).
- Collectively, predisposing, reinforcing, and enabling factors (the "PRE") account for public health challenges that are best addressed by behavioral theory. Thus, the PRE analysis is critical.
- **ADMINISTRATIVE AND POLICY ASSESSMENTS AND INTERVENTION ALIGNMENT** (phase 4) is important. Policy, regulation, and organization changes can have an important effect on program delivery as well as enabling factors (and possibly reinforcing factors). Political savvy is an important aspect of public health planning.

and procedures developed during the planning stages; thus, monitoring is required, followed by corrective feedback. This process of monitoring and correction is iterative and ongoing, ending only when the program comes to a close.

Once the program has reached maturity, the key question is, "Were the behavioral and environmental subobjectives (as developed in phase 2) met?" This is known as the impact evaluation (phase 7). Impact evaluation determines whether the intervention achieved its intermediate outcomes, which typically are more readily measurable than the long-term health outcome determined in the outcome evaluation (phase 8). The impact evaluation may show, for example, that behaviors did change at the population level.

Equally important (if not more so), the impact evaluation may also show that targeted environmental structures were successfully changed. Sustained success on one or both of these fronts is theoretically an indicator of eventual declines in the disease outcome or condition that was initially targeted (i.e., the primary objective of the intervention program). Unfortunately, with chronic disease prevention, the effects

Unfortunately, with chronic disease prevention, the effects of behavioral and environmental changes on actual health outcomes may take a decade or more to materialize.

BOX 3-4 A Phase-by-Phase Summary of the Action Processes in the PRECEDE–PROCEED Model

Specific Monitoring and Improvement Phases

PROCEED:

- **IMPLEMENTATION** (phase 5) means the program has been developed and goals have been established that will meet objectives identified in the epidemiologic and behavioral assessments.
- Budget, policy, regulation, and organizational resources must be considered for implementation to occur.
- A timetable is established that is reasonable.
- **PROCESS EVALUATION** (phase 6) is an ongoing procedure. Data should be collected on an ongoing basis to confirm progress.
- Process objectives, the process of completing the project, are evaluated according to the timeline created. For example, a process objective would read: by December of this year, target areas of education programs will be identified. Also, by December of next year, 1000 adolescents will attend the risk-reduction program.
- **IMPACT EVALUATION** (phase 7) and **OUTCOME EVALUATION** (phase 8) are also ongoing processes. Clear and concise objectives are the foundation for the evaluation of the project.
- An objective needs to have a measurable component. The evaluation of the objectives becomes part of both planning and implementation.
- An impact objective, or immediate behavior change, for individuals in the target audience, could be: by May of this year, 70% of the adolescents who attended the program will not engage in unsafe sex.
- The outcome objective, a long-term effect of changes in the target population, would be: STD rates among adolescents will decrease by 15% in our target area by 2020.

---

of behavioral and environmental changes on actual health outcomes may take a decade or more to materialize. Thus, it is indeed a challenge, even with success in achieving the subobjectives, to produce a favorable outcome evaluation (meaning that the primary objective was achieved). See **BOX 3-4** for more information.

▶ An Applied Example

Effective use of the PPM requires that you truly understand the entire process. To this end, a bit of applied practice using a hypothetical example can be very useful.

Phase 1: Little Fork, Iowa, has been experiencing a severe shortage of hospital beds. This problem has necessitated the transport of new patients to distant cities. As director of the local health department, you have been asked to help solve the problem. You meet with several community agencies and advisory boards and you quickly learn that building rooms is not an affordable solution. You also learn that much of the space crunch is attributable to an overflow from the neonatal care unit, caused by the long stays necessitated by premature birth and full-term babies with a low birth weight (LBW; LBW is less than 5.5 pounds). You learn that both issues are common concerns among residents of the community and you find support to change things. At this point you form a community coalition comprising key stakeholders that begins to meet on a monthly basis.

Phase 2: You conduct an epidemiological diagnosis and determine that the incidence of LBW has indeed escalated over the past several years. Using local data, you find that about 60% of the LBW babies born in the past year were full term, so you develop the following primary objective: In the next 2 years, the incidence of LBW in the community hospital will decrease by 75%. Next, you identify behavioral risk factors for LBW; these include tobacco use, teen pregnancy, and poor nutrition during pregnancy. Then you identify the environmental risk factors for LBW.

Two factors were identified: lack of access to prenatal care and lack of subsidized food to low-income pregnant women. Consequently, you develop five subobjectives:

- Behavioral Subobjective 1: In the next 12 months, reduce the rate of tobacco use (cigarette use) among pregnant women by 50%.
- Behavioral Subobjective 2: In the next 12 months, reduce the rate of teen pregnancy by 20%.
- Behavioral Subobjective 3: In the next 12 months, increase mean daily calorie intakes (with an emphasis on protein consumption) among pregnant women by 25%.
- Environmental Subobjective 1: In the next 12 months, increase the availability of pregnancy testing and prenatal care services to women residing in Little Fork.
- Environmental Subobjective 2: In the next 12 months, increase the availability of programs that provide free or reduced-cost food to pregnant women residing in Little Fork.

Phase 3: For each behavioral subobjective you conduct a PRE analysis, meaning that you identify all relevant predisposing, reinforcing, and enabling factors. An example of one PRE analysis is shown here.

Behavioral Subobjective 1: In the next 12 months, reduce the rate of tobacco use (cigarette use) among pregnant women by 50%.

Identified predisposing factors were:

   a. Belief that smoking "keeps you thin" during pregnancy and that "thin is good."

      Subobjective = Pregnant women will understand that gaining approximately 40 pounds during pregnancy is desirable.

   b. Belief that smoking during pregnancy cannot possibly harm the fetus.

      Subobjective = Pregnant women will understand the multiple negative effects of smoke and nicotine on fetal development.

   c. Access to cigarettes is very easy in Little Fork, and the rate of tobacco use is very high.

      Subobjective = Decrease access to teens by enforcing existing purchasing laws. Subobjective = Decrease access to adults by lobbying for higher state taxes on cigarettes.

Of course, this one PRE analysis needs to be repeated for each of the other four identified subobjectives. As you can easily envision, the cumulative product of these five PRE analyses will be a large number of subobjectives that must each be considered in the planning process. Because you now have so many PRE-related subobjectives, you prioritize these based on importance and changeability.

Phase 4: At the conclusion of your work pertaining to all necessary PRE analyses, you conduct the administrative and policy assessment. As a result, you determine that your available resources will be adequate to achieve the vast majority of the behavioral subobjectives, but you have serious doubts about your capacities as they pertain to many of the environmental subobjectives. Consequently, you rely on members of your community coalition to leverage the help of others who can mobilize the efforts needed to leverage PRO changes at the local level (Little Fork) and even the state level (Iowa).

Next, you engage in the process of intervention alignment. You begin by selecting two behavioral theories that will best guide your education programs and that are designed to achieve the behavioral subobjectives. Education plans (curricula) are developed and you begin to make the administrative arrangements to implement these plans. You also decide to "target" local obstetricians, gynecologists, and family practice physicians in the community with an educational program designed to persuade them to address the barriers experienced by low-income teens to receiving timely and adequate prenatal care. As part of this effort, you quickly learn that the same people are quite willing to help the program by promoting state-funded contraception options to teens seen in their clinics.

Phase 5: After an extensive process of intervention alignment (lasting more than 6 months), the education programs are implemented and you find yourself constantly engaged in full-time efforts to change policy. Almost immediately, you realize that the critically valuable process of evaluation must be initiated.

Phase 6: Working through the community coalition, you begin to conduct process evaluation. You find yourself counting the number of hours a given curriculum was delivered to a given number of teens and the number of meetings (as well as the number of attendees) held by the community coalition. As this process evaluation matures, you soon learn to use the results as an indicator of breakdowns that occur relative to the plans made, in contrast to the actual programs being conducted (see Chapter 13 for an extensive treatment of program evaluation). The ultimate question you continually seek to answer in this sixth phase is whether the PRE-related subobjectives were met.

Phase 7: As the program matures, you conduct the impact evaluation. At this point you are determining whether the behavioral and environmental subobjectives were met. You found that three of these five subobjectives were met: teen pregnancy rates dropped (although slightly), prenatal nutrition was generally improved in Little Fork, and the environmental goal of improved access to prenatal care was realized.

Phase 8: Finally, you conduct the outcome evaluation to determine whether your primary health objective was met. You find that the incidence of low–birth weight babies born in Little Fork hospital decreased (a small but significant decrease was observed).

A summary of this applied example is provided in **TABLE 3-2** for your quick reference.

TABLE 3-2 Applied Example of PRECEDE–PROCEED Model to Hospital Bed Shortage

PRECEDE–PROCEED Phases	Action Taken	Result
Social assessment:	Meetings with key stakeholders	Overflow from neonatal care unit causing space issues
Assess shortage of hospital beds		High rates of premature births and low–birth weight babies
Epidemiological assessment: Determine extent of premature births and low–birth weight babies born in community	Identify sources of data and collect data about incidence of preterm and low birth weight in community Set objectives for improvement	Low–birth weight incidence has risen in past 5 years; preterm births not the problem Decrease rate of low–birth weight births by 75%
	Identify potential genetic, behavioral, and/or environmental risk factors	Tobacco use, teen pregnancy rate, poor nutrition, lack of access to prenatal care, low awareness of food stamp program
	Set behavioral and environmental subobjectives	Decrease tobacco use, reduce teen pregnancy, enhance nutrition for pregnant women, increase access to prenatal care, increase accessibility of food stamp program

PRECEDE–PROCEED Phases	Action Taken	Result
Educational and ecological assessment:	Identify predisposing, enabling, reinforcing factors	Lack of knowledge that smoking harms fetus, tax on cigarettes too low, lack of awareness of how to get food stamps, lack of support for teens who are pregnant
Administrative and policy assessment:	Identify resources	Department of Public Health, community coalition members
	Align intervention to meet objectives	Health belief model as framework, target healthcare providers and teens, lobbying efforts to change tobacco policies
Implementation	Create timeline and mobilize resources to implement strategies	Education program implemented at local healthcare conferences, medical and nursing school seminars, community-based organizations; multiple contacts initiated with local state and city elected officials
Process evaluation	Ongoing assessment of activities	Counted number exposed and meetings with elected officials
Impact evaluation	Assess effectiveness of strategy in meeting immediate objectives	Teen pregnancy rate decreased, women accessing prenatal care increased, women using food stamps increased
Outcome evaluation	Low–birth weight rates	Low–birth weight rate decreased slightly

▶ Take Home Messages

- The PPM framework is capable of being your primary method of orchestrating and planning your health-promotion program. The program itself is always the key focus, with theory being an important part of the program planning process.
- An implicit and all too often forgotten part of this framework is community involvement.
- Within this context, the initial goal is a social assessment, followed by an epidemiological assessment. From that starting point you will always be "guided by the goal" and you will have a measurable outcome that can be used to evaluate your success.
- Multiple subobjectives (in phase 2 and phase 3) will be developed to help ensure that the larger goal is achieved. It is the phase 3 subobjectives that require the application of theory to ensure a successful programmatic plan.
- Theory, in essence, becomes the lynchpin in translating the efforts of a program into changes in the identified mediators that will, in turn, foster behavior change.

▶ **References**

Feinberg, M. E., Greenberg, M. T., Osgood, D. W., Sartarious, J., & Bontempo, D. (2007). Effects of the Communities That Care model in Pennsylvania on youth risk and problem behaviors. *Prevention Science, 8,* 261–270.

Green, L., Richard, L., & Potvin, L. (1996). Ecological foundations of health promotion. *American Journal of Health Promotion, 10*(4), 270–281.

Green, L. W., & Kreuter, M. W. (2005). *Health program planning: An educational and ecological approach* (4th ed.). New York, NY: McGraw-Hill.

Green, L. W. (2017). Retrieved from http://lgreen.net/precede%20 apps/preapps-NEW.htm

Jones, L., & Wells, K. (2007). Strategies for academic and clinician engagement in community-partnered research. *Journal of the American Medical Association, 297,* 407–410.

Kahn, B., Grouix, D., & Wong, P. (2009). The interactive domain model approach to best practices in health promotion. In R. J. DiClemente, R. A. Crosby, & M. Kegler (Eds.), *Emerging Theories in Health Promotion Practice and Research* (2nd ed, pp. 511–534). San Francisco, CA: Jossey-Bass Wiley.

Salinero-Fort, M. A., de-Santa Pau, E. C., Arrietta-Blanco, F. J., Abanda-Herranz, J. C., Martin-Madrazo, C., Rodes-Saldevia, B., & Bugos-Lunar C. (2011). Effectiveness of PRECEDE model for health education on changes and level of HbA1c, blood pressure, lipids, and body mass index in patients with type 2 diabetes mellitus. *BMC Public Health, 11,* 267, doi 10.1186/1471-2458-11-267

Workgroup for Community Health and Development. (2017). The Community Toolbox. Retrieved from http://ctb.ku.edu/en/table-contents/overview/other-models-promoting-community-health-and-development/preceder-proceder/main

Chapter Opener: © MeskPhotography/Shutterstock; © Hero Images/Getty Images; © lzf/Shutterstock; © Henrik Sorensen/Getty Images

SECTION II

Conceptual and Theoretical Perspectives for Public Health Research and Practice

▶ Introduction

The next eight chapters of this book introduce you to a broad spectrum of theories and approaches that have been widely used in health-promotion practice and research. These chapters may well be some of the most important chapters you will read in preparing yourself to effectively improve public health through the promotion of health-protective behaviors. We have carefully sequenced these chapters so you can observe the progression from theories that focus mostly on proximal influences of behavior to those that emphasize distal influences. The progression from proximal to distal as shown in this section is quite similar to the history of theory development in health promotion. We begin first by introducing the value–expectancy models; each of these maintains the basic premise that people are essentially rational actors working on a "stage" based largely on their perceptions. We then move into models that incorporate the idea that perceptions toward a particular health outcome are important, but so too are the specific perceptions regarding the severity of that outcome and the perceived susceptibility of acquiring that outcome. For example, even if people have positive attitudes toward exercising to avoid being overweight, they may not act on that without perceiving their being overweight as severe or that they are vulnerable to being overweight.

A development parallel to the value–expectancy theories/models was based on the concept of producing stage-matched interventions. The basic premise behind this concept is that various levels of readiness to change will exist across any given population of people. The next chapter then shifts the perspective somewhat to include the robust utility of social influences on health behavior. Given that humans are social beings, you will be able to quickly find the eloquence in applying theories that harness social influence in order to promote health-protective behaviors at the population level. A particularly prominent theory in this regard is known as social cognitive theory. Developed by Albert Bandura, social cognitive theory greatly expanded original thinking in health behavior by emphasizing the point that the social environment (including economics, policy, law, and even culture) interacts with cognitive influences to ultimately determine behavior. Social cognitive theory has been widely applied to health behavior, and as you learn more about this theory we are confident that you will soon be able to apply it to health promotion.

As this section of the textbook progresses, you will be introduced to persuasion and communication techniques, as well as social marketing, to promote health-protective behaviors across large populations. These approaches to health promotion fall under the discipline known as health communication. Even though you will notice elements of value–expectancy theories and social influence theories interwoven in this chapter on health communication, please be alert to somewhat of a paradigm shift, as the thinking will be centered upon approaches rather than theory per se.

Moving even farther into this next section of the textbook, you will learn about the Diffusion of Innovations Theory as popularized by Everett Rogers. In many ways, this theory embodies all that you will have learned earlier in this section of the textbook and then extends those concepts by posing a framework that describes how a population adopts novel health behaviors. We anticipate that you will find Diffusion Theory to be an extremely valuable asset in your professional repertoire.

Finally, the last chapter of this section introduces the rapidly emerging theories generally referred to as ecological approaches. In many ways, these population-based approaches are quite the opposite of the value–expectancy theories that you will learn about in the opening of this section. A major difference lies in the reliance on changing entire systems to produce the ecological advantages needed to optimally enable people to adopt and maintain health-protective behaviors.

As you sequentially read the chapters in this section, please know that we (the authors) have successfully guided scores upon scores of students through what may first appear to be a quagmire of theory. Be assured that we recognize the inherent complexities in learning about the theories and ultimately choosing among them to develop an effective health-promotion program. Even the most accomplished students in fields of study such as medicine, dentistry, pharmacy, and biology, have indeed struggled to master these theories, and these students eventually came to understand that changing health behavior is rarely a straightforward process and that theory can be an indispensable tool to aid you in the process of preventing disease. Given this basic observation as a starting point, we urge you to embrace the seemingly subtle differences between theories and to become comfortable with the idea that a vast arsenal of theory is a necessity to understanding and changing health behaviors.

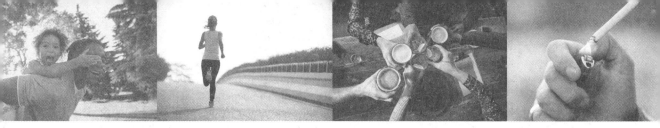

CHAPTER 4
Value–Expectancy Theories

Richard A. Crosby, Laura F. Salazar, and Ralph J. DiClemente

The awareness that health is dependent upon habits that we control makes us the first generation in history that to a large extent determines its own destiny.

—Jimmy Carter

PREVIEW

Understanding health behavior is the first step to affecting change in a positive direction. A specific category of theories has been instrumental in explaining how individuals make health-behavior decisions in terms of their expectations or beliefs regarding the health behavior and the value attached to the behavioral health outcome.

OBJECTIVES

1. Understand value–expectancy as a general theoretical concept.
2. Understand the constructs and overall propositions of the theory of reasoned action, the theory of planned behavior, and the Information–Motivation–Behavioral Skills (IMB) model.
3. Be able to articulate similarities between the theory of reasoned action, the theory of planned behavior, and the IMB model.
4. Be able to identify key differences between the theory of reasoned action, the theory of planned behavior, and the IMB model.

▶ Introduction

One effective way to begin to learn about health behavior is to think about examples in your own life. Consider, for example, a recent health behavior that you wanted to alter, such as diet or exercise. Chances are good that while contemplating whether you really wanted to make this change, you asked yourself questions such as, "What will I gain as a result of this change?" This type of thinking may be common among people who are in the midst of deciding to adopt a given health-protective behavior. This thinking is emblematic of a basic class of theories known as value–expectancy theories. At their core, these theories assume that people will change a behavior if they anticipate the personal benefits derived from the outcome will outweigh any "costs" incurred through enacting the behavior. In essence, it is anticipated that people will opt for behaviors that maximize benefits in comparison to costs. An intuitive logic is thought to operate, which might be termed "mental math." In this mental math, costs (in sum) are subtracted from benefits and the remaining value (if positive) serves as the basis for an adoption decision (see **FIGURE 4-1**).

So, thus far, it seems that value–expectancy is a rather simple concept. The initial simplicity has an unfortunate tendency to fade when the concept of cost is defined in more detail. Costs may be social, emotional, physical, or financial. For example, consider a woman who feels that her new male sex partner may be infected with HIV. Although they have had sex several times already, condoms have not been used. She may contemplate the adoption of condom use to gain relief from her anxiety about contracting HIV from him. The benefit is relatively clear: reduced anxiety/fear and possibly avoiding HIV. The costs, however, may not be immediately apparent and her perceptions may become the basis for decision making. She may imagine, for instance, that asking her partner to use condoms might seem like an accusation that he was harboring HIV or some other sexually transmitted infection. She may further imagine that this could lead him to end their relationship, an outcome with a cost that may potentially be counted so high by her that the mental math will leave a remainder of zero or less, thereby negating the behavior change.

The initial simplicity also fades somewhat when you consider that benefits may also be social, emotional, physical, or financial. All too often, health-promotion programs focus only on the physical benefits of a given health behavior. This approach may be an artifact of the training and orientation of health-promotion professionals to avert morbidity and mortality; however, the question that begs to be asked is, "Do people typically adopt health behaviors to gain a physical benefit?" Think again about yourself. Have you ever adopted a health-protective practice for social reasons? For example, have you practiced good dental hygiene to improve appearance? Have you adopted a diet and exercise program to improve sex appeal? And, if you smoke, have you attempted cessation to be more compatible with a growing number of friends who do not smoke? Like costs, the benefits of any given health behavior are not always clear, and therefore perceptions may be an important aspect of the mental math that accounts for behavior.

A final observation about value–expectancy theories involves yet another form of perception, one that deals with immediate versus delayed benefit. Again, think about examples in your own life, such as losing weight. The social benefit of losing weight to increase sex appeal may indeed materialize relatively soon in comparison to the physical benefit of delaying heart disease or avoiding adult-onset diabetes. In fact, the event of looking thin (and receiving social praise/approval for this look) is a benefit in the form of

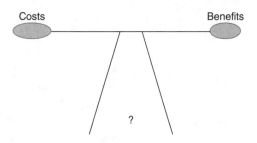

FIGURE 4-1 Weighing costs and benefits

something added—a gain—whereas the benefit of averting heart disease or diabetes is in the form of avoiding—a loss. Thus, perceptions pertaining to benefits may take the form of prospective gains or averted losses.

Given the basic concepts of value–expectancy theory just described, you are now well positioned to develop an understanding of several individual-level theories of health behavior that are based on value–expectancy. This chapter presents three theories that are essentially predicated on value–expectancy assumptions. First, you will learn about the theory of reasoned action, a very common application of a value–expectancy theory. Subsequently, you will learn how the theory of planned behavior serves as an effective expansion of the theory of reasoned action. Next, you will learn about the Information–Motivation–Behavioral Skills Model, this model will provide you with an approach that is distinct from the two theories presented first.

▶ Key Concepts

The Theory of Reasoned Action

The theory of reasoned action (TRA) was developed by Ajzen and Fishbein (1980) and was derived from their previous research, which started out as a theory of attitude and led to the study of attitude and behavior. Behavioral intention is the primary construct of this theory—intention is posited to subsequently lead to the adoption of health-protective behaviors. The TRA has a dual focus. First, it suggests that beliefs about health behaviors will largely shape behavioral intent, and second, it suggests that social influences are an equally important influence on behavioral intent. Even with the added dimension of social influences, the same value–expectancy undertone will be apparent to you as you learn about this theory. With the construct of social influences, the idea that benefits and costs are vital determinants of subsequent behavior is clearly applicable. The social benefits, for example, of smoking cessation are likely to carry a great deal of weight in the context of recently passed ETS (environmental tobacco smoke)

laws. However, these social benefits may be sparse in communities where smoking is widely accepted. Social costs are also likely to be a robust determinant of behavior change, as going against the grain of prevailing social norms is never easy and seldom reinforcing. A few examples of situations with a potentially high social cost include college students abstaining from alcohol, eating a vegetarian diet in rural farming communities where meat in used every meal, and taking exercise breaks at a worksite where everyone else consumes soft drinks or coffee during their breaks. You can, of course, easily think of many more health-behavior examples that involve social benefits and social costs, and so the value–expectancy theme is clear in the TRA.

> *Social costs are also likely to be a robust determinant of behavior change, as going against the grain of prevailing social norms is never easy and seldom reinforcing.*

Behavioral intent is a key construct in the TRA as it is the cognitive endpoint of the theory. In essence, the formation of intent is the last step in the theory before the actual behavior. The two independent constructs that precede intent are: (1) the overall **attitude toward the health behavior** and (2) **subjective norms**. The first construct is centered on beliefs. The TRA posits that multiple beliefs combine to form attitudes toward a specified behavior. An example may be helpful.

Consider a person (let's call him George) who wants to lower his cholesterol levels. George has a few options. He can change his diet, exercise, or take cholesterol-lowering drugs. Imagine that you (as a health professional) inform George that his best bet is to change his diet. The task for George is now to formulate an attitude toward the behavior of eating a diet low in cholesterol-producing foods.

According to the TRA, however, predicting intention with such a universal attitude as "eating a diet low in cholesterol producing foods" is difficult at best. Instead, the TRA recommends that attitudes toward very specific behaviors be assessed. George, for example, may first form an attitude toward the health behavior of forgoing all meat products from now on (going vegetarian). Next, George would consider his beliefs relative to becoming a vegetarian. He might first conclude that doing so would certainly lower his cholesterol, but he must also consider all of the other possible outcomes that could stem from going vegetarian. For example, he may believe that he will have a difficult time finding enough food to eat. This perception about not finding enough meat-free food is considered a **behavioral belief**. Next, the TRA would suggest that George will evaluate this behavioral belief relative to "good versus bad." Let's assume that George is a bit on the skinny side, thus he attaches the evaluation of "very bad" to the belief that he may not find enough meatless food alternatives. For someone who is rather obese, however, the behavioral belief of having less food to select from may be viewed as "good" simply because weight loss may follow.

The TRA suggests that the degree of "good versus bad" could be assessed on a 7-point scale ranging from -3 to $+3$, with 0 being the point of indifference. So, in this case it may be fair to say that George would rate the behavioral belief of not finding enough meatless food as a -3. Let's say that George next thinks about the social outcomes of not eating meat. He first thinks about the fact that so many of his business and social meals comprise a primary meat dish and he concludes that going vegetarian could be socially awkward. Here, of course, the assessment will most likely pertain only to the degree of "badness," as being socially awkward is never a good thing. This behavioral belief could then also be assessed on the same 7-point scale perhaps, in this case, yielding a value of -1 (not so bad but certainly not a positive thing). The next behavioral belief that George comes up with may be that not eating meat would be very positive in terms of averting colorectal cancer, so he is likely to evaluate this belief in a very positive manner (perhaps a $+3$).

According to the TRA, once a person such as George considers all relevant behavioral beliefs toward a very specific health behavior

and evaluates each belief as being good or bad, then attitude formation regarding the health behavior takes place. It is vital that you understand the point made earlier; that attitudes are about highly specific behaviors. For example, imagine that George later learns about the value of drinking modest amounts of red wine to favorably alter his cholesterol profile (this will increase the HDL cholesterol levels, which are actually protective against heart disease). This behavior (drinking modest amounts of red wine) then requires the formation of second attitude, one that is formed in the same manner (i.e., behavioral beliefs are identified and evaluated by George). In summary, it is not enough to measure what George believes about a vaguely defined health behavior such as changing diet; an attitude toward a specific health behavior must be identified, and that attitude is composed of behavioral beliefs and an accompanying evaluation of the "goodness" corresponding with the expected outcome.

The second construct in the TRA (subjective norms) comes from sociology and entails the idea that people are motivated by their perceptions of what is considered normative and acceptable to others. Subjective norms suggest that "gains" may be viewed as social and not strictly personal. Note that people make decisions about health based not only on their values about health, but also on the basis of their values with respect to relationships, family ties, cultural practices, and the like. So, again, using George and his cholesterol problem as an example, please consider the health behavior of taking medication to lower cholesterol. According to the TRA, George would likely think about what other people might want him to do relative to taking these drugs; specifically, TRA suggests that the people who are most central to George will be considered first. He may, for example, first consider whether his wife would think that taking cholesterol-lowering drugs is a good thing to do. He may then

> *People are motivated by their perceptions of what is considered normative and acceptable to others.*

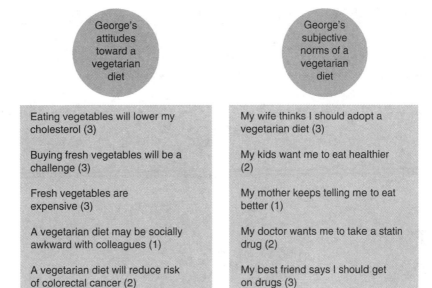

FIGURE 4-2 George's attitudes toward and subjective norms of a vegetarian diet

consider what his close friends or family members may think about this health behavior. The perceptions that George has about what others think he should do regarding the behavior of using medication to lower cholesterol are known as **normative beliefs**.

The TRA suggests that George will have several normative beliefs. Further, the TRA goes on to speculate that each normative belief will be "weighted" by a person's motivation to comply with the **referent source**. The term "referent source" refers to the source of the normative belief; for example, George may consider what his doctor would want him do to relative to taking cholesterol-lowering drugs, and so the doctor would then be the referent source. Assuming that George has a regular doctor that he sees, we might guess that the normative belief held by George about this referent source is that "George should take the medication." The "weighting" comes into play next by considering how motivated George is to act in a way that pleases his doctor. Again, the TRA suggests this level of motivation could be measured by a seven-point scale; this time ranging from one to seven. In summary, to arrive at a subjective norm toward the health behavior of taking cholesterol-lowering

medication, a two-step process occurs: (1) identify all relevant normative beliefs and (2) weight each normative behavior by the motivation to comply with the referent source. George's attitudes toward and subject norms about adopting a vegetarian diet are presented in **FIGURE 4-2**.

According to the TRA, both of these primary constructs (attitude toward the health behavior and the subjective norms) independently contribute to the formation of behavioral intent. Intent is defined very specifically in the TRA, necessitating that measures of intent include: (1) *time frame* for performance of the behavior, (2) an exact description of the *action* composing the behavior, (3) the desired outcome (*target*) of the behavior, and (4) the *context* of the behavior. For example, intent to use condoms may be specifically defined as "intent to use condoms for STD prevention (target) in the next 6 months (time) for every act of penile–vaginal sex (action) with people other than your primary sex partner (context)." Continuing with our example of George and his cholesterol problem, we illustrate in **TABLE 4-1** how George can be more specific according to time, action, target, and context with adopting his vegetarian diet.

TABLE 4-1 Specifics of Health Behaviors for George

Action	Target	Context	Time
Get	Prescription for Lipitor®	Internist office	Next 2 months
Use Take	Fresh vegetables Lipitor®	In meals cooked at home Unspecified	Always Daily
Order	A salad	Eating out	Always

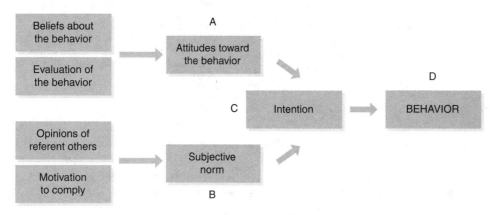

FIGURE 4-3 Essential constructs in the theory of reasoned action

Modified from Ajzen, I., & Fishbein, M. (1980). *Understanding attitudes and predicting social behavior*. Englewood Cliffs, NJ: Prentice-Hall.

The TRA is diagrammed in **FIGURE 4-3**. Again, for ease of presentation the constructs are labeled "A" through "D." Also, the endpoint of the theory (i.e., behavior) is emphasized by capitalization. The theory is somewhat elaborate; however, the heart of the theory is relatively easy to understand. To begin, the theory asserts that the decision to adopt a given health-protective behavior (i.e., **intent** or construct "C") is partly a function of the **attitudes that people hold toward the behavior** (construct "A"). In the parlance of this theory, attitudes are a person's evaluation of the anticipated positive or negative outcomes associated with engaging in a given behavior. Consider, for example, smoking cessation. The TRA suggests that attitudes toward smoking cessation are influenced by the belief that stopping smoking would decrease the risk of heart disease, cancer, and other smoking-related problems and also the value placed on those outcomes. However, outcomes are not limited to health outcomes. For example, they may also include having more money, an improved ability to taste food, or less annoyance of nonsmokers. The value placed on the outcomes is essentially an assessment of *goodness*, meaning that people will decide whether the outcome is rated favorably or unfavorably. Ultimately, the person develops an overall evaluation of the behavior (smoking cessation) and this evaluation then drives (in part) the level of intent to quit.

According to theory of reasoned action, the other influence on intent is the **subjective norm toward the behavior** (construct "B"). This construct is predicated on the notion that people will hold varying perceptions relative to how strongly valued people in their lives would advocate adoption of the health-protective behavior in question. For example, imagine a 17-year-old male (Joe) who is contemplating smoking cessation after 5 years of tobacco use. He may consider whether (and how strongly) the following people would think that he should quit:

- His father and mother
- His brothers (neither of whom smoke)
- His friends at school (many of whom smoke)
- His older friends at his part-time job (all of whom smoke)
- His favorite uncle (a person he admires and who does not smoke)
- His teachers at school
- His girlfriend (she does not smoke)

According to the theory, Joe will form an impression of what these significant others in his life would want him to do relative to smoking cessation. He will then temper each impression by his *level of motivation to comply* with what these people may think he should do. For example, his friends at work may be perceived as people who do not think Joe needs to quit (after all, "he's only 17; he is a long way from having any problems") and Joe may hold these older friends in high esteem, thus wanting to please them. His girlfriend, on the other hand, may have outwardly expressed to Joe that she doesn't like it when he smokes and she desperately wants him to quit. Joe, however, is not enamored by his current girlfriend and is no hurry to make changes in his life just to please her.

As you might imagine, this process of summing all of the normative beliefs in Joe's life culminates in the creation of his subjective norms toward the behavior of smoking cessation. At this juncture it is important to note that the term "subjective" is not merely a name—it implies that perceptions are the critical component of this concept. Because perceptions may or may not be an accurate reflection of reality, one intervention implication is that sometimes altering perceptions alone may foster positive intent to adopt a given health behavior. In Joe's case, for example, his perception that his friends do not think he should quit may be false in reality. His friends who smoke may have already tried quitting or may privately want to try quitting. If Joe were to see these realities, his original perception may change.

Given the mutual influence of constructs "A" and "B" on the intent to quit smoking, the last "leg" of the theory posits that level of intent will be associated with actual behavioral efforts to quit. This last leg generally becomes a breaking point for the theory. The often weak connection between intent and actual behavior is most likely attributable to external circumstances; that is, perceptions of environmental factors, or the actual reality of environmental barriers, may heavily confound the translation of behavioral intent. For example, Joe may develop a relatively strong intent to quit smoking, but he may perceive a lack of access to an affordable cessation program to help him break the strong physical addiction created by nicotine dependence. In the absence of this professional assistance, his intent may remain as nothing more than "a good idea for someday." Again, the term "perceived" is vital here, as it may well be that Joe could easily access a free smoking cessation program but he is unaware that this possibility exists. The intervention implication is clear: in some cases, raising awareness of existing resources and programs pertaining to health behaviors may catalyze the translation of intent into behavior. Of course, the converse is not true: in the absence of environmental supports for behavior change, simply altering perceptions is ineffective. It is at this juncture that an extension to the theory of reasoned action becomes warranted. The extension is the theory of planned behavior.

The Theory of Planned Behavior

The theory of planned behavior (TPB) is simply the theory of reasoned action with another construct added: an overall comparison of perceptions related to external factors, as well as objective realities that may facilitate and inhibit the adoption of the health behavior. The construct is known as **perceived behavioral control** (Ajzen, 2002), and it is primarily concerned with the extent to which a person or a group of people perceive that they are able to control the outcome, meaning that change is within their control. According to

> *A facilitating factor is any actual or perceived external factor that increases the likelihood of the occurrence of the behavior in question.*

the theory of planned behavior, if a behavior is perceived to be important (favorable attitudes) and subjective norms seem to support the behavior, then people are more likely to engage in that behavior if they also *perceive* that it is within their control. This perception of control is based on an intersection of factors external to the person making the decision and their cognitive evaluation of those external factors. External factors that serve to facilitate a given behavior or those that act to inhibit a given behavior are based on personal *perceptions* (these may or may not reflect an objective reality).

These perceptions include the existence of **facilitating factors**. A facilitating factor is any actual or perceived external factor that increases the likelihood of the occurrence of the behavior in question. Pap testing serves as an excellent example. One factor that may facilitate Pap testing is the existence of easily accessible clinics that offer expanded hours for women who work from 9:00 AM to 5:00 PM. Other facilitating factors may include a "user-friendly" clinic environment and the availability of childcare services.

These perceptions also include factors that may inhibit performance of the behavior. **Inhibiting factors** are, again, external to the person, and perceptions and reality may not always coincide. For example, one inhibiting factor relative to Pap testing, for some women, may be their belief that a positive Pap result indicates "full-blown cancer" and that cancer can only be treated through hysterectomy. This perception is, of course, not aligned with reality and correcting this perception may be a useful objective of health-promotion intervention. Another perceived inhibiting factor may be the out-of-pocket costs for the Pap test and the accompanying pelvic exam. In this case, for the millions of U.S. women who are uninsured, the perception may align perfectly with reality, thereby rendering education-based intervention useless.

In addition to facilitating and inhibiting factors, the theory of planned behavior suggests that the **perceived power** of these factors is considered by people in the process of adopting a health-protective behavior. Perceived power pertains to the strength of the facilitating and inhibiting factors. A single but strong inhibiting factor, for example, may negate translation of behavioral intent. Consider, again, the out-of-pocket expense for a Pap test among uninsured women. Despite the existence of multiple facilitating factors, this single inhibiting factor may preclude the formation of a positive intent or the translation of the positive intent into behavior.

FIGURE 4-4 displays the added construct that represents the extension of the theory of reasoned action to the theory of planned behavior. The added construct, perceived behavioral control, is somewhat more complex than its counterpart found in the theory of reasoned action. It is very important that you first understand that this construct is not identical to self-efficacy. Self-efficacy is a task-specific perception of personal ability, while, in contrast, perceived behavioral control is much broader in scope. To begin, the construct is assessed by considering all of the environmental factors that may facilitate the action. Then, the relative power of each facilitating factor is considered. Again, for example, one identified factor that might apply to Joe's smoking cessation would be the existence of a freely available cessation program through Joe's school. Joe's perception of the power of this cessation program to facilitate his successful transition to a nonsmoker then becomes paramount. Joe may see the program as a "big joke" and place very little stock in its value, or he may see the program as being an important factor in his decision (given that he believes it would help him quit successfully). The second part to this added construct is simply asking

> *In addition to facilitating and inhibiting factors, the theory of planned behavior suggests that the **perceived power** of these factors is considered by people in the process of adopting a health-protective behavior.*

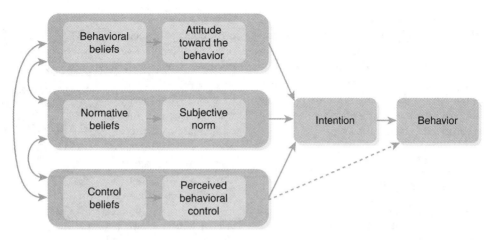

FIGURE 4-4 The theory of planned behavior

Modified from Ajzen, I., & Madden, T. J. (1986). Prediction of goal-directed behavior: Attitudes, intentions, and perceived behavioral control. *Journal of Experimental Social Psychology, 22*, 453–474. With permission.

TABLE 4-2 Potential Facilitating and Inhibiting Factors Relative to Condom Use	
Facilitating Factors	**Inhibiting Factors**
Condoms are affordable The skills needed are easily obtained Condoms that enhance eroticism are available Condoms can be acquired 24 hours a day	Buying condoms is embarrassing Comfortable condoms are hard to get Partners may object to condom use

the reverse of this first question. Whereas the first question may have been, "What are the facilitating factors?," the second would be, "What are the barriers?" (i.e., the inhibiting factors). The assessment process, however, is the same. Inhibiting factors are identified and the power of each relative to performing (or not performing) the behavior in question is considered.

Before proceeding to the next section of this chapter, we feel it is essential for you to thoroughly understand the perceived behavioral control construct of the theory of planned behavior (as this is where many students first become confused). To help enhance your understanding, **TABLE 4-2** displays a listing of potential facilitating factors and inhibiting factors relative to yet another example of a health-protective behavior: condom use. As shown, seven factors are listed—each is external to the person and therefore none are redundant

with the other two constructs of the theory of planned behavior (i.e., attitudes toward the behavior and the subjective norm toward the behavior). If you were actually assessing this construct for a population, you would also need to know how much "power" each factor held for people making decisions about condom use. For example, the final inhibiting factor listed in Table 4-1 (partners may object to condom use) may be so strong that it carries far more weight than the combined advantages of all four facilitating factors.

At this point, you should be able to piece together this construct with the other two constructs from the TRA (attitudes toward the behavior and subjective norms) to form a prediction of behavioral intent to use condoms. According to the TRA, high intent would be predicted by an overall favorable evaluation (attitude toward the behavior) of condom use combined with an overall perception that significant others (when motivation to comply is high) would endorse the person's decision to use condoms (subjective norm toward the behavior). According to the TPB, it is also critical to consider perceptions and objective realities relevant to the strength of all applicable facilitating factors and all applicable inhibiting factors (perceived behavioral control).

The Information–Motivation– Behavioral Skills Model

Unlike the TRA and the TPB, the **Information– Motivation–Behavioral Skills (IMB) Model** is a somewhat more recent innovation in the behavioral sciences. Grounded in the value–expectancy tradition, the IMB model (Fisher & Fisher, 1992) was initially developed for and applied to HIV risk behaviors among various populations of adults and adolescents, both domestically and internationally. Subsequently, it has been successfully applied to promote breast self-examination, use of motorcycle safety gear, and medication adherence Its tenets and constructs are not unique in comparison with other value–expectancy theories; however, they expand upon and are combined with other constructs. Thus, the IMB has sufficient integrity for widespread application in health promotion.

Understanding the IMB model is relatively easy given what you have already learned about other value–expectancy theories. The first construct of the IMB, information, is simple and fairly self-explanatory. Having a high degree of relevant knowledge pertaining to the health behavior is considered a prerequisite to behavior change. As a rule, while information is necessary, it alone is not sufficient for some behaviors to evoke change. We wish to emphasize here that the information must indeed be highly relevant to the adoption of a given behavior. Information, for example, about how losing excess weight can ease problems such as lower-back pain, knee issues, and a host of other musculoskeletal problems may be very useful.

In explaining the next construct, it would be helpful to think about the theory of planned behavior. The TPB includes a construct (attitudes) that is consistent with the concept of seeking a positive net gain with regard to a perceived threat. Also included is the concept of social influences (subjective norms). Collectively, these constructs could be classified as motivation, which is one of the main constructs of the IMB. Motivation in this model is conceived as a construct that embodies a range of perceptions related to the behavior in question. These perceptions also include outcome expectations and outcomes expectancies (both of which are described in detail as part of Chapter 7, Social Cognitive Theory).

Motivation in this model is conceived as a construct that embodies a range of perceptions related to the behavior in question.

The third construct, **behavioral skills**, is based on the construct of self-efficacy. As noted previously in this chapter, self-efficacy can be thought of as a task-specific perception of personal ability. Although self-efficacy is a perception, it is linked strongly to actual task-specific ability (i.e., skill). Behavioral skills, as defined in the IMB model, are an integration of both actual skill and self-efficacy. The placement of this construct within the flow of the model is critical. As you examine the model, please note that this construct is located between the "I" and "B" and similarly between the "M" and the "B." This middle ground represents a mediation effect, meaning that, for example, Information acts on behavior through the mediating variable of behavioral skill. Please note that the model also includes pathways that by-pass behavioral skill: these pathways would apply when a behavior is fully volitional (i.e., when levels of self-efficacy and skill are universally high in a population).

FIGURE 4-5 displays the IMB model. As shown, the model has five pathways (i.e., five connections among constructs). First, as noted in the previous paragraph, observe that the outer two pathways bypass the construct of behavioral skills entirely. The model speculates that information can directly influence the health behavior and, further, that motivation can do the same. Next, please observe that the remaining three pathways (inner pathways) form two indirect routes from information and motivation to the actual behavior through behavioral skills. The routes are indirect because behavioral skills

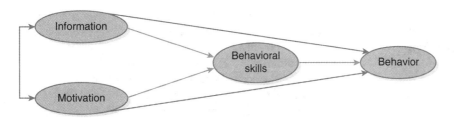

FIGURE 4-5 Representation of the Information–Motivation–Behavioral Skills Model

mediates (comes between) the influence of both information and motivation on behavior.

The concept here is simply that increased relevant information leads to improved behavioral skills, which, in turn, may promote increased odds of actually performing the behavior. Similarly, increased motivation would lead to improved behavioral skills, which, in turn, promotes the behavior. In examining the differences between the direct pathways and the inner pathways comes down to a single question: does the behavior involve skill? The idea is that, for many health behaviors, skill is often required to perform the behavior, but not always—hence the two outside pathways. Yet, it is important to note that skill acquisition is more likely when the person has the right information and attitudes.

On the surface, behaviors such as wearing a seat belt would not seem to be skill based, yet consider that adolescents tend not to wear their seat belt, especially when the driver of the car does not. This suggests that the driver exerts social influence on the behavior of the other adolescents in the car. One could argue that skill is needed to deal with the peer pressure. Thus, in this context, some skill is necessary to wear a seat belt.

Sometimes no skill is needed and, as indicated by the outer pathways, behavior is dependent mainly on information and motivation. Upon reflection, however, you may soon realize that the indirect pathways are more common, as most health-protective behaviors do indeed require perceived and actual skill.

Now that you have a basic working knowledge of the IMB model, it is worth learning more about the basic constructs. First, it should be noted that information pertains only to highly relevant knowledge that is potentially linked to the decision point of performing the health behavior in question. This point is vital to preserving the integrity of the model, as not all knowledge is of equal value. Consider, for example, the health behavior of eating a low-fat diet to prevent atherosclerosis. Would you classify knowledge about the physical process of atherosclerosis as being vital to the behavior? How about knowledge relevant to the three major categories of dietary fat (saturated, monounsaturated, and polyunsaturated) and the health behavior? Of these two options, the latter would actually be far more compatible with the intent of the IMB because managing a low-fat diet actually translates into avoiding saturated fats (as these are the fats that play a key role in atherosclerosis). Maybe all people need to know is that eating fruits and vegetables is healthful and eating meat and other foods high in saturated fat can be bad for health. In essence, knowledge without direct relevance to the health behavior in question is not the focus of the information construct; instead, the construct is built on behavior-specific information. Several examples pertaining to a low-fat diet for the prevention of atherosclerosis follow:

- Saturated fats are typically found in the same foods (animal products) that also produce elevated blood cholesterol levels.
- Polyunsaturated fats may be protective against some forms of cancer, and monounsaturated fats may be partially protective against stroke.
- Cooking oils may be high in saturated fats, and these types of oils should be avoided in favor of those that contain either polyunsaturated fats or monounsaturated fats.

As you can see by looking at these few examples, the assessment of behavior-specific knowledge held by people in your target audience can be a very important aspect of understanding, and therefore changing, a health behavior.

Like the information construct, motivation must be assessed on a behavior-specific basis.

The next construct to consider is motivation. Simply stated, motivation is the combined influence of a person's attitude toward the behavior and his/her socially inspired motives to perform the behavior (please note here the very clear resemblance to the theory of reasoned action). Like the information construct, motivation must be assessed on a behavior-specific basis. For example, using a condom to prevent pregnancy may produce a very different level of motivation than using a condom to prevent the acquisition of sexually transmitted diseases.

The final construct to consider is behavioral skills. As noted previously, this construct is actually a combination of self-efficacy and actual skill. As you might well imagine, measuring either of these components can be a tricky proposition. Given the introductory nature of this chapter, we have chosen not to provide instruction relevant to the complexities of assessing this (or other) IMB constructs; however, you can easily read more about the model and its application (see Fisher & Fisher, 1992; Fisher, Fisher, Amico, & Harman, 2006; Fisher, Fisher, Bryan, & Misovich, 2002).

Once you have a basic understanding of the three constructs, the next step is learn how the IMB can be used to first understand a health behavior and then to inform the design of intervention efforts. The model specifies that an **elicitation phase** should precede the intervention phase. The elicitation phase may involve qualitative investigation (i.e., collecting data that does not involve numbers, such as face-to-face interviews or focus groups) as well as quantitative investigation (i.e., collecting data that is numerical, such as frequency counts). The goal is to assess each of the constructs so that analytic associations between the "I," "M," and "BS" constructs (see Figure 4-5) can be revealed.

FIGURE 4-6 displays an example of the IMB model applied to the health behavior of correct condom use (Crosby et al., 2008). To understand this figure, it is first important to understand that the coefficients shown on each pathway may have a potential value ranging from -1.0 to $+1.0$. A negative value (that is also significant) represents an inverse association (meaning that as the magnitude of one construct increases, the magnitude of the other decreases). For example, the direct pathway between information and the health behavior (condom use errors) has a significant coefficient of -0.14. This means that as information increases, the number of condom use errors decreases. However, it must be noted that the strength of this association is relatively weak (strength increases as the value approaches 1.0 in either direction).

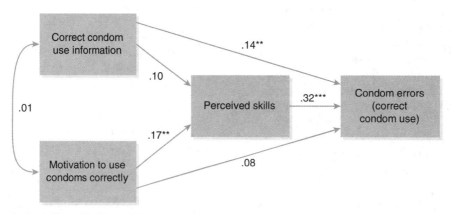

*p 0.05. **p 0.01. ***p 0.001.

FIGURE 4-6 An example of the IMB model applied in a study of correct condom use.

With kind permission from Springer Science + Business Media: Crosby, R. A., Salazar, L. F., Yarber, W. L., Sanders, S. A., Graham, C. A., Head, S., & Arno, J. N. (2008). A theory-based approach to understanding condom errors and problems reported by men attending an STI clinic. *AIDS & Behavior, 12,* 412–418.

A positive value (that is also significant) represents a direct association (meaning that as the magnitude of one construct increases, the magnitude of the other also increases). For example, the indirect pathway between motivation and perceived behavioral skills has a significant coefficient of 0.17. Thus, as you might expect, as motivation to use condoms correctly increases, one's level of self-efficacy to achieve correct condom use also increases. Given this basic understanding of the pathway coefficients, you should now be able to look at the remaining significant value of -0.32 and determine what that means. The answer is that a significant inverse relationship exists between the perceived skills construct and the health behavior. As you might have guessed, increasing amounts of self-efficacy lead to decreased errors in condom use.

Given the data in Figure 4-6, imagine what you would conclude from a study designed to initially assess the IMB constructs in a sample of people who will eventually become recipients of your health-promotion program. The best conclusion would be twofold: (1) information (as it was assessed) about correct condom use is an important predictor of the health behavior, and (2) motivation (as it was assessed) to use condoms correctly is an important predictor of increased self-efficacy which, in turn, predicts the health behavior. As you can see, the elicitation exercise essentially informs the design of the intervention phase. In this case, effort expended on increasing all three constructs is warranted. Once the intervention has been designed and delivered, the model specifies an **evaluation phase**. One part of the evaluation phase may involve collecting follow-up data that is subsequently analyzed for associations between the IMB constructs.

▶ Summary

In sum, the theories described in this chapter provide clear models describing the relationships among information, cognitions, and behavior that can be used in developing and evaluating the success of health-promotion programs. For example, evaluations can ask questions such as the following: Did the program favorably influence changes in attitudes toward the behavior? Did the program favorably alter perceptions of social norms? Did the program minimize people's perceived barriers to performing the recommended health behavior? Was the program effective in increasing knowledge and skills related to the behavior? These types of questions compose a systematic evaluation of program effects on the hypothesized mediators of behavior change.

▶ An Applied Example

Now that you have a working knowledge of value–expectancy theories, please consider the following scenario.

Juanita is a clerical worker in a large company (about 4000 employees). She is 39 years old and in reasonably good health. Juanita has never known anyone who has been hospitalized with or died from the flu. She has received the flu vaccine twice in the past, and both times she experienced fever and malaise lasting more than 24 hours. Her job is very demanding and work much be completed on time, so she often works extra hours. Juanita has recently learned that a new strain of flu (Avian flu) may become a public health problem, but she does not intend to take time off from work to be vaccinated. One day, however, as she routinely goes to meet with friends for lunch, Juanita discovers that her friends do intend to be vaccinated and that some have already done so by taking advantage of the 1-day vaccination station set up in the company cafeteria. A few of her friends who have not yet been vaccinated invite Juanita to go with them to be vaccinated that day. Juanita gladly accepts this offer.

The scenario is probably common (in many different forms). The question that is posed by this example is, "How do the value–expectancy theories you have learned about in this chapter apply to people like Juanita?" After taking a moment to think this through, please read the following few paragraphs for some insights regarding this question.

First, it is well worth noting that, from a strict cost-versus-benefit analysis, it would be unlikely that people like Juanita would take the vaccine. She has clearly experienced negative consequences of being vaccinated in the past and there is no question that she finds even the minor time commitment required for vaccination to be an inconvenience. But, as you have learned in this chapter, the concept of benefits is one that extends far beyond personally experienced physical gains. The reason Juanita so easily accepted vaccination appears to be focused on the simple concept of social benefit—she was simply doing something in harmony with her friends.

Second, consider for a moment that some very smart healthcare administrator had "engineered" the environment to make the act of getting vaccinated extremely easy for Juanita and making the entire social aspect of vaccination possible. Thinking about the theory of planned behavior, you can quickly connect the construct of perceived behavioral control (specifically, facilitating factors) to the idea of making the vaccine easy to obtain. You can also quickly identify that the same theory would indeed predict that a conducive social environment would capitalize on the construct of subjective norms, thereby increasing the odds of vaccine acceptance.

Finally, think about the practical implications of using value–expectancy theories to promote relatively simple, one-time health behaviors such as vaccination. From a value–expectancy perspective, one aspect of a program might include a media campaign that seeks to improve people's overall evaluation of the vaccine, perhaps by dispelling misconceptions that the vaccine can actually cause the flu or by convincing people that the flu can indeed be quite serious, even deadly. Indeed, a value–expectancy intervention could produce a seemingly endless number of benefits that could become targets of intervention efforts and an equally long list of costs that could be addressed through intervention efforts. One of the true joys that you will experience in your career is the creative pleasure entailed in analyzing what people need to persuade their behavior change and then designing strategies that will meet those needs. Thus far in this textbook you have this one set of tools (value–expectancy theories) firmly in your grasp!

▶ Take Home Messages

- The value–expectancy theories are centrally focused on decision making and cognitive processes. The endpoint of these cognitive processes is a decision about a particular behavior.

- The decisional process is based largely on information (or cues) obtained from various sources and interpreted by the individual based on past experience and personality.
- Value–expectancy theories share the common assumption that people have agency (control) over their health-related behaviors; engage in cognitive evaluation processes to decide what, if anything, to do; and are motivated by the result of these processes.
- Value–expectancy implies that perceptions are paramount and can be modified by health-promotion activities.
- The value–expectancy theories provide a wealth of potential modifiable factors (e.g., behavioral beliefs, normative beliefs, social norms, self-efficacy, and the potential barriers to and benefits of performing a given health behavior) that may be addressed through education.
- Environmental conditions are also important in their influence on perceptions, attitudes, and norms, which are all key constructs to these theories.

▶ References

Ajzen, I. (2002). Perceived behavioral control, self-efficacy, locus of control, and the theory of planned behavior. *Journal of Applied Social Psychology, 32,* 665–683.

Ajzen, I., & Fishbein, M. (1980). *Understanding attitudes and predicting social behavior.* Englewood Cliffs, NJ: Prentice-Hall.

Crosby, R. A., Salazar, L. F., Yarber, W. L., Sanders, S. A., Graham, C. A., Head, S., & Arno, J. N. (2008). A theory-based approach to understanding condom errors and problems reported by men attending an STI clinic. *AIDS & Behavior, 12,* 412–418.

Fisher, J. D., & Fisher, W. A. (1992). Changing AIDS risk behavior. *Psychological Bulletin, 111,* 455–474.

Fisher, J. D., Fisher, W. A., Amico, K. R., & Harman, J. J. (2006). An information–motivation–behavioral skills model of adherence to antiretroviral therapy. *Health Psychology, 25,* 462–473.

Fisher, J. D., Fisher, W. A., Bryan, A. D., & Misovich, S. J. (2002). Information–motivation–behavioral skills model-based HIV risk behavior change intervention for inner-city high school youth. *Health Psychology, 21,* 177–186.

Section Opener: © lzf/Shutterstock; © Henrik Sorensen/Getty Images; © MeskPhotography/Shutterstock; © Hero Images/Getty Images
Chapter Opener: © Hero Images/Getty Images; © lzf/Shutterstock; © Henrik Sorensen/Getty Images; © MeskPhotography/Shutterstock

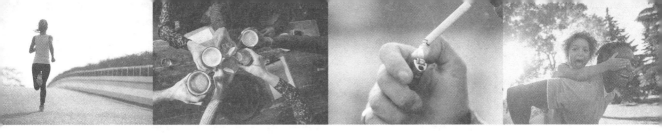

CHAPTER 5

Models Based on Perceived Threat and Fear Appeals

Laura F. Salazar, Richard A. Crosby, Seth M. Noar, Anne Marie Schipani-McLaughlin and Ralph J. DiClemente

Just as courage imperils life; fear protects it.

—**Leonardo Da Vinci**

PREVIEW

Fear can be a great motivator to avoid adverse health outcomes. A group of theoretical models suggests that instilling fear of a disease or condition, combined with enhancing skills to avoid it, may be an effective approach to changing risk behaviors.

OBJECTIVES

1. Understand perceived threat as a theoretical concept.
2. Understand the constructs and overall propositions of the health belief model, the protection motivation theory, and the expanded parallel process model.
3. Be able to articulate similarities among the health belief model, the protection motivation theory, and the expanded parallel process model.
4. Be able to identify key differences among the health belief model, the protection motivation theory, and the expanded parallel process model.
5. Describe how fear appeals can motivate behavior change and understand how to design effective persuasive messages.

▸ Introduction

Imagine that you are home alone and it is nighttime—it is dark out and you're watching a show about famous theoretical physicists. The house is very quiet other than the sound of Dr. Neil deGrasse Tyson's voice discussing Einstein's general theory of relativity. All of a sudden, you hear a loud crash coming from one of the bedrooms upstairs. You think someone must be up there. Your breathing speeds up, your heart is pounding, and your muscles tighten. You grab a knife from the kitchen and proceed slowly up the stairs to investigate what caused the noise. You are terrified. When you reach the top of the stairs, you look into your bedroom. A shelf containing books and trophies had fallen down from the wall. You let out a nervous laugh as you realize that no one is in the house. You reassure yourself, "The shelf was just too heavy—I shouldn't have put my science fair trophy on there." But, for 1 or 2 minutes, you were so afraid that you reacted as if your life were in danger, your body initiating the fight-or-flight response. But in reality, there was no danger. What happened to cause such an intense reaction? What exactly is fear?

At a very basic level, fear is a chain reaction in the brain that starts when faced with a stressful stimulus and ends with the release of chemicals that cause your heart to race, your breathing to escalate, and your muscles to energize (see **FIGURE 5-1**). This physiological reaction is known as the fight-or-flight response. For humans, fear may be expressed physiologically (as arousal), but also through language behavior (verbal self-reports) or through overt acts (facial expressions) (Lang, 1984). However

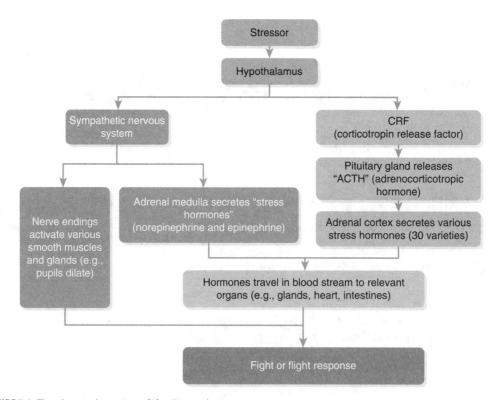

FIGURE 5-1 The chemical reaction of "fear" in our brain

Without fear and the associated fight-or-flight response, our life expectancy would be greatly reduced.

fear is expressed, it begins when you are exposed to a scary stimulus and ends with this intense physiological response.

One important aspect when discussing fear is that fear is relative. What people consider "scary" varies. For most of us, a scary stimulus would be crossing paths with a king cobra or having a gun pointed at us while walking home from the train station; for some of us, however, it might be a classroom full of people waiting for us to deliver a speech, having to do statistics, or even a sudden, loud crash heard late at night of which the cause is unknown. No matter what the stimulus is, if it is perceived as being scary, it will result in the fear response. These physiological responses are intended to help you survive a dangerous situation by preparing you to either fight for your life or run for your life (hence the term "fight or flight"). Fear and the fight-or-flight response are considered instinctual and virtually every animal possesses them. Without fear and the associated fight-or-flight response, our life expectancy would be greatly reduced. Essentially, fear protects us.

Some public health professionals hypothesized early on that it might be possible to harness the power of the instinctual fear response to change health-risk behaviors. If people feared certain disease outcomes, then perhaps they would take action to avoid them. The action might not be in the form of fight or flight per se, but maybe, if sufficiently afraid, they might order the steak but then take a statin drug to lower their cholesterol afterwards (fight), quit smoking (flight), or refrain from that third alcoholic beverage (flight). However, an important point for public health professionals to consider is, as stated earlier, that people perceive stimuli differently. One person may not be afraid of the possibility of getting emphysema in 10 years, whereas another person may view emphysema as the worst thing that could happen to them. Also, some people view themselves as being invulnerable to many diseases; thus, perceptions regarding susceptibility differ as well. To create an effective response,

To create an effective response, the stimulus must be perceived as scary to the people being exposed and they must perceive that they will be affected.

the stimulus must be perceived as scary to the people being exposed and they must perceive that they will be affected. If these two conditions are not met, then no fear and no fight-or-flight response. For public health professionals who want to evoke a fear response to change health-risk behavior, perceptions of their target audience must be considered.

These two conditions, perceived scary stimulus plus perceived vulnerability, when taken together add up to form a theoretical construct called **perceived threat**. Perceived threat is a construct that is common to several theories used in public health research and practice and is the inspiration for fear appeals. This chapter presents three of these theories. First, you will learn about a behavioral theory, the health belief model, which was one of the first psychological theories to describe this construct. The health belief model was developed in the 1950s by researchers at the U.S. Public Health Service to explain why some people were willing to get an X-ray to screen for tuberculosis; they found that high perceived threat equated with a greater likelihood of getting the X-ray.

With the introduction of the perceived threat concept into the public health field, public health campaigns were subsequently developed that tried to use fear appeals (sometimes referred to as scare tactics) to affect perceived threat and motivate people to change their negative behaviors. For example, many fear appeals have targeted teens, especially in the area of drug and alcohol use. However, many of the early fear appeals were not effective. Showing teens' grim and dramatic reenactments of alcohol-related automobile crashes, or exposing them to messages that warned them their brains would get fried if they did drugs ("this is your brain—this is your brain on drugs"), did not work.

There are several reasons why some fear appeals work and some do not; however, it is important to remember that health behaviors are much more complex than simple behaviors such as a person running away if they come face-to-face with a dangerous snake. When faced with a health threat, which may not be imminent, making the decision to not engage in a particular health-risk behavior clearly involves cognitive processes. This brings us to our second theory, the protection motivation theory. The protection motivation theory is considered a communication theory and was developed to better understand the specific cognitive processes underlying how fear appeals motivate people to change their behavior. Protection motivation theory acknowledges that fear appeals, to be effective, must consider the cognitive complexities involved when motivating people to change their behavior in addition to perceived threat. Finally, the most contemporary theory in this chapter is the third theory described, the extended parallel process model. The extended parallel process model is an integrative model in that it starts with protection motivation theory and expands upon it by incorporating another theory called the parallel process model. All three of these theories have commonalities, such as the inclusion of perceived threat; however, the health belief model is considered a behavioral theory, which attempt to explain why people engage in particular behaviors, whereas the protection motivation theory and the expanded parallel process model are communication theories, which help to understand why people respond or fail to respond to fear-arousal messages. We present all three because of the commonalities and implications for public health.

▶ Key Concepts

The Health Belief Model

Initially used to identify determinants of being screened for tuberculosis, the health belief model (HBM) has been part of public health practice for more than 50 years. The model is logical, well-articulated, and simple. It is very much a value–expectancy model, in that the primary construct is predicated on the basis that behavior change will occur only when sufficient benefits remain after subtracting the costs incurred by performing the behavior. As you read about the HBM, please keep in mind this essential benefit-versus-cost comparison.

At its heart, the model suggests that two constructs have an independent influence on health behavior. The first construct is perceived threat (described previously) and the second is the **expected net gain** of adopting the health-protective behavior. **FIGURE 5-2** displays a representation of how the HBM might be applied to a relatively simple health behavior (being vaccinated against influenza). For ease of presentation, we have labeled the diagram with letters that could conceivably correspond with a sequence of mental operations that may occur when contemplating whether to be vaccinated. Two main constructs (labeled "D" and "E") are bold for emphasis. We will begin by building up to the first of these, "D": perceived threat. The endpoint of the diagram is the box labeled "F"; this is the likelihood of the actual behavior in question (shown in italic for emphasis). Ultimately, the likelihood of action is determined by the perceived gains in something that a person values/desires, hence the term value–expectancy. This concept was covered in the previous chapter on value–expectancy theories. As discussed in Chapter 4, perceived benefits and barriers are the primary elements of the "mental math" that exemplify value–expectancy theories. In essence, all value–expectancy theories assume that people desire to maximize their outcomes while minimizing the costs. This is a rational process; however, it is important for the health-promotion professional to appreciate that the value of the process depends on the quality of the perceptions used

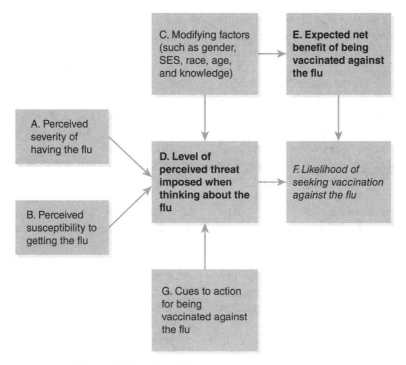

FIGURE 5-2 A representation of the health belief model

in the mental math. Decisions may be rational, but they can lead to unintended outcomes when based on faulty beliefs. Nevertheless, value–expectancy theory suggests that inconsistencies between beliefs and behavior create cognitive dissonance that can be uncomfortable or even threatening, and therefore motivate people to seek or restore a sort of balance between beliefs and behavior.

At first blush, constructs "A" (**perceived severity**) and "B" (**perceived susceptibility**) often appear to students as being redundant. However, the two constructs are actually quite distinct.

*At its heart, the model suggests that two constructs have an independent influence on health behavior. The first construct is perceived threat (described previously) and the second is the **expected net gain** of adopting the health-protective behavior.*

Consider perceived severity in relation to influenza. From the prospective of any one person in the population, the primary question would be, "If I got the flu, how bad would it be?" It is easy to imagine that responses to this question might range from slightly worse than a cold to terrible (with most people falling in between these extremes). So, already the health belief model (HBM) sheds some light on health behavior—it is logical, for example, that people at one extreme (slightly worse than a cold) may be substantially less likely than those at the other extreme (terrible) to seek vaccination. Indeed, it is already clear that people responding more toward "terrible" may be much more likely to seek the vaccination. But is this really the case?

Next, consider the construct labeled "B" (perceived susceptibility). Here, the question that might apply is, "How likely am I to catch the flu?" This is a much different question than the first one and there may be very little correspondence between the way people answer the first question and the way they answer the second. For example, a person who tends toward the "terrible" end of the continuum may feel that the odds of him or her catching the flu are extremely low. In contrast, someone who falls closer to the "slightly worse than a cold" end of the continuum may feel the odds of him or her catching the flu are actually quite high.

The ultimate "mixing" of constructs "A" and "B" creates the construct of perceived threat for influenza acquisition (construct "D"). Perceived threat, then, essentially is defined as a compound of the two elementary constructs (severity and susceptibility). The HBM suggests that this combined construct of perceived threat directly influences the likelihood of engaging in the protective behavior. However, the HBM also suggests that perceived threat may be moderated (i.e., differentially affected) by a host of factors such as age, race, socioeconomic status, and knowledge pertaining to the disease in question. Construct "C" (**modifying factors**) is included in the model to account for these influences in perceived threat, as well as likely influences on the expected net gain.

The challenge to public health professionals is in the process of "taking apart" the reasoning that leads to perceptions creating low perceived threat. As might be expected, a low level of perceived threat is unlikely to advance people into further mental effort pertaining to influenza vaccination. Indeed, when perceived threat is low, the question of adopting a health-protective behavior may become a nonstarter and the entire process of contemplating the expected net gain of the behavior may be lost entirely. Thus, the health belief model sets up an initial focus for the efforts of a health-promotion program: the program must find a way to inspire realistic perceptions of threat among the target population.

> *The challenge to public health professionals is in the process of "taking apart" the reasoning that leads to perceptions creating low perceived threat.*

Another example is educating young female college freshmen about their risks of sexual assault. When young women learn that alcohol use can affect their cognitive abilities where they are less likely to pick up on dangerous cues in their environment, this awareness (a modifying factor) may lead to greater perceived levels of threat. The increased threat would, however, be attributable to an increase in perceived susceptibility. Most young women already perceive being raped as severe, thus, severity is a constant and may not need messaging. Indeed, a recent study demonstrated that college women who were exposed to an alcohol abuse intervention that, along with sexual assault risk reduction messaging, demonstrated the concept of alcohol myopia, which is a cognitive effect of alcohol and posits that *alcohol reduces a person's risk perceptions*. Alcohol myopia explains how some women who drink may not pick up on peripheral environmental cues that are associated with an increased risk of being a victim of sexual assault. The authors found that women in the treatment group who reported higher incidence and severity of sexual assault at baseline experienced less incapacitated attempted or completed rapes, less incidence/severity of sexual assaults, and engaged in less heavy episodic drinking compared to women in the control condition at the 3-month follow-up (Gilmore, Lewis, & George, 2015).

Another form of public health intervention, which we briefly touched upon in the introduction to this chapter and that has been used widely to increase perceived threat, is called a **fear appeal**. Fear appeals are persuasive messages designed to scare people by describing the terrible things that will happen to them if they do not do what the message recommends (Witte, 1992). Thus, a fear appeal campaign designed for the human papillomavirus (HPV) vaccination, for example, could create ads that utilize actors who resemble young people who are not getting the HPV vaccine while highlighting the debilitating effects of combating cervical, throat or anal cancer in the future (see **FIGURE 5-3**).

As discussed previously, modifying factors exert influence on perceived threat; thus, according to the HBM, a fear appeal campaign would have to be targeted to different subgroups to account for these modifying factors. Thus, for an HPV vaccination fear appeal campaign to be effective, different ads should be developed that

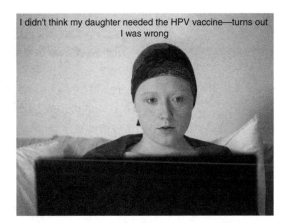

I didn't think my daughter needed the HPV vaccine—turns out I was wrong

FIGURE 5-3 Perceived fear appeal for HPV vaccine campaign
© KatarzynaBialasiewicz/iStock /Getty Images

would appeal to subgroups that differ by gender, age, and religious or political affiliation.

Of note, measuring the construct of perceived susceptibility requires the use of conditional statements. A conditional statement simply means that a behavior is included. For example, consider the question that follows: "In your lifetime, how likely are you to be infected with Human Papillomavirus (HPV)?" Suppose that people are asked to respond using a scale ranging from (1) "very unlikely" to (5) "very likely." A person who answers by selecting "very unlikely" could be doing so because they truly feels invulnerable to HPV, but alternately, that same person could be selecting "very unlikely" because they has recently been vaccinated against HPV. The solution to this problem is simply to include the behavior in the question stem, for example, "In the next year, if you were vaccinated against HPV, how likely are you to become infected with HPV?" The question would be better framed as follows: "Assuming you were vaccinated, how likely are you to be infected with HPV?" By asking the question using this structure, and then asking the question again but rephrasing it to include "assuming you were not vaccinated . . .," it may be possible to correctly determine perceived susceptibility.

Thus far, you have learned that perceived threat is a primary driving force of the decision to adopt a given health-protective behavior. The remaining primary force is the expected net gain of the behavior (construct "E"). Here, the term

FEAR APPEAL CAMPAIGN TO PREVENT DISTRACTED DRIVING

A recent online fear appeal campaign called, "It Can Wait" (itcanwait.com) was developed to get people to stop looking at their cell phone while driving. The campaign encourages people to make a pledge to not look at their phone, but the campaign also has several components including videos of real life stories that incorporate fear appeals. For example, in one video, young people, who regularly look at their phone while driving, are asked "why do you look at your phone"? They are then brought together with a young woman, who experienced a horrific car accident at the hands of a driver distracted by their cell phone. Her narrative describes the death of her parents while her person shows the severe, painful, and permanent injuries that she must live with. In another campaign video, a beautiful young woman tells her story of what her life was like before her car accident including actual photos that show her as beautiful, popular, hanging out with her friends, engaging in school activities, etc. and then she describes her life in the present. Her face is extremely disfugured and she describes other permanent and severe injuries she sustained. For example, she was blinded in one eye, her tear ducts are permanently damaged, and she has lost her sense of smell. Most disturbing to her is that she has no friends anymore—her friends gave up on her because of all of her problems. Her car accident occurred when she was distracted by a text message. Although the campaign has not been evaluated yet, the messages are designed to increase young and old drivers' perceptions of guilt (i.e., looking at your cell phone while driving can cause serious consequences to *other*, innocent people) but also to increase drivers' perceived threat of looking at their cell phone while driving (i.e., by conveying the severity of causing or experiencing death and/or permanent and acute injury combined with the likelihood of these outcomes happening to them).

The term "net" is used just as it would be from an economic perspective: in economics, the net is what remains after resources to defray expenses have been allocated.

"net" is used just as it would be from an economic perspective: in economics, the net is what remains after resources to defray expenses have been allocated; it is what is leftover. From a behavioral viewpoint, expenses may be financial (e.g., the price of the vaccine), but they may also be related to time investment and inconvenience associated with vaccination. Think about, for example, a parent who believes that his or her child's HPV shot will mean taking time out of a busy work day to wait in an endless line while filling out forms that may be required. In essence, the "costs" of time loss and hassles become barriers to a favorable net gain. A common cost that may be perceived by many people is the mistaken belief that being vaccinated for HPV will cause serious illness and even death. The vaccine is composed of proteins (surface antigens) found on the HPV virus; these proteins may rarely trigger an immune response that includes fever and malaise, but the body is not infected by the HPV virus. Unfortunately, attempts to convince people of this reality may be difficult at best, and the result is that a significant cost is charged against any perception of benefit a person may hold. Again, the model stipulates that modifying factors (construct "C") may be critical in determining the perceptions that people hold relative to the expected net gain.

Because people are unlikely to act (adopt a health-protective behavior) in the absence of a clear expected net gain, understanding this construct is essential to the design of health-promotion programs. A positive net gain can be achieved by:

- Increasing the perceived value of benefits that can be expected from the action
- Decreasing the perceived barriers (i.e., expenses) to performing the action
- Both of the above

Here you can clearly see a second practical implication of the health belief model. The model

tells you that effective health promotion must make the benefits of the suggested health behavior highly salient to people in the target population, while at the same time the model suggests that programs should also include provisions to minimize barriers (costs) that may detract from any inherent appeal of the benefits. Thus, needs assessments that precede the development of HPV vaccine programs should identify barriers and benefits that people in a defined population may perceive about the vaccine and vaccination.

In fact, a recent study applied the HBM to understand the factors impacting Pap screenings for cervical cancer among sub-Saharan African immigrant women in the United States (Adegboyega & Hatcher, 2016). Disparities in cancer diagnosis and survival among racial and income groups are well documented, and programs to reduce disparities have become a national priority (Bradley, Given, & Roberts, 2004). Twenty-two immigrant women participated in qualitative focus groups in Lexington, Kentucky to learn the motivators and barriers to getting Pap screenings. Perceived barriers to getting screened included: lack of knowledge about screenings for cervical cancer; costliness of the procedure; cultural norms and religious beliefs regarding privacy and embarrassment for sexual health services; fear of experiencing discomfort during the procedure; and issues communicating with providers. The perceived motivators of getting screened were: the known benefits of getting Pap screenings considering this procedure can detect cervical cancer; provider recommendations; family support; enlightenment about screening from members of the African community; and, for those who had insurance, coverage for Pap screenings served as a source of encouragement to obtain this procedure. These known benefits and barriers can help healthcare providers address these challenges and improve cervical cancer screenings among sub-Saharan African immigrant women (Adegboyega & Hatcher, 2016).

The model tells you that effective health promotion must make the benefits of the suggested health behavior highly salient to people in the target population

At this juncture, the construct of modifying factors deserves a bit more explanation. Modifying factors are typically demographics such as age, race, gender, and socioeconomic status. Whether a given theoretical construct (e.g., perceived threat of a disease) has a strong influence on health behavior is often a function of one or more modifying factors; for example, the perceived threat of HPV infection and the resulting cancer may be a function of a modifying factor such as race, gender, income and education level of the parents.

One final look at Figure 5-2 is warranted. Looking at construct "F" (**likelihood of action**) you will see that both perceived threat and net gain act upon this endpoint. This endpoint is essentially a measure of behavioral intent, meaning that it assesses the degree of motivation a person may have to engage in a given health-protective behavior. Although the model represents the action of constructs "D" (perceived threat) and "E" (expected net gain) as being independent, it may be that the actual relationship is far more complex. Consider, for example, the relationship depicted by **FIGURE 5-4**.

As shown, when perceived threat reaches a certain level it may alter the mental math used to calculate expected net gain. The level of perceived threat alters the balance between the perceived gains of reducing the threat, assuming the costs associated with obtaining a vaccine do not outweigh the anticipated benefits. Conversely, the level of gain obtained may not be so highly valued when the perceived threat is low or only modest. Regardless of the exact relationship that may exist among the constructs shown in Figure 5-4, the implications for planning health-promotion

programs are clear: create a realistic sense of perceived threat, reduce costs, and foster perceptions of positive net gain. Figure 5-4 also suggests that a simple one-to-one correspondence between net gain and the endpoint is questionable. Indeed, most health behaviors are either "do" or "do not." Thus, the question is, "How much net gain is needed to find the tipping point, from 'do not' to 'do'?" These concepts are known to be associated with vaccination behavior on a group basis, but, of course, may not explain any specific person's behavior.

Finally, you may have noticed that up until now no mention has been made of construct "G" in Figure 5-2. This construct is known as **cues to action**. The model posits that these cues may be events (e.g., watching a news broadcast that highlights a celebrity's throat cancer diagnosis and how it stemmed from HPV infection), or *reminders* provided by a credible source (e.g., email or notice from physician's office or the health department reminding people that their child is due for the HPV vaccine). In essence, events and reminders can each be viewed as forms of intervention, and so cues to action may be planned as part of a health-promotion program. For example, the common event of a health fair may serve to remind people that they have indeed resolved to quit smoking; thus, these people may be motivated to sign up for a cessation program during the event.

One final note on the HBM is that the HBM was altered in 1988 when self-efficacy was added to the model (Rosenstock, Strecher, & Becker, 1988). Self-efficacy is confidence in one's ability to take action or to change a health-related behavior. Self-efficacy as a construct was introduced by

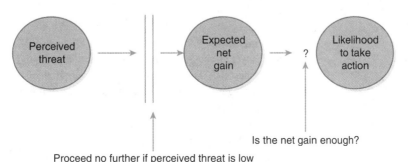

FIGURE 5-4 Alternative relationship between key constructs of the health belief model

Bandura (1977) and will be explored in depth in Chapter 9. However, the main point is that people generally will not try a new behavior unless they are confident that they can perform the behavior. If someone perceives that a health behavior will be useful (perceived benefit), but does not perceive that they are capable (perceived barrier), then they will most likely not try it. Thus, low self-efficacy results in less likelihood of engaging in the behavior.

Protection Motivation Theory

Protection Motivation Theory (PMT) is similar to the HBM in that at its core is the concept of perceived threat along with an analysis of rewards and costs for engaging in either maladaptive or adaptive responses. The PMT was originally conceptualized to explain the specific processes that explain the effects fear appeals have upon attitude change. As mentioned previously, fear appeals are often used in public health campaigns to affect perceived threat of a disease (see **FIGURE 5-5**) or condition and to show the negative consequences of not adopting a health-protective behavior (e.g., not getting vaccinated) or of engaging in a health-risk behavior (e.g., doing drugs). In simple terms, the premise of how they work is that when faced with fear-arousing stimuli, individuals can either adopt positive, adaptive responses to avoid the threat or, instead, choose maladaptive, negative behaviors that ignore the risk. This choice is made following several cognitive mediating processes. The PMT is often used in designing messages for health awareness campaigns that utilize fear as a primary motivator for positive behavior, such

> *In simple terms, the premise of how they work is that when faced with fear-arousing stimuli, individuals can either adopt positive, adaptive responses to avoid the threat or, instead, choose maladaptive, negative behaviors that ignore the risk.*

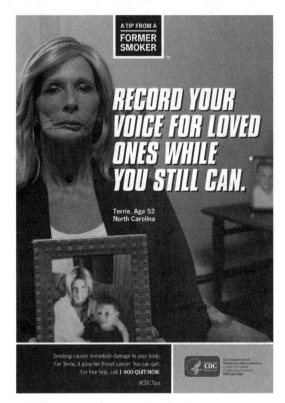

FIGURE 5-5 An antismoking fear appeal advertisement
Courtesy of the Centers for Disease Control and Prevention (CDC), 2013 Tips From Former Smokers® campaign.

as antismoking advertisements (Pechmann, Zhao, Goldberg, & Reibling, 2003), exercise and cardiovascular health concerns (Tulloch et al., 2009), and communications about HIV risk behavior (Van der Velde & Van der Pligt, 1991). In this next section, we provide the history and an overview of the PMT.

History of the PMT

Dr. R. W. Rogers (1975) originally proposed the PMT in his 1975 paper to explain the cognitive effects of fear appeals. Much prior thinking had conceptualized fear to be an emotional trigger for trial-and-error type responses in an attempt to escape the experience of fear (Hovland, Janis, & Kelley, 1953). Rogers, however, understood fear to be an initiator of a cognitive mediating process (fear leads to cognitive assessments that lead to

People differ in sensitivity and vulnerability to certain types of events, as well as in their interactions and reactions.

behavior change), taking into account both a threat appraisal and a response appraisal and resulting in either an adaptive or maladaptive behavioral change (Rippetoe & Rogers, 1987). Much of Rogers's work was founded upon principles established by Richard Lazarus and Howard Leventhal, both of whom related fear and coping responses to cognitive processes (Lazarus & Launier, 1978; Leventhal, 1970). Lazarus recognized that fear triggers an automatic appraisal: a cognitive assessment of the situation and how it can affect the individual in the long term (Lazarus & Launier, 1978) and that people differ in sensitivity and vulnerability to certain types of events, as well as in their interactions and reactions. Leventhal further divided the fear reaction into two processes: danger control (from environmental cues) and fear control (an internal process) (Leventhal, 1970). It is from the environmental factor danger control of Leventhal's parallel response model that Rogers derived his first three factors of the PMT: threat severity, threat vulnerability, and response efficacy. Rogers later extended the theory to include self-efficacy and to be a more generalized persuasive communication theory that emphasizes the cognitive processes, which motivate either adaptive or maladaptive behavioral responses (Rogers, 1983).

Components of the PMT

The PMT is depicted in **FIGURE 5-6** and illustrates how two appraisal processes, the threat appraisal and the coping appraisal, are in close proximity to protection motivation. Protection motivation is defined as a mediating variable whose function is to direct protective health behavior. Each of these two processes is further divided into several components. The threat appraisal process involves an assessment of the seriousness of the health threat by estimating the probability of a negative outcome (i.e., vulnerability) and the severity of the negative outcome if no remedial action is taken. Using the health threat example of type 2 diabetes, let's imagine that a doctor informs a patient that their blood glucose level is very high and they must lose weight to bring their glucose levels down or they might develop type 2 diabetes. The doctor further explains the consequences of type 2 diabetes. This person would first assess how severe these consequences would be for them and then try and estimate the likelihood of actually becoming a type 2 diabetic.

Severity and vulnerability constructs are similar to the perceived severity and perceived susceptibility constructs from the HBM; however, threat appraisal from the PMT posits that another aspect—rewards, both intrinsic and extrinsic—plays a role in the threat appraisal process. Rewards are positive consequences for a maladaptive behavioral response, whether the response is engaging in a health-risk behavior or not adopting a protective behavior. Staying with the type 2

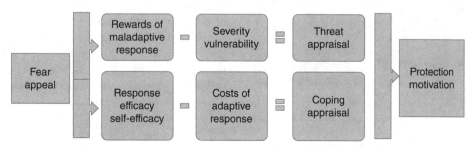

FIGURE 5-6 Protection motivation theory

Reproduced from Rogers, R.W. (1983). Cognitive and physiological processes in attitude change: A revised theory of protection motivation. In J. T. Cacioppo (Ed.), *Social psychophysiology: A sourcebook* (pp. 153–176). New York, NY: Guilford Press. With permission.

diabetes example, a person may be experiencing some rewards for not eating healthily and not exercising, such as the pleasure derived from eating high-fat foods and the extra time saved by avoiding exercising to do other things (see **FIGURE 5-7**).

Thus, according to the PMT, the entire threat appraisal process suggests that a maladaptive response (e.g., eating unhealthily) is likely when considering the rewards (tastes great), but that the severity and vulnerability of the negative outcomes reduce the attractiveness of the rewards so that an adaptive response is likely to occur.

As shown in Figure 5-6, the second cognitive process, coping appraisal, includes the response efficacy of the recommended behavior, which is an evaluation of how effective the behavior will be in protecting the individual from harm. In other words, the patient believing, "If I exercise strenuously every day, I will lose weight and I won't get type 2 diabetes." Coping appraisal also involves perceived self-efficacy, which is the individual's evaluation of their capacity to perform the recommended behavior ("I am confident / not confident that I can

exercise daily"). However, the coping appraisal process factors in the costs of the adaptive response. Costs incurred in this context would involve physical, social, or psychological consequences for engaging in the adaptive response. Thus, coping with a health threat involves the perception that engaging in the protective behavior will lead to averting the threat, the assumption that the individual can confidently engage in the behavior to avert the threat, and the consideration that the costs are not too great for engaging in the behavior.

In a recent study, researchers used the PMT to understand willingness to use pain medication to treat pain using a cross-sectional survey with 123 randomly selected U.S. adults (Hong, Cagle, Van Dussen, Carrion, & Culler, 2016). They examined the threat appraisals and coping appraisals as cognitive factors that may impact individuals' willingness to use pain medication. Findings indicate that threat appraisals, coping appraisals, and attitudes were common factors that affected participants' willingness to use pain medication. Thus, participants could be concerned about the threats of using pain medication, such as worsening pain (threat appraisal), but may be curious about how well pain medication works (coping appraisal). Specific factors affecting willingness to take pain medication included income, awareness of hospice care, threat appraisal, and attitudes. Overall, results indicate that the PMT can be used to understand the underlying mechanisms behind health decision-making, such as individuals' willingness to use pain medication (Hong et al., 2016).

In sum, the PMT suggests that when faced with a fear appeal that makes someone aware of a health threat, such as the fact that smoking will lead to lung cancer, an individual takes into account these four cognitive considerations in sequence: evaluating the chances of harm to themselves (e.g., probability of lung cancer if one continues to smoke), the severity of the outcome (mortality or morbidity of disease), the efficacy of response (such as the effect smoking cessation would have on cancer prevention), and the self-efficacy of the individual (the subject's evaluation of their own ability to quit smoking).

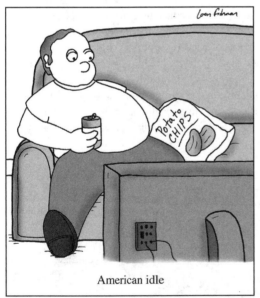

American idle

CartoonStock.com

FIGURE 5-7 "Rewards" of unhealthy eating and not exercising

Courtesy of Fishman, Loren/Cartoonstock

The rewards of continuing to smoke (e.g., nicotine fix, weight control, psychological feeling of euphoria) can be reduced given the severity and vulnerability of getting lung cancer, while the costs of quitting (e.g., withdrawal, weight gain, depression) are considered given the effectiveness of quitting in averting lung cancer and the ability to successfully quit to arrive at an overall state of protection motivation. In addition to these two main cognitive processes, which affect behavior, other important contributors are an individual's past experiences (learning theory), environmental factors, and personality variables.

Protection Motivation Theory is especially useful when applied to health communication, though it has also been applied to injury prevention, political issues, environmental concerns, and many other issues (Rogers & Prentice-Dunn, 1997). Many observational studies have utilized the PMT in order to discover which part of message design has the greatest impact on message efficacy (often measured by rate of desired outcome behavior). Generally, it is observed that all four parts of the PMT—severity, vulnerability, response efficacy, and self-efficacy—should be addressed to maximize the desired effect (Boer & Seydel, 1996). That is, for a health awareness message to be a successful fear appeal, it should communicate effectively that the disease or negative outcome is sufficiently severe (perhaps graphically) and that the observer has a significant vulnerability to the negative result. This activates the threat appraisal process in the subject. The message should also, however, indicate an appropriate behavioral response and stress the efficacy of this response in preventing the disease, as well as highlight the individual's personal adaptive capability to perform the desired response. The strength of these four factors is positively correlated with the magnitude and frequency of an adaptive response in the target audience. This has been tested in case-control studies by varying one or more of the factors and observing the given response (Floyd, Prentice-Dunn, & Rogers, 2000). These factors are also observed to function in an additive manner, though the possibility of synergy and further interaction certainly cannot be ruled out.

The Extended Parallel Process Model

The extended parallel process model (EPPM) is the newest theory among the group of theories covered in this chapter. By the EPPM developer's own description (Witte, 1992), it is not so much a new theory as it is an integration of several previous theories, most notably the PMT and Leventhal's parallel process model (Leventhal, 1970, 1971). In addition, many of its constructs, such as perceived efficacy (from Social Cognitive Theory [SCT]) and perceived threat (from the HBM) will be familiar to one who is versed in behavioral theory. From the perspective of the EPPM, each of these theoretical perspectives contributes a critical component to our understanding of effective risk messages, but only the EPPM brings these components together into an integrated model (Witte, Meyer, & Martell, 2001).

The key theoretical question that the EPPM attempts to answer is the following: "How do individuals respond to fear-arousing communications?" Similar to the PMT, the EPPM is, in many ways, a communication theory more than a behavioral theory; that is, the EPPM attempts to explain how and why individuals respond to and act (or do not act) in response to fear-arousing messages. This can be contrasted with a behavioral theory such as the HBM, which is focused more on helping us understand which factors predict engagement in particular health behaviors.

The first test of the EPPM was in the HIV prevention context (Witte, 1994); however, the EPPM has never been conceptualized as an

> *For a health awareness message to be a successful fear appeal, it should communicate effectively that the disease or negative outcome is sufficiently severe (perhaps graphically) and that the observer has a significant vulnerability to the negative result.*

CASE STUDY OF OPIOID CAMPAIGN MESSAGE USING THE PMT

Let's take a look at a recent campaign message (**FIGURE 5-8**) and figure out if it uses the four PMT components. Recently, the American Academy for Orthopaedic Surgeons (AAOS) launched a campaign to address the national opioid addiction crisis (American Academy for Orthopaedic Surgeons, 2017). The multimedia campaign uses a fear appeal with the tagline, "Painkillers are easy to get into. Hard to escape" and urges doctors and patients to exercise caution in prescribing and taking painkillers. This campaign highlights the severity and susceptibility to the opioid epidemic, activating the threat appraisal process. Its sub-message also addresses the response efficacy by addressing how minimizing opioid use will contribute to opioid addiction prevention. However, it does not include messaging on self-efficacy by offering doctors an alternative to opioid pill prescription and patients an alternative to taking painkillers (American Academy for Orthopaedic Surgeons, 2017).

In fact, the PMT has been tested widely in observational studies as a means to elucidate the factors governing its efficacy. Several studies have shown that the coping variables show slightly stronger relationships with the adaptive behaviors than the threat variables, but that all variables are still positively correlated with adaptive behavior and that specific health issues differ in the message components that prove most vital. In tests of antismoking message efficacy, it was observed that threat variables showed a lower association with smoking cessation than coping variables, with the biggest detriment to adaptive behavior being low perceived vulnerability (especially among youth). Healthy diet, exercise, cardiovascular disease risk, and medical-treatment adherence showed especially strong association between coping variables and positive behavioral change, with self-efficacy being the most crucial predictor of healthy outcomes (Grindley, Zizzi, & Nasypany, 2008). In studies of HIV-risk communication, the efficacy of high magnitudes of the threat appeal was quite strong, but the most important component was again self-efficacy, indicating that describing the severity and vulnerability of individuals at risk of HIV is important (and quite common in such interventions), but also that emphasizing the capability of individuals to protect themselves from infection is the most crucial factor (Lwin, Stanaland, & Chan, 2010).

These studies show that the PMT is an effective predictor and model of adaptive responses to fear-based messages. These types of communications have at their heart an attempt to elicit a desired, beneficial health action in the target audience. Social marketing of this type is especially effective because of its unique ability to change behaviors on a widespread, population-based scale. The use of the PMT can improve the efficacy of such health awareness campaigns, and thus should always be taken into account when designing messages. For maximum effectiveness, health awareness messages should effectively communicate the vulnerability of the target population to negative health outcomes, the severity of these outcomes, recommendations of prophylactic (preventive or protective) responses, and guarantees of their response efficacy, as well as encouragement that the target audience has the means, will, and motivation to perform the desired response.

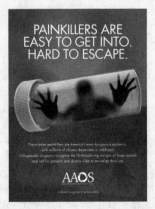

FIGURE 5-8 Opioid campaign image AAOS campaign against opioid addiction

© American Academy of Orthopaedic Surgeons

HIV-specific theory. Rather, the theory was originally conceptualized as one that explains reactions to fear-arousing communications in general (Witte, 1992). Since that initial application, the EPPM has been applied to smoking cessation (Wong & Cappella, 2009), breast cancer prevention (Hubbell, 2006), skin cancer prevention (Stephenson & Witte, 1998), stroke awareness (Davis, Martinelli, Braxton, Kutrovac, & Crocco, 2009), asthma prevention/management (Goei et al., 2010), kidney disease testing (Roberto & Goodall, 2009), and public health workers' response willingness in an influenza pandemic (Barnett et al., 2009), among other areas (McMahan, Witte, & Meyer, 1998). It has additionally been tested in several HIV prevention studies (Roberto et al., 2007; Smith, Ferrara, & Witte, 2007; Witte, Cameron, Lapinski, & Nzyuko, 1998; Witte & Morrison, 1995), as well as used as a theoretical basis for a meta-analysis of fear appeals across a number of health behaviors (Witte & Allen, 2000).

To understand the constructs and tenets of the EPPM, it is in many ways easiest to begin at the far right of the EPPM figure (see **FIGURE 5-9**). Provided that a fear appeal elicits some level of perceived threat on the part of the individual, the EPPM posits that individuals will either accept a fear appeal message and engage in a danger-control process, or reject a message and engage in a fear-control process (Witte, 1992; Witte et al., 2001). The **danger-control process** is what the designers of the health message are hoping to achieve, as this means the individual will engage in strategies to avert the threat (i.e., protection motivation). For example, if a fear appeal message makes the case that exposure to radon in one's home can lead to lung cancer, a danger-control response would be for the homeowner to order a radon test, and if high levels of radon are found, to have a mitigation system installed. Thus, danger-control responses in the EPPM can be measured in terms of changes in beliefs, attitudes, intentions, and behavior that are consistent with the position being advocated in the message.

In contrast to the danger-control process, the **fear-control process** is characterized by an individual's belief that they are either unable to engage in the recommended response or they believe the response to be ineffective.

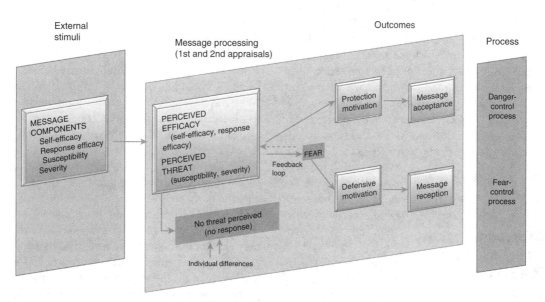

FIGURE 5-9 Expanded parallel process model

Reproduced from Witte, K. (1992). Putting the fear back into fear appeals: The extended parallel process model. *Communication Monographs, 59*(4), 329–349. © National Communication Association, reprinted by permission of Taylor & Francis Ltd., (http://www.tandf.co.uk/journals) on behalf of The National Communication Association.

Danger-control responses in the EPPM can be measured in terms of changes in beliefs, attitudes, intentions, and behavior that are consistent with the position being advocated in the message.

The fear-control process is what designers of the health message need to be careful of, as individuals apply fear control by engaging in coping responses that reduce fear but also prevent a danger-control process from occurring (i.e., defensive motivation). In other words, the individual is controlling the fear rather than controlling the threat. Again using the radon example, an individual may not be able to afford the cost of radon testing or mitigation or may not believe that radon mitigation achieves its purported goal. Fear-control responses can be measured by levels of cognitive and affective response to the message, such as denial, defensive avoidance, and reactance. It should be noted that the EPPM explains both fear appeal successes and failures, rather than only focusing on factors and processes related to successful fear appeals, as much previous work had done (Witte, 1998). The additional constructs described as follows attempt to explain which message factors increase or decrease the chances of danger or fear-control processes taking place, and thus whether a fear appeal is ultimately a failure or a success.

As can be seen in Figure 5-9, the positive outcomes of protection motivation, message acceptance, and danger control are predicted by certain types of message processing, while the negative outcomes of defensive motivation, message rejection, and fear control are also predicted by particular types of message processing. The ways in which messages are processed is influenced by the content of the message, or its **message components**, as well as any key individual differences. The message components, at the far left of the figure, are the theoretical building blocks of messages developed from an EPPM perspective. As mentioned earlier in this chapter, these components were originally derived from other theories, and they reside in two sets of constructs. The first construct, perceived threat, is made up of both perceived susceptibility and perceived severity. This construct is exactly the same as that from the HBM, and thus is concerned with an individual's perception both of whether they are at risk, as well as how serious or severe they perceive that potential negative outcome to be. Using the radon example, this would be conceptualized as the perceived risk of getting lung cancer as a result of radon exposure in one's home (susceptibility), as well as how severe one believes getting lung cancer would be (severity). The second group of constructs is referred to as perceived efficacy, which is made up of both self-efficacy and response efficacy. These concepts are derived from SCT. Self-efficacy is defined as an individual's perceived ability to perform a behavior necessary to achieve a particular outcome, while response efficacy is an individual's belief that engaging in the protective behavior will avert the threat that has been identified. Thus, self-efficacy would involve an individual's belief that he or she could schedule and pay for a radon test, while response efficacy would focus on the extent to which an individual believes conducting radon mitigation would ultimately reduce the risk of lung cancer from this source.

If we now work from the left to right of the EPPM figure, we can see that these theoretical constructs make up the message components in the theory. Thus, when designing messages using the EPPM, a message designer should base their messages on the concepts of perceived threat and efficacy. The extent to which these variables are used successfully in message design is theorized to impact how individuals process those messages.

A critical goal of EPPM-based intervention is to design messages that increase both perceived threat and perceived efficacy of the

Fear-control responses can be measured by levels of cognitive and affective response to the message, such as denial, defensive avoidance, and reactance.

issue/behavior at hand. It should also be noted that individual differences come into play in the message processing realm as well, as such variables may impact how an individual processes messages. For example, an individual who has high anxiety as a personality trait may require a slightly lower threat message in order to feel at risk, while someone with a sensation-seeking personality may require a higher-than-average threat message in order to feel at risk. Thus, when designing messages for particular audience segments, individual differences should be taken into account where possible and as appropriate.

As can be seen in Figure 5-9, there are several possible responses that an individual can have to a message. If in response to the message the individual does not perceive a threat at all (no threat), then he or she is unlikely to have a tangible response to the message. For example, if an individual lives in a home or neighborhood where radon is not present, then he or she may have no response to a radon message. On the other hand, if an individual perceives a threat, but either a clear response is not depicted in the message or the person has low efficacy to engage in the recommended response (high perceived threat, low efficacy), then the person is likely to engage in a fear-control process and the message will likely fail. This particular individual may engage in **defensive avoidance**, where he or she blocks further thoughts or feelings about the health threat (Witte, 1998), and may also avoid exposure to any further information about the topic. A person in this circumstance will thus conclude that radon is a threat, but that they simply cannot do anything about it (e.g., "I can't afford radon mitigation, so why would I even bother to have my house tested and know if it's there").

Finally, if a person feels increased threat in response to the message, and also high efficacy to engage in the recommended response (high threat, high efficacy), then the EPPM suggests that this individual is likely to engage in a danger-control process where the danger (e.g., radon) is controlled. This person would feel fear by the health threat posed by radon, but would also feel efficacious in their ability to avert the threat, so the person would engage in the recommended response—in this case, ordering a radon test and mitigating the radon if it existed at unacceptably high levels. The EPPM thus has a very clear and easy-to-follow message for public health practitioners: for a fear appeal to be successful, it must increase not only a sense of perceived threat, but also an individual's sense of efficacy to successfully engage in the recommended response. This is a very important lesson for those interested in using fear-arousing communications to change health behavior, as a large meta-analysis of fear

APPLYING THE EPPM TO THE TRUTH CAMPAIGN

The truth campaign exposes the lies and manipulations of the tobacco companies. A recent study analyzed television ads in the truth campaign using theoretical components of the EPPM (LaVoie & Quick, 2013). Researchers conducted a content analysis of truth campaign videos, analyzing visual and audio content to learn if messaging used the four components of the EPPM: severity, susceptibility, self-efficacy, and response efficacy. Out of 86 television video ads analyzed, the majority of ads used severity ($n = 72$) whereas a moderate amount of ads used susceptibility ($n = 31$) messages. None of the ads analyzed used self-efficacy or response efficacy messaging. Similarly, the audio analysis revealed that the majority of audio in the ads used severity ($n = 51$), a moderate amount used susceptibility ($= 17$), and none used self-efficacy or response efficacy. McNemar tests revealed that severity is used significantly more than susceptibility, self-efficacy, or response efficacy in the messaging and in the audio components of the ads ($p < 0.001$). These results indicate that the truth campaign relies heavily on fear appeals without communicating the recommended response. According to the EPPM, the truth campaign may not be successful using solely severity and susceptibility messaging without any self-efficacy or response efficacy message (LaVoie & Quick, 2013).

For a fear appeal to be successful, it must increase not only a sense of perceived threat, but also an individual's sense of efficacy to successfully engage in the recommended response.

appeals suggests that such messages do, in many cases, increase defensive responding such as reactance and denial (Witte & Allen, 2000). It is likely that many of those fear appeal messages that increased perceived threat did not have convincing efficacy messages built into them. This same meta-analysis found that fear appeal messages that increase both perceived threat and perceived efficacy are more successful in stimulating behavioral change than messages that do not increase perceived levels on both constructs.

▶ An Applied Example

Smoking serves as an excellent example of a maladaptive behavior and for applying the EPPM to develop a campaign to prevent teens from smoking. Although there are ecological factors that help to prevent tobacco use (e.g., no-smoking policies), many ecological factors also promote smoking (e.g., media, advertising efforts, low taxes, accessibility, availability), especially in certain geographic areas of the United States. Thus, one challenge in attempting to prevent teens from ever starting is creating an effective fear appeal that may counter some of these influences. As highlighted earlier, the truth campaign albeit provocative, did not include messaging for response efficacy or self-efficacy to not smoke. The EPPM can be used as a guide to develop an effective approach for the prevention of tobacco use in this population and perhaps diminish the glamorization and appeal (i.e., rewards) of smoking created by the media and tobacco advertising; however, messaging focused on self-efficacy and response efficacy must be included.

According to the EPPM, an effective fear appeal will include four aspects:

- Threat of harm if the message's recommendations are not followed.
- Threat that is personalized to the target of the message.
- Response efficacy, in which the recommendation given will both eliminate the threat and demonstrate that this elimination is positive.
- Personal efficacy or self-efficacy; the belief that an individual can perform the recommended action.

Regarding the first three aspects, there has been research that shows it is possible to manipulate perceived threat and response efficacy in many fear appeals (Witte 1992, 1994); however, many fear appeals fail to adequately address self-efficacy in their messages. For this practice example, self-efficacy can potentially be increased through vicarious experiences that involve the person observing someone perceived to be similar to them successfully performing a behavior and also being rewarded as a result.

Another avenue to enhance self-efficacy is through social persuasion. In fear appeals, the characters are often punished, not rewarded; however, having others tell us we can do something or that we have control over something can increase our self-efficacy. Keeping this in mind, another challenge will be to adequately address self-efficacy in the messages, in addition to perceived threat and response efficacy. Addressing all four aspects of an effective fear appeal will be a challenge, especially given that the fear appeals campaign will consist of 30-seconds and 60-seconds public service announcements (PSAs). Thus, building self-efficacy may indeed require personal-level intervention approaches.

First, to enhance perceived severity, a fear appeal must convey that the consequences of smoking will be severe and truly scary. One possible idea is to show graphic, enhanced images of teens with mouth tumors, yellowing teeth, a cigarette in their mouth, and virtually no lung capacity—similar to zombies—slowly stumbling through the halls of their school while the other students run from them in fear. The zombie smokers actually bypass the students and head for the graveyard out in back of the school, where their coffins and open graves are waiting for them. Another potential idea is to start with a young group of teens and fast-forward to their 10-year reunion, where some of their friends who smoked in high school are showing up with oxygen tanks because of their emphysema, some have had heart attacks, and others are coughing and hacking away while trying to dance. For each table at the reunion, one chair remains empty, signifying that one out of three people who smoke will die from it. Of course, creativity here is critical and the possibilities for enhancing perceived severity are almost infinite. The main point is to convey the severe consequences of smoking in a way that resonates to the teen audience.

Second, it is important to consider how to personalize the threat of smoking. Teens in general perceive themselves to be somewhat invulnerable to many health threats. One way to overcome this would be to use teen actors from diverse ethnic, racial, geographic, and socioeconomic backgrounds (see **FIGURE 5-10**) for the television ads. By using members of the target audience in the PSAs, the threat can be personalized and teens can see other, similar teens experiencing the negative consequences of smoking.

The third aspect involves efficacy. Because high self-efficacy can have an effect on response efficacy, and the PSAs are of short duration, it may be easier to focus on self-efficacy with the idea that if self-efficacy to NOT smoke can be enhanced,

then teens will think that not smoking will result in avoiding negative consequences, which is valued positively. The idea is to convey to teens that they can avoid smoking and that they have control over whether they decide to smoke. One idea to enhance self-efficacy in an antismoking fear appeal campaign was through the addition of directed tag lines (e.g., "You can control your future," "You can make the right decision") placed at the end of several PSAs (Hively, 2006). This is a simple way to enhance self-efficacy and, playing on the idea of the zombie smokers, a possible tag line could be, "Don't be a zombie." Another potential idea is to play with the concept of peer pressure and perhaps do a role reversal of the typical scenario using social persuasion. A PSA could depict teens putting pressure on other teens to not smoke and telling them "good job" for not smoking, while taunting the teens who do smoke.

Finally, it is important to note that although we described potential ideas for a fear appeals campaign using the EPPM as a framework, for any fear appeals campaign to be truly effective, messages must be developed based on extensive formative research with the target audience and on previous research that shows what works and what doesn't. Nevertheless, fear appeals have a certain "appeal" to many public health researchers and practitioners who are in touch with their creative side and are interested in overcoming maladaptive health behaviors and countering many of the environmental and personal determinants of those behaviors.

▶ **Take Home Messages**

- ▪ Fear is a powerful reaction that has both emotional and cognitive components and can be utilized to motivate health behavior.
- ▪ Fear is an emotional reaction to a threatening stimulus and results in the fight-or-flight response.
- ▪ Evoking fear in messages has been used to increase perceived threat of a health condition or disease and to change maladaptive or adaptive behaviors.

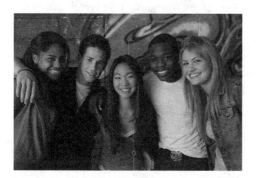

FIGURE 5-10 Diverse teens for antismoking fear appeal
© Jupiterimages/Comstock/Thinkstock.

- The Health Belief Model describes the fear process as a value–expectancy combination of two driving forces: the perceived threat of the fear appeal and the expected net gain of a protective health behavior.

- The Protection Motivation Theory describes the response to a fear appeal as based upon four sequential cognitive evaluations: personal susceptibility to the threat, potential severity of the threat, expected efficacy of any prophylactic response, and personal evaluation of self-efficacy to enact the desired response.

- The Extended Parallel Process Model combines the previous theories and addresses the way people respond to fear appeals, by either a danger-control process (addressing the threat and enacting beneficial behaviors to reduce the danger), or by a fear-control process (denying the threat or ignoring the danger in order to reduce the emotion of fear).

- The job of the health professional or public health communicator is to design messages of maximum efficacy, and the proper manipulation of fear appeals is key to this design.

- Effective messages should emphasize accurate threat, vulnerability, and severity, as well as provide suitable solutions and encourage self-efficacy in enacting these solutions.

- Understanding the proper audience is critical in appropriate message generation, as different emphasis must be given to different message components depending on both audience characteristics and the intended behavioral adaptation.

▶ References

Adegboyega, A., & Hatcher, J. (2016). Factors influencing Pap screening use among African immigrant women. *Journal of Transcultural Nursing, 28*(5), 479–487. http://doi.org/10.1177/1043659616661612

American Academy for Orthopaedic Surgeons. (2017). New AAOS public service campaigns tackle opioid misuse, childhood obesity. Retrieved October 5, 2017, from http://newsroom.aaos.org/media-resources/news/opioid-abuse-childhood-obesity.htm

Bandura, A. (1977), *Social Learning Theory.* Englewood Cliffs, NJ: Prentice-Hall.

Barnett, D. J., Balicer, R. D., Thompson, C. B., Storey, J. D., Omer, S. B., Semon, N. L., ... Links, J. M. (2009). Assessment of local public health workers' willingness to respond to pandemic influenza through application of the extended parallel process model. *Plos One, 4*(7), e6365.

Boer, H., & Seydel, E. R. (1996). Protection motivation theory. In M. Conner & P. Norman (Eds.), *Predicting health behaviour.* Buckingham, England: Open University Press.

Bradley, C. J., Given, C. W., & Roberts, C. (2004). Health care disparities and cervical cancer. *American Journal of Public Health, 94*(12), 2098–2103.

Davis, S. M., Martinelli, D., Braxton, B., Kutrovac, K., & Crocco, T. (2009). The impact of the extended parallel process model on stroke awareness: Pilot results from a novel study. *Stroke: A Journal of Cerebral Circulation, 40*(12), 3857–3863.

Floyd, D. L., Prentice-Dunn, S., & Rogers, R. W. (2000). A meta-analysis of research on protection motivation theory. *Journal of Applied Psychology, 30*(2), 407–429.

Gilmore, A. K., Lewis, M. A., & George, W. H. (2015). A randomized controlled trial targeting alcohol use and sexual assault risk among college women at high risk for victimization. *Behaviour Research and Therapy, 74*, 38-49. doi:10.1016/j.brat.2015.08.007

Goei, R., Boyson, A. R., Lyon-Callo, S. K., Schott, C., Wasilevich, E., & Cannarile, S. (2010). An examination of EPPM predictions when threat is perceived externally: An asthma intervention with school workers. *Health Communication, 25*(4), 333–344.

Grindley, E. J., Zizzi, S. J., & Nasypany, A. M. (2008). Use of protection motivation theory, affect, and barriers to understand and predict adherence to outpatient rehabilitation. *Physical Therapy, 88*(12), 1529–1540.

Hively, M. H. (2006). *The effects of self-efficacy statements in anti-tobacco fear appeal PSAs.* Unpublished master's thesis, Washington State University.

Hong, S., Cagle, J. G., Van Dussen, D. J., Carrion, I. V., & Culler, K. L. (2016). Willingness to use pain medication to treat pain. *Pain Medicine, 17*, 74–84. http://doi.org/10.1111/pme.12854

Hovland, C. I., Janis I. L., & Kelley G. H. (1953). *Communication and persuasion.* New Haven, CT: Yale University Press.

Hubbell, A. P. (2006). Mexican American women in a rural area and barriers to their ability to enact protective behaviors against breast cancer. *Health Communication, 20*(1), 35–44.

Lang, P. J. (1984). Cognition in emotion: Concept and action. In C. E. Izard, J. Kagan, & R. B. Zajonc (Eds.), *Emotions, cognition, and behavior* (pp. 192–226). Cambridge, England: Cambridge University Press.

LaVoie, N. R., & Quick, B. L. (2013). What is the truth? An application of the extended parallel process model to televised Truth® Ads. *Health Communication, 28*(1), 53–62. http://doi.org/10.1080/10410236.2012.728467

Lazarus, R. S., & Launier R. (1978). Stress related transactions between person and environment. In L. A. Pervin & M. Lewis (Eds.), *Perspectives in interactional psychology* (pp. 287–327). New York, NY: Plenum Press.

Leventhal, H. (1970). Findings and theory in the study of fear communications. In L. Berkowitz (Ed.), *Advances in experimental social psychology* (Vol. 5, pp. 119–186). New York, NY: Academic Press.

Leventhal, H. (1971). Fear appeals and persuasion: The differentiation of a motivational construct. *American Journal of Public Health, 61*(6), 1208–1224.

Lwin, M. O., Stanaland, A. J., & Chan, D. (2010). Using protection motivation theory to predict condom usage and assess HIV health communication efficacy in Singapore. Health *Communication, 25*(1), 69–79.

McMahan, S., Witte, K., & Meyer, J. A. (1998). The perception of risk messages regarding electromagnetic fields: Extending the extended parallel process model to an unknown risk. *Health Communication, 10*(3), 247.

Pechmann, C., Zhao, G., Goldberg, M. E., & Reibling, E. T. (2003) What to convey in adolescents: The use of protection motivation theory to identify effective message themes. *Journal of Marketing, 67*, 1–18.

Rippetoe, P. A., & Rogers, R. W. (1987). Effects of components of protection–motivation theory on adaptive and maladaptive coping with a health threat. *Journal of Personality and Social Psychology, 52*(3), 596–604.

Roberto, A. J., & Goodall, C. E. (2009). Using the extended parallel process model to explain physicians' decisions to test their patients for kidney disease. *Journal of Health Communication, 14*(4), 400–412.

Roberto, A. J., Zimmerman, R. S., Carlyle, K. E., Abner, E. L., Cupp, P. K., & Hansen, G. L. (2007). The effects of a computer-based pregnancy, STD, and HIV prevention intervention: A nine-school trial. *Health Communication, 21*(2), 115–124.

Rogers, R. W. (1975). A protection motivation theory of fear appeals and attitude change. The *Journal of Psychology, 91*, 93–114.

Rogers, R. W. (1983). Cognitive and physiological processes in attitude change: A revised theory of protection motivation. In J. Cacioppo & R. Petty (Eds.), *Social psychophysiology* (pp. 153–176) New York, NY: Guilford Press.

Rogers, R. W., & Prentice-Dunn, S. (1997). Protection motivation theory. In D. S. Gochman (Ed.), *Handbook of health behavior research: Vol. 1. Determinants of health behavior, personal and social* (pp. 113–132). New York, NY: Plenum.

Rosenstock, I. M., Strecher, V. J., & Becker, M. H. (1988). Social learning theory and the health belief model. *Health Education Quarterly, 15*(2), 175–183.

Smith, R. A., Ferrara, M., & Witte, K. (2007). Social sides of health risks: Stigma and collective efficacy. *Health Communication, 21*(1), 55–64.

Stephenson, M. T., & Witte, K. (1998). Fear, threat, and perceptions of efficacy from frightening skin cancer messages. *Public Health Reviews, 26*(2), 147–174.

Tulloch, H., Reida, R., D'Angeloa, M. S., Plotnikoff, R. C., Morrina, L., Beatona, L., ... Pipe, A. (2009). Predicting short and long-term exercise intentions and behaviour in patients with coronary artery disease: A test of protection motivation theory. *Psychology and Health, 24*(3), 255–269.

Van der Velde, F. W., & Van der Pligt, J. (1991). AIDS-related health behavior: Coping, protection motivation, and previous behavior. *Journal of Behavioral Medicine, 14*(5), 429–451.

Witte, K. (1992). Putting the fear back into fear appeals: The extended parallel process model. *Communication Monographs, 59*(4), 329–349.

Witte, K. (1994). Fear control and danger control: A test of the extended parallel process model (EPPM). *Communication Monographs, 61*(2), 113–134.

Witte, K. (1998). Fear as motivator, fear as inhibitor: Using the extended parallel process model to explain fear appeal successes and failures. In P. A. Andersen & L. K. Guerrero (Eds.), *Handbook of communication and emotion: Research, theory, applications, and contexts* (pp. 423–450). San Diego, CA: Academic Press.

Witte, K., & Allen, M. (2000). A meta-analysis of fear appeals: Implications for effective public health campaigns. *Health Education & Behavior, 27*(5), 591–615.

Witte, K., Cameron, K. A., Lapinski, M. K., & Nzyuko, S. (1998). A theoretically based evaluation of HIV/AIDS prevention campaigns along the trans-Africa highway in Kenya. *Journal of Health Communication, 3*(4), 345–363.

Witte, K., Meyer, G., & Martell, D. P. (2001). *Effective health risk messages: A step-by-step guide.* Thousand Oaks, CA: Sage.

Witte, K., & Morrison, K. (1995). Using scare tactics to promote safer sex among juvenile detention and high school youth. *Journal of Applied Communication Research, 23*(2), 128–142.

Wong, N. C. H., & Cappella, J. N. (2009). Antismoking threat and efficacy appeals: Effects on smoking cessation intentions for smokers with low and high readiness to quit. *Journal of Applied Communication Research, 37*(1), 1–20.

Chapter Opener: © Izf/Shutterstock; © Henrik Sorensen/Getty Images; © MeskPhotography/Shutterstock; © Hero Images/Getty Images

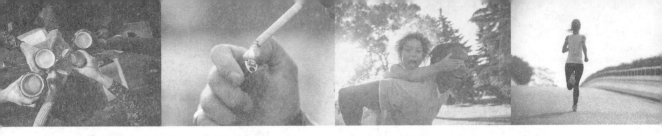

CHAPTER 6

Stage Models for Health Promotion

Ralph J. DiClemente, Richard A. Crosby, and Laura F. Salazar

Timing is the essence of all things.

—**François de La Rochefoucauld**, French Author (1613–1680)

PREVIEW

Understanding *why* individuals may or may not engage in health behaviors is critical; however, understanding *when* individuals are ready to change their behavior, the catalyst promoting change, and *how* they change their behavior is equally important. The first step toward this understanding is acknowledging that any type of behavior change will involve a process.

OBJECTIVES

1. Apply the transtheoretical model of change (TMC) to a variety of health behaviors.
2. Distinguish between each stage of the TMC and describe how the processes of change can best be applied to promote movement across these stages.
3. Apply the precaution adoption process model (PAPM) to a variety of health behaviors.
4. Identify similarities and differences between the TMC and the PAPM.

▶ Introduction

Stage theories are a subset of value–expectancy theories. Stage theories share the same underlying principles and assumptions as value–expectancy theories (see Chapter 4), but they are distinguished from these theories by suggesting that change occurs as a result of individuals passing through a series of sequential stages that culminate either in the elimination of a health-risk behavior (e.g., smoking) or the long-term adoption of a health-protective behavior (e.g., exercise). Characteristically, these theories suggest that an individual's trajectory through a hierarchy of stages is dependent on the successful completion of the tasks of the previous stage in order to achieve lasting or durable behavior change. The eloquence of stage models is that they allow intervention programs to be matched or targeted to a particular stage, meaning that the objective is to intervene "where people are" in the behavior change continuum and move them one step (one stage) closer to lasting behavior change. This type of approach to behavior change implies that a single intervention is not be the optimal approach to promoting behavior change across any given population. This is the case because people comprising a population are typically distributed across the spectrum of stages (i.e., people are "located" at different points on the change continuum). To be most effective at facilitating behavior change, stage theories recommend that interventions, be "matched" to an individual's specific stage of change. This **targeted** approach maximizes the likelihood that the intervention can facilitate moving individuals from their current stage to the next one. Stage theories also assert that asking individuals to move one stage forward will be more acceptable and more efficacious in the long run than asking them to simply take action (change their behavior) regardless of their level of readiness of change that specific behavior, which is characteristic of most traditional action-oriented programs. The term **stage-matched (or stage-targeted) intervention** is therefore applicable to stage theories.

To understand stage theories or, for that matter, any theory, you have to recognize that theories are like puzzles: all the pieces are designed to fit smoothly and seamlessly together, and once they do, a picture emerges. Applied to health behavior theories, the "pieces" are called constructs, the "fit" is the integration of these constructs, and the picture that emerges is an understanding of how these constructs interact to influence people's health behavior. The proverbial key to understanding theory—in this case, stage theory—is to identify its core underlying principle, that is, the central principle that threads throughout the theory. To illustrate one core principle of stage theories, we would like to recount a children's story. This may sound unusual, but rest assured that a core principle of stage theories will shortly become patently clear.

The story we use to illustrate this core principle is that of "Goldilocks and the Three Bears." This is the story of a precocious young girl going into the woodland home of three very neat, anthropomorphic bears and tasting their porridge, sitting in their chairs, and resting in their beds until she found the one **bed** that fit her "just right." There is a theme that threads through this tale, namely, finding what is "just right." This is one core principle of stage theories. Another metaphor would be in medicine, where finding the right medication for specific conditions is important; in stage theories, finding the constructs or process variables that are "just right" for someone at a particular stage of change is also important. Matching intervention constructs to an individual's stage of change can optimize the potential for progress to the next stage and, working systematically, to higher stages, until achieving lasting behavior change. So, to come full circle, stage theories are concerned with finding scientifically "what is just right" for people in terms of promoting behavior change.

> *Matching intervention constructs to an individual's stage of change can optimize the potential for progress to the next stage and, working systematically, to higher stages, until achieving lasting behavior change.*

There are two stage theories that predominate in health-promotion research and practice: the Transtheoretical Model of Change (TMC), developed by James O. Prochaska and colleagues (Prochaska & DiClemente, 1983; Prochaska DiClemente, & Norcross, 1992; Prochaska, Redding, & Evers, 2008) and the Precaution Adoption Process Model (PAPM), developed by Weinstein and Sandman (2002). Both theories have been used successfully to change a diverse array of health behaviors, either facilitating the elimination of health-risk behaviors or the adoption of health-protective behaviors. The TMC, however, was the original stage theory in the field of health promotion and it has been used significantly more often than the PAPM to provide the theoretical foundation guiding a range of health-promotion interventions.

▶ Key Concepts

Origins of the Transtheoretical Model of Change

The TMC is a model of intentional behavior change that describes the phases that people go through (stages of change) and the mechanisms that people use (processes of change, decisional balance, efficacy) when they adopt or modify new health-promoting behaviors or eliminate old health-risk behaviors. This model provides a description of how people change their behaviors. Of note, the question of how people change is quite different than questions pertaining to why people change. In Chapter 5 you learned, for example, that people may adopt a health-protective behavior in response to a sufficient level of perceived threat if they feel they are capable of the new behavior and that the new behavior will produce more benefit than cost. These and other constructs are addressing *why* people change. The "*how* of behavior change" is much different, as it also involves understanding what happens after people decide to change.

Consider that therapists are essentially in the business of understanding and helping people change their behaviors. People do, for example, seek the assistance of skilled therapists to help them quit smoking or to control problem-drinking behavior. Although the notion of using therapy to promote a health-protective behavior is somewhat removed from the long-standing practice of eliminating risky behaviors, the assumption is that underlying processes are similar, if not identical. The TMC integrates processes and principles of individual-level behavior change from across major theories of psychotherapy, hence the name *transtheoretical*. James O. Prochaska and his colleagues have noted that the intellectual impetus for developing the TMC was "the lack of an overall guiding theory, the search for the underlying principles, the growing acknowledgement that no single therapy is more 'correct' than any other, and general dissatisfaction with their often limited approaches" (Prochaska et al., 1992). Thus, this model emerged from a comparative analysis of leading theories of psychotherapy and behavior change. The search was for a systematic integration in a field that had fragmented into more than 300 theories of psychotherapy (Prochaska, 1979, 1986). The comparative analysis identified 10 processes of change among these theories, derived from psychological approaches developed by prominent theoreticians such as Freud, Skinner, Rogers, and others. Later studies with smokers both confirmed the measurement structure of the processes of change applied to smoking cessation (Prochaska, Velicer, DiClemente, & Fava, 1988) and supported the TMC idea that different constructs were important for smokers at different stages of change (Prochaska, Velicer, Guadagnoli, Rossi, & DiClemente, 1991).

The Stages of Change

The TMC, like all theories and models of health promotion, is predicated on a set of core assumptions or principles of how people intentionally change their behavior (Prochaska et al., 2008). Understanding these assumptions can be valuable in selecting a theory to guide a particular behavior change intervention. The core assumptions of the TMC are delineated in **TABLE 6-1**.

TABLE 6-1	Underlying Assumptions of the Transtheoretical Model of Change
Assumption 1	No single theory can account for all the complexities of behavior change. Therefore, a more comprehensive model will most likely emerge from integration across major theories.
Assumption 2	Behavior change is a process that unfolds over time through a sequence of stages. Stages are both stable and open to change, just as chronic behavioral risk factors.
Assumption 3	Behavior change is both stable and open to change.
Assumption 4	Without planned interventions, populations will remain mired in early stages. There is no inherent motivation to progress through the stages of intentional change as there seems to be for stages of physical and psychological development.
Assumption 5	The majority of at-risk populations are not prepared for action and will not be well served by traditional action-oriented prevention programs. Health promotion can have much greater impact if it shifts from an action paradigm to a stage paradigm.
Assumption 6	Specific processes and principles of change need to be applied at specific stages if progress through the stages is to occur. In the stage paradigm, intervention programs must be matched to each individual's stage of change.
Assumption 7	Behavior is not random, inevitable, or uncontrollable. Chronic behavior patterns are under some combination of biological, social, and psychological influences. Stage-matched interventions have been designed primarily to enhance self-control.
Assumption 8	Behavior change typically consists of several attempts where the individual may progress, backslide, and cycle and re-cycle through the stages of change a number of times before they ultimately implement a behavior change. (This is a key assumption and one that is absent from other health-promotion theories that do not acknowledge this change process.)

The TMC originally assumed six sequential stages through which individuals proceed to affect lasting behavior change. However, further refinements of the model often omitted the last stage, **termination**, as this reflected its origins in the field of psychotherapy and applied mainly to addictive behaviors. The five stages of the TMC are: **precontemplation** (PC), **contemplation** (C), **preparation** (PR), **action** (A), and **maintenance** (M). The sequence of stages is important, because it represents the progression that describes how people change. The explicit goal of health promotion becomes one of moving people successfully through the stages until they ultimately achieve maintenance. Each stage has its own set of unique challenges, thus any intervention program can more appropriately be construed as being, in reality, four programs rather than one. This is true simply because facilitating someone's advancement from "PC" to "C" is clearly a much different task, for example, than facilitating the advancement of someone from "A" to "M." In essence, the five stages create at least four distinct transition challenges, thereby leading to the concept of stage-matched or stage-targeted interventions. We describe the five stages of change as follows:

Precontemplation. This is the stage in which people have no intention to take action in the foreseeable future (usually defined as within the next 6 months). People may be in this stage because they are uninformed or under-informed about the consequences of their behavior, they may have tried to change a particular behavior a number of times and have become demoralized about their capability to change, or they may not even recognize that they need to change a particular behavior. Both uninformed and under-informed groups tend to avoid reading, talking, or thinking about their high-risk behaviors. They are often characterized in other theories as resistant or unmotivated individuals or as "not ready" for health-promotion programs.

Contemplation. This is the stage in which people engage in cognitive processes. The challenge of this stage is to arrive at an affirmative resolution to adopt a health-protective behavior or to eliminate a health-risk behavior. This resolution is the impetus for personal intent to change behavior in the near future (again, most often defined as being within the next 6 months). One especially valuable construct for this stage is known as **decisional balance**, which represents a mental weighing of the importance of the pros and cons associated with changing behavior (this concept is similar to the concept of "benefits and barriers" described in value–expectancy theories in Chapter 4). Simply stated, the process always begins with the relative difference between the pros and cons, favoring the cons. The pros of changing may be small, whereas the cons of changing are large; hence, people are ambivalent and have reasons for not yet adopting the health-protective behavior. Successfully passing through higher-level stages results in a reversal of this initial relation of pros to cons, meaning that the pros will become relatively more important in comparison to the cons. Clearly, implications for behavior change interventions are based on: (1) enhancing perceptions of the advantages of changing behavior, and (2) minimizing perceptions of the barriers to adopting these behavior changes. Because of the importance of decisional balance, it is described in greater detail in a subsequent section of this chapter.

Preparation. In this stage, people intend to adopt a new behavior in the immediate future, usually defined as within the next month. They may have already taken some steps in preparation to change their behavior, such as joining a health club or participating in a health education class, consulting a counselor or life coach, or talking to their physician. A primary assumption of this stage is that lasting change will require some combination of skills and resources, both of which take time to acquire.

Action. In this stage, people have made specific overt modifications in their lifestyles within the past 6 months. Behavioral change has often been equated with action; however, not all behavioral changes qualify as action. People must achieve a level of behavior change that scientists and professionals agree is sufficient to reduce the risk of disease. For example, in promoting smoking cessation, abstinence would be the appropriate and most effective endpoint for reducing risk of disease. The use of electronic cigarettes (e-cigarettes) would not, for example, be considered a valid form of behavior change. As another example, in watching one's diet, there is a consensus that one should consume no more than 30% of calories from saturated fats and no fewer than five to nine servings of fruits and vegetables per day. Regardless of the behavior, the action criterion should reflect the degree of behavior change that is significant from a public health (epidemiological) standpoint to reduce the risk of adverse health outcomes or, conversely, enhance the likelihood of improved health outcomes.

Maintenance. In this final stage, people still work to prevent relapse, but they do not need to apply change processes as frequently as do people in the action stage. They are less tempted to relapse and increasingly more confident that they can maintain their behavior change. Typically, maintenance of behavior is defined as sustaining that specified behavior for 6 months or longer. Based on data from a variety of sources (e.g., U.S. Department of Health and Human Services, 1990), it is estimated that maintenance lasts from 6 months to about 5 years for smoking cessation, and may be ongoing for some behavior changes (alcohol or substance abuse).

Movement Across the Stages of Change

Unfortunately, a neat progression through the five stages may rarely occur for any one person. Thus, the stages of change have often been schematically represented as a spiral staircase, as depicted in **FIGURE 6-1**.

This is a useful analogy because it both pictorially represents a sequence of steps and because the spiral model reflects the principle that behavior change is neither a binary, all-or-nothing phenomenon, nor a unidirectional, linear process. A key underlying assumption of the TMC is that the amount of time that an individual is in a particular stage varies greatly within and across populations and across various behaviors. However, because behavior change may not be linear for any individual, individual paths across the stages can be highly variable, including relapse to earlier stages and/or re-cycling through the stages.

Although the depiction of Figure 6-1 is a useful representation of movement across the stages in the TMC, it does not adequately convey the concept that behavior change typically involves multiple efforts, meaning that people may revert, at any time, to a previous stage, or they may revert entirely to the precontemplation stage; that is individuals may fall back to a previous stage, subsequently move forward again, and fall back again. The process of cycling and re-cycling through the stages a number of times is a critical concept of the theory and is often a central characteristic of behavior change efforts. Indeed, the TMC was originally developed to aid people in their efforts at smoking cessation and, as you might expect, the model needed to accommodate the prevalent event of backsliding among people newly entering the action stage and then suddenly experiencing physiological effects of nicotine withdrawal. You can easily imagine that some people may revert to preparation ("Maybe I wasn't ready just yet"), while others may revert two stages to contemplation ("I need to think

> *In effect, the TMC supports the idea that the process of behavior change is "evolutionary, not revolutionary."*

this through again—is it right for me?") and others may revert all the way to precontemplation ("I am no longer willing to even think about quitting"). In effect, the TMC supports the idea that the process of behavior change is "evolutionary, not revolutionary" (Prochaska et al., 2008).

The relapse itself may be less important than the actual stage to which the individual relapses. Depending on the stage, the health-promotion intervention may have to remobilize efforts to maximize their chances of further progress. Remobilizing individuals after a relapse (when the individual may be feeling disappointed or demoralized), although difficult, may benefit from harnessing their capacity to learn from their experiences, build upon that learning, and thereby improve their readiness for the next behavior change effort.

The implication that behavior change typically involves failed efforts (backsliding or relapse) is critical for intervention planning and the evaluation process. From a public health perspective, for behavior change to be meaningful, it must be enduring. Thus, long-term maintenance of a health-protective behavior has the most value (e.g., eating a low-fat diet or a low-sodium diet daily, exercising regularly, or consistently practicing proper oral hygiene). On the other hand, even in the absence of overt behavior change, from an intervention perspective, some movement across stages in a health-positive direction is certainly better than no movement at all. Because each stage is associated with a desired behavior change, forward progress is also associated with some reduction in unhealthy behaviors or some increase in healthier behaviors, even though the person is not yet meeting the action criterion. This is an important point because it suggests that health-promotion efforts may include stage movement as a goal. Furthermore, baseline stage of change is predictive of subsequent lasting behavior change across a range of health behaviors (Blissmer et al., 2010; Evers, Harlow, Redding, & LaForge, 1998; Velicer, Redding, Sun, & Prochaska, 2007).

From an evaluation perspective, stage-matched interventions can be deemed successful even in the absence of lasting behavior change if stage progression is achieved. Thus, stage progression thus becomes a useful outcome in evaluating

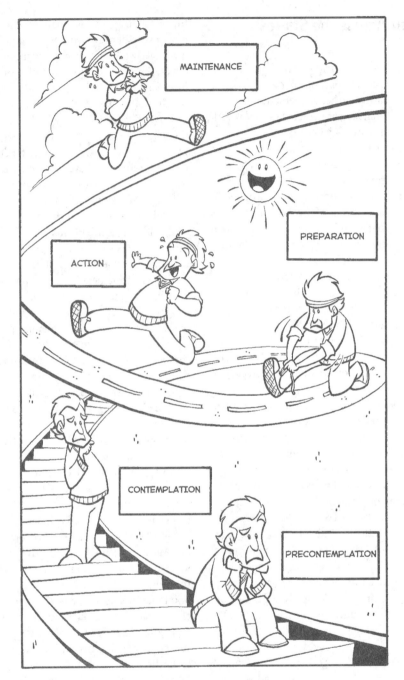

FIGURE 6-1 Stages of change for exercise behavior

Copyright 2011 by Justin Wagner. With permission.

public health efforts. Stage-matched interventions seldom work in grand sweeping motions; instead, they catalyze people's movement on the road to lasting change—each new stage represents a milestone of eventual overall success, despite failed efforts.

Stage Matching

A major premise of the TMC is that people can be "staged"; that is, they can be assessed and categorized at a particular stage of change for a specific behavior. The staging process is critical as it provides valuable information about a person's readiness to change a health behavior and therefore how best to design an intervention to eliminate health-risk behavior or adopt health-protective behavior. It is this specificity that is one of the hallmarks of stage models: the capacity to intervene at a specific stage of change, which makes stage models appealing, effective, and valuable in the health-promotion armamentarium. This is an important concept and one that may benefit from a brief illustration. For example, two people, Joe and Sally, both smoke a comparable amount of cigarettes per day and they would like to change (eliminate) this health-risk behavior, we could assess their readiness to quit smoking and "stage" them. This staging would determine the most appropriate strategies to help them progress through the subsequent stages of change. However, people differ in their desire, willingness, and level of perceived threat pertaining to various health behaviors and, thus, they may be at different stages in the change process. For example, Joe

may have thought about quitting smoking, but perhaps he has not made any active effort to seek professional help. On the other hand, Sally has tried repeatedly to quit smoking to no avail. Joe would be staged in contemplation: he's thought about changing his smoking behavior, but has not taken any active steps. Sally would be staged in preparation: she has made some attempts to quit smoking, although none have been successful. Thus, both people smoke, but they are at different stages in terms of their readiness to quit smoking. With that information, a health-promotion practitioner can determine which strategies are the most likely to be effective at achieving movement to the next stage. For Joe, the next stage is preparation (i.e., taking active steps, such as a practice 24-hour quit) whereas for Sally, the next stage is action (i.e., actually quitting).

Although staging has an intuitive appeal and utility for health-promotion practitioners and researchers, an important question is "How do you determine a person's stage of change?" The simple answer is through a staging algorithm. Specifically, an algorithm is defined as a computable set of steps to achieve a desired result. Although this process seems complex, in practice, it is relatively straightforward. Let's use an example from DiClemente et al. (1991). Following the algorithm in **FIGURE 6-2**, you can see

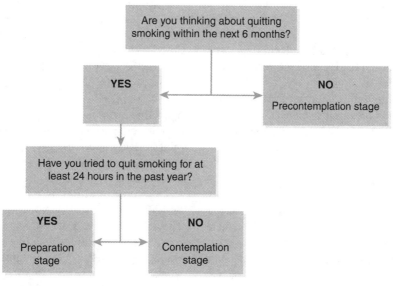

FIGURE 6-2 Illustration of a staging algorithm

that a person's stage of change for smoking cessation is quickly determined by asking a few questions that assess readiness to change.

Identifying a person's stage of change is the initial step in intervening to promote behavior change. Once we know a person's stage, we will use a diverse array of strategies to promote a person's willingness and motivation to progress through the stages until the desired behavior change is achieved. These strategies are referred to as the **processes of change**.

Processes of Change

Processes of change (POC) are defined as essential principles that promote change. Intervention strategies that help modify a person's thinking, feeling, or behavior constitute a change process. Processes are the actual mechanisms or drivers, propelling forward progression through the stages of change and, ultimately, the elimination/adoption of behavior(s). Processes lay the framework for the design of the ensuing behavior change intervention. In effect, health-promotion practitioners and researchers can use these processes to promote progression through the stages of change and, ultimately, lasting behavior change. Ten processes that have received substantial empirical support are shown in **TABLE 6-2**.

Consciousness raising involves increasing awareness about the health-damaging effects of a particular behavior (for instance, sun exposure increasing the risk of developing skin cancer) and ways to reduce these adverse health consequences (i.e., use appropriate SPF sunscreen to block out harmful UVA/UVB rays).

Dramatic relief produces increased emotional awareness or anxiety, followed by relief if appropriate action is taken. For example, seeing pictures of skin cancer lesions or sun-damaged skin may produce affective reactions to sun exposure. Also, knowing that using sunscreen can reduce the risk of skin cancer and sun-damaged skin may reduce negative affect.

Intervention strategies that help modify a person's thinking, feeling, or behavior constitute a change process.

Self-reevaluation combines both cognitive and affective assessments of one's self-image in conjunction with a given health behavior. A good example is having obese people visualize their life as a sedentary person who is obese or as an energetic person who is physically fit.

Environmental reevaluation combines both affective and cognitive assessments of how the presence or absence of a certain health behavior affects one's social environment. An assessment of the effects of secondhand smoke on others is one example. It can also include the awareness that one can be a positive or negative role model for others; for example, obese parents may be motivated to change their diet and initiate a regular exercise routine by focusing on the example they set for their children. If their children see them watching television and not eating well or exercising, then they are modeling health-threatening behaviors that may be acquired by their children, leading to adolescent obesity.

Self-liberation is both the belief that one can change and the commitment and recommitment to act on that belief. For example, let's say that Joe has decided he needs to start eating a healthier diet. By publicly announcing his intentions to change his diet in multiple forums (e.g., family, work colleagues, neighbors, on social networking websites), he may feel empowered to initiate and maintain that healthy diet.

Helping relationships combine caring, trust, openness, and acceptance, as well as support for the healthy behavior change. Helping relationships can be a highly influential process of change and can be used across all the stages of change to foster sustainable behavior change. For example, Joe wants to lose weight but cannot seem to maintain an aerobic workout regimen. Joe would benefit from partnering with a buddy or trainer to reinforce the importance of regular exercise and provide an impetus for him to maintain his workout schedule.

Counterconditioning means substituting healthier coping strategies for unhealthy ones. This often requires learning new behaviors that can serve as substitutes for unhealthy behaviors. For example, Joe has been thinking about quitting smoking for a number of months, but he has been reluctant to quit because he believes that smoking

TABLE 6-2 Processes of Change

Processes of Change	Description/Definition
Consciousness raising	Enhance awareness of health risks and protective behaviors
Dramatic relief	Enhance emotional reaction to health-risk behaviors
Self-reevaluation	Visualize oneself and life without the health-risk behavior
Environmental reevaluation	Understand how the health habit may adversely affect others in one's social environment
Self-liberation	Foster the belief that one can change and the reinforce the commitment to change
Helping relationships	Utilize supportive others to promote behavior change
Counterconditioning	Substitute healthier behaviors for unhealthy behaviors
Contingency management (sometimes referred to as reinforcement management)	Provide reward for positive behaviors or punishment for health-threatening behaviors
Stimulus control	Remove cues for unhealthy behaviors and add cues that support health-promoting behaviors
Social liberation	Change or transcend socially designated norms and practices to adopt health-protective behaviors

Data from Prochaska, J. O., Redding, C. A., & Evers, K. (2008). The transtheoretical model and stages of change. In K. Glanz, B. K. Rimer, & K. V. Viswanath (Eds.), *Health behavior and health education: Theory, research and practice*, 4th ed. (pp. 170–222). San Francisco, CA: Jossey-Bass Inc. pp. 97–122.

has been important in controlling stress. However, Joe can learn other, more effective coping strategies for dealing with his stress, strategies that are health promoting rather than health damaging. Some possible strategies might be for Joe to learn meditation or yoga or to channel his stress into physical activities.

Contingency management (also known as reinforcement management) provides consequences for taking steps in a particular direction. Although contingency management can include the use of punishments, relying on rewards is likely to be more effective; reinforcements are

emphasized because a philosophy of this model is to work in harmony with people's natural ways of changing. Contingency contracts, overt and covert reinforcements, and group recognition are procedures for increasing the probability that healthier responses will be repeated. For example, once Joe decides to quit smoking, he could save up all the money he would have spent on cigarettes and use it to go on a vacation or buy something else special to him.

Stimulus control removes cues for unhealthy behaviors and adds cues that support the adoption and maintenance of healthy behaviors.

One example might be changing the route you travel to avoid walking past the ice-cream shop or French bakery. By avoiding these eateries, you may reduce the likelihood that you would be tempted to stop in for a snack. Another example would be to keep your exercise bag/shoes in your office or car as a reminder to use them.

Social liberation focuses on utilizing/ increasing social opportunities that support health-promoting behavior change. On a societal level, the proliferation of smoke-free restaurants and bars (and, in some cases, entire cities) and the elimination of trans fats from food have been instrumental in supporting health-promoting behavior change. Continued advocacy at the national, state, and local levels is needed to maintain these changes and further strengthen public health efforts.

Stage-Matched Interventions

We noted in a previous section of this chapter that one advantage of a TMC-based intervention approach is that we can determine what stage a person is in and apply those strategies most likely to help promote movement to the next stage in the change process. This is called a stage-matched or stage-targeted intervention—essentially, we match the strategies that are most likely to produce movement through the stages of change given the current level of a person's readiness. Stage-matching is a critical aspect of stage theories that allows for more precise targeting of the intervention, thus enhancing the likelihood that the intervention will be effective in promoting the desired behavior change. In **TABLE 6-3**, we describe the alignment of stage transitions and change processes.

This point is critical and must not be misunderstood or ignored, as doing so greatly reduces the application of the model and the effectiveness of the health-promotion intervention. The systematic relationship between stage transitions and the processes used to promote that transition is important because the change processes are not universally applicable across stages. Indeed, each stage comes with its own set of unique challenges, therefore demanding a wide variety of available change processes. In general, the research suggests that in early stages, people apply cognitive, affective, and evaluative processes to progress through the stages, while in later stages, people rely more on commitments, conditioning, contingencies, environmental controls, and support for

> *Each stage comes with its own set of unique challenges, therefore demanding a wide variety of available change processes.*

TABLE 6-3 Alignment of Stage Transitions and Process of Change	
Stage Transition	**Process of Change**
Precontemplation → Contemplation	Consciousness raising, dramatic relief, self-reevaluation, environmental reevaluation
Contemplation → Preparation	Self-reevaluation, environmental reevaluation, self-liberation, self-efficacy, stimulus control
Preparation → Action	Self-liberation, self-efficacy, stimulus control, counterconditioning, helping relationships
Action → Maintenance	Stimulus control, counterconditioning, helping relationships, reinforcement management

progressing toward maintained behavior change. For example, dramatic relief may be effective to move someone from "PC" to "C," but it will have little if any value for moving someone from "PR" to "A" or from "A" to "M." Conversely, contingency management is effective in moving someone from "A" to "M" but has little if any effectiveness in moving someone from "PC" to "C."

At this juncture, an important question needs to be raised and addressed: what are the practical implications of this systematic relationship between the stages of change and the processes of change? Quite simply, health-promotion interventions delivered in communities need to be inclusive of all potential stages of readiness to change and thus apply the change processes in accordance with those stages. In essence, the population can be segmented into stages, and interventions can then be designed for each segment. For people in precontemplation, for example, practitioners need to apply such processes as consciousness raising and dramatic relief to help promote their progress to the contemplation stage. Applying processes of change such as contingency management, counterconditioning, and stimulus control to people in precontemplation would not be as effective in promoting transition from "PC" to "C" or from "C" to "PR." In fact, mismatching of the processes of change could be counterproductive, hindering progress toward behavior change. As further research evolves, researchers will be able to more precisely delineate when to apply a particular process of change in a particular stage to maximize the likelihood of stage progression.

Differentiating Processes of Change from Techniques

As we noted, there are 10 POCs. However, students are sometimes uncertain of how to distinguish between the POC and the techniques used to articulate a particular process. It is important to avoid equating the processes of change with the techniques used to enhance/promote each of the processes, as the two concepts are not identical. First, techniques are strategies, methods, or planned activities that are used to amplify a process of change. There is a broad

array of techniques used for each POC, which can be best clarified by presenting each POC and its concomitant techniques. **TABLE 6-4** provides some brief examples of techniques used to enhance each POC. Please note that the list of techniques is illustrative, not exhaustive.

> *It is important to avoid equating the processes of change with the techniques used to enhance/promote each of the processes, as the two concepts are not equivalent.*

Additional TMC Constructs

In addition to the stages of change, the processes of change, and the techniques used to enhance/promote each process, there are two other key constructs in the TMC: **decisional balance** and **self-efficacy**. Decisional balance is a construct that we discussed earlier as especially relevant for those in the contemplation stage. Self-efficacy has been described in previous chapters, as it is a central construct in many other theories. Now we will describe each construct in greater detail.

Decisional balance. This construct is derived from the seminal work of Janis and Mann (1977) on decision making and reflects an individual's relative weighing of the pros and cons of changing his or her behavior. Let's refer to an earlier example about our friend Joe who wants to quit smoking. Imagine that Joe feels that smoking cigarettes provides a measure of stress reduction and a way of coping with stress that would no longer be available to him if he did not smoke. Joe is aware that smoking increases his risk for myriad adverse health outcomes, including a variety of cancers and heart disease. However, he is weighing the pros of being healthier in the future with the cons of not being able to effectively cope with stress in the present. This simplistic illustration does not adequately capture the complexity, intricacies, or careful calibration involved in the internal weighting of the pros and cons of changing behaviors, as people are usually (though not always) aware of the threat posed by most health-risk behaviors,

TABLE 6-4 Techniques Associated with Processes of Change

Processes of Change	Techniques
Consciousness raising	Educational brochures; exposure to information on the Internet; personal feedback from friends, family, healthcare professionals; and media campaigns.
Dramatic relief	Role-playing; personal testimonies from people experiencing the adverse health consequences associated with a risk behavior; media campaigns that target emotional aspects of a health-risk behavior; and emotionally arousing, threatening, or motivational images.
Self-reevaluation	Using values-clarifying exercises and visualization exercises of a "healthy self" without a particular risk behavior.
Environmental reevaluation	Empathy training, family interventions, and worksite interventions with colleagues.
Self-liberation	Personal pronouncements, such as resolutions to initiate a new, healthy behavior or eliminate a current health-damaging behavior; public testimonies to family, friends, and work colleagues stating willingness and commitment to change a health-risk behavior.
Helping relationships	Support groups, health-promotion practitioner contacts, use of a "buddy system" to provide social support and reinforce healthy behaviors.
Counterconditioning	Relaxation or desensitization exercises, or replacement of unhealthy behaviors with healthy substitutes, such as nicotine replacement therapy for cigarette smokers or low-fat/skim milk for whole milk.
Stimulus control	Activities that promote avoidance of cues that stimulate risk behaviors by modifying one's personal environmental (simply removing unhealthy foods from the cupboard and replacing them with healthy foods or removing all the ashtrays/lighters from the house on quit day).
Social liberation	Advocacy to change health policies that would support a person's behavior change—for example, providing free condoms in school-based clinics to reduce the risk of teen pregnancy and sexually transmitted diseases, including HIV. Also, strategies to normalize condom use and to reduce any stigma associated with them.

but these behaviors are often difficult to change because they serve some purpose; in Joe's case, smoking helps him cope with stress. The goal of intervention is to maximize the pros of adopting a new, healthier behavior or eliminating a health-threatening behavior, and minimize the cons associated with adopting that behavior.

Decisional balance and its relationship to the stages of change have been validated meta-analytically for diverse different health behaviors, across different languages, and countries (Hall & Rossi, 2008;). This meta-analytic evidence supported the **strong principle of progress**, which means the pros of the health behavior change must increase by about one standard deviation (SD) from "PC" to "A" (Hall & Rossi, 2008; Prochaska, 1994). The same evidence also supported the **weak principle**, which means the cons of the health behavior change must decrease by one-half SD from "PC" to "A" (Hall & Rossi, 2008; Prochaska, 1994). This theory and the cumulative evidence support the concept that there is a "tipping point" when an individual's internal scales weighing the pros and cons tip in favor of the pros (i.e., behavior change). When this occurs, a person is more likely to progress to the next stage of change. As you can see, this construct is nearly identical to the construct of expected net gain as described in Chapter 5.

Self-efficacy. This construct is derived from the groundbreaking research of Albert Bandura (1986), a giant in the field of behavior theory (self-efficacy is discussed in greater detail in Chapter 7). As conceptualized in the TMC, self-efficacy consists of two components: confidence and temptation (DiClemente & Prochaska, 1982; Velicer, DiClemente, Rossi, & Prochaska, 1990). **Confidence** is the primary construct in self-efficacy and refers to individuals' perceived ability to cope with high-risk situations without relapsing to unhealthy behaviors. **Temptation** describes the intensity of urges to engage in a specific behavior when confronted with challenging situations. Thus, confidence and temptation interact in a way that makes the most demanding situation one in which confidence is low and temptation is high. This scenario is more likely to occur for people in precontemplation or contemplation; however, someone just entering the action stage could be affected. For example, Emily has just started eating a low-fat diet, so she has not built up a high level of confidence yet. Imagine that she finds herself immersed in the holiday season (cakes, cookies, lavish meals and desserts) while she is still learning how to cope with the "loss" of high-fat foods. Her lack of confidence in this high-temptation circumstance may spell the end of the action stage and signal backsliding to a previous stage. Conversely, high confidence and low temptation interact to provide optimal conditions favoring successful progress

to lasting behavior change. The term **resilient self-efficacy** has been used to describe people with sufficiently high levels of self-efficacy, such that the behavior can be performed despite extremely challenging circumstances.

Application Across Diverse Health Behaviors

From the initial studies of smoking **cessation**, the TMC has rapidly evolved to include application to myriad other health, addictive, and affective behaviors. The diversity of studies and health behaviors has provided robust empirical support for the TMC core constructs (Noar, Benac, & Harris, 2007; Prochaska et al., 2008). There are several different types of TMC interventions that can be developed. Some include stage-matched peer advisors (Cabral et al., 1996), motivational interviewing or enhancement (DiClemente & Velasquez, 2002) and stage-matched or stage-targeted materials. This allows for tailoring of intervention materials to help "meet people at their current level of readiness to change." A meta-analysis summarizing results across numerous studies examining health behavior change interventions supported the efficacy of tailoring on each TMC construct (stages, decisional balance, efficacy, and processes) across a wide range of problem behaviors (Noar et al., 2007). A highly tailored computer-based intervention, also called an expert system, provides individually tailored feedback on each TMC construct both at baseline and as changes happen over time (Redding et al., 1999; Velicer et al., 1993). Such highly tailored systems have been found effective (Prochaska et al., 2008) in changing a range of health-risk behaviors including, but not limited to:

- smoking cessation
- dietary-fat reduction
- stress management
- sun protection
- mammography screening
- weight management
- bullying prevention

One assumption of the TMC is that a common set of change processes can be applied across a broad range of behaviors; however, application of the different processes across behaviors has been less consistent compared to the staging and the pros and cons of changing (Hall & Rossi, 2008). Also, more research is needed to better understand the relationships between the processes of change and the stages of change within the TMC. An important implication is that the processes of change should be matched to a particular stage; however, the number and type of processes is dependent on the specific target behavior. Often, when designing a TMC intervention, data are collected to examine the relationships between the stages and processes of change within a specific problem behavior area. There is some evidence, for example, that people use fewer change processes with more episodic behaviors, such as a yearly Pap or mammography screening exams, requiring utilization of fewer processes to change behavior (Pruitt et al., 2010; Rakowski, Dube, & Goldstein, 1996; Rakowski et al., 1998).

▶ Global Application of the TMC

Research based on the TMC has been applied across international borders in countries like Australia, Taiwan, Turkey, and France. In Australia, Taiwan, and Turkey, the TMC has focused on smoking cessation and avoiding secondhand smoke, while in France, research focused on physical activity (Bernard et al., 2014; Campbell et al., 2013; Ergul & Temel, 2009; Huang, Guo, Wu, & Chen, 2011).

The implementation of different TMC constructs varies by study and behavior, showcasing its wide-use and flexibility on a global scale. A study by Huang and colleagues focused on avoiding secondhand smoke among pregnant women and women with young children—it applied all of constructs of the theory: SOC, POC, decisional balance, and self-efficacy (2011). This study also combined an additional theoretical construct: knowledge, demonstrating the feasibility

of complementing the TMC with other theories. Another study carried out among 539 indigenous Australians in North Queensland focused on stage matching to assess where individuals were on the change continuum. Results demonstrated that because 80% of the participants are matched to the precontemplation and contemplation stages, it would be most beneficial to allocate resources to individuals in these stages (Campbell et al., 2013).

The Precaution Adoption Process Model

An important maxim when thinking about theory is that theories are seldom static—that is, they are constantly evolving. In some cases, the evolutionary process stems from entirely new theories that contain potential improvements over previous theories. The precaution adoption process model (Weinstein & Sandman, 2002) is an example of this evolutionary concept. The precaution adoption process model (PAPM) is the second major stage theory in the field of health promotion. This model provides a somewhat different and, perhaps, more fine-grained approach to the concept of the five classic stages in the transtheoretical model (see Figure 6-1).

This theory, like the TMC, asserts that people pass through a sequence of stages (also known as stage progression) before ultimately achieving sustainable behavior change. Although the PAPM resembles the TMC in that they are both stage models, there are also important theoretical differences that have health-promotion research and practice implications. Close examination shows that the number of stages is different, and even stages that have similar names are actually defined quite differently. Perhaps the key difference is the emphasis placed on intrapsychic concepts in the PAPM and the greater emphasis on environmental factors in the TMC (e.g., stimulus control, environmental reevaluation, social liberation). It is this difference in emphasis that differentiates these two stage theories. We will review the stages in the PAPM, identify key underlying assumptions of the model, and make comparisons and contrasts with the TMC.

Stages in the PAPM

The PAPM consists of seven distinct stages as shown in **FIGURE 6-3** and described in **TABLE 6-5**. The PAPM asserts that these stages represent qualitatively different patterns of behavior, beliefs, and experience and that the factors that produce transitions between stages vary depending on the specific transition being considered.

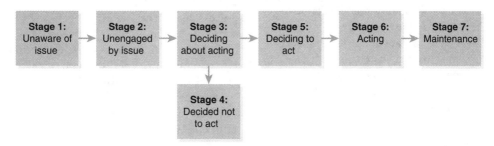

FIGURE 6-3 Stages of the precaution adoption process model
Modified from Weinstein, N. D. (1988). The precaution adoption process. *Health Psychology, 7*, 355–386.

TABLE 6-5 Stages of the Precaution Adoption Process Model

Stages	Definition/Description
Stage 1: Unaware of health risk	If people have never heard about a particular health risk, they may not have formed an opinion about it. Forcing these people to state an opinion (surveys, etc.) makes them reluctant to respond. Often times, they "don't know" and results are ignored.
Stage 2: Unengaged by the health risk	Have heard about the health risk and are starting to form opinions about it. They are aware of the health risk but do not think it applies to them.
Stage 3: Deciding about acting	Important to distinguish between those who have never thought about personally taking action, and those who ARE thinking about it, but haven't decided to take action yet. These people may have had some personal experience with the health risk.
Stage 4: Decided not to act	These people have considered the available information and have decided not to act, perhaps because they do not feel it is necessary to take any protective action. They tend to engage in actions that protect their decision/ position (this tendency is often referred to confirmation preservation or hypothesis preservation).
Stage 5: Deciding to act	Considered the available information and decided that they needed to take action.
Stage 6: Acting	Detailed implementation information can be dealt with now, which is information they weren't ready to hear before they had decided to act. Information will influence what they choose to do.
Stage 7: Maintenance	Similar to all other theories: behavior change has occurred. The change has to reach the point of being ingrained.

The primary differences in the conceptualization of the PAPM stages and the TMC stages can be traced back to the four basic assumptions of stage theories as proposed by Weinstein and Sandman (2002). Stages theories must include:

1. A classification system to define stages
2. An ordering of stages
3. Stages that are defined such that common barriers to change are faced by people in the same stage
4. Stages that are defined such that different barriers to change are faced by people in different stages

The last two assumptions represent the primary departure points between the TMC and the PAPM. Consider, for example, a person who would be classified in the TMC as a precontemplator. Thinking carefully about the stage of precontemplation, you may recall that these people have not yet begun to consider changing the health behavior in question. According to the PAPM, this precontemplation stage can be further divided into two sub-stages: (1) unaware of the issue, and (2) unengaged by the issue. The difference between the two stages is simply described by the concept of perceived susceptibility (see Chapter 4). According to Weinstein (1989), people typically have an optimism bias when it comes to their health-related behaviors. **Optimism bias** means that people do not see themselves as being as vulnerable to the adverse consequences of health-risk behaviors as their peers who engage in the same risk behaviors. This is a relatively common phenomenon. For example, drivers on an interstate highway may be delayed for hours as they are slowly motioned around the scene of a fatal accident, but they quickly accelerate past the speed limit to make up for lost time, not recognizing that their behavior could

> **Optimism bias** means that people do not see themselves as being as vulnerable to the adverse consequences of health-risk behaviors as their peers who engage in the same risk behaviors.

also result in a fatal accident. Similarly, cardiac surgeons and operating room personnel may conduct dozens of bypass procedures, yet still sit down to a meal of steak and baked potatoes (complete with copious portions of butter and sour cream) at the end of the day. Optimism bias defines the unengaged stage of the PAPM; people in stage 2 are aware of the threat (stage 1), but feel it does not apply to them. Now, the important question: why is this seemingly minor distinction so important?

The distinction between the "unaware" and "unengaged" stages is important because the intervention implications for each are markedly different. Again, think about the last two of the four assumptions of stage theories. If all people in the same stage face common barriers, then the intervention can be targeted efficiently to those people by addressing the common barriers of that stage. This holds for stages 1 and 2 in the PAPM. In contrast, this does not hold for the TMC stage of precontemplation. In fact, the barriers may be quite different because this stage includes both individuals who are "unaware" and who are "unengaged." Awareness of the potential health threat may be the objective for people who are unaware, but the intervention materials designed to create this awareness may not necessarily consider optimism bias. As such, an intervention to raise awareness for people in precontemplation may not be effective for all the people in this stage, and to reach all people in this stage intervention efforts also need to help people overcome optimism bias (thereby becoming engaged by the threat). Such programs may require people to accept personal vulnerability for events that may seem quite unlikely (e.g., fatal car accidents, myocardial infarctions). The reason that this fine-grained distinction is made in the PAPM is based entirely on the rationale for using stage theories: to create stage-matched interventions, thereby optimizing the "fit" between intervention objectives, strategies, and activities and the recipient population.

A second key difference between the TMC and the PAPM involves, once again, this same principle of targeting interventions to optimize fit. Consider the TMC relative to someone who progresses through preparation to action, only to later relapse and reverse his or her initial decision regarding the adoption of a health-protective behavior. The TMC would classify this person as a precontemplator because they do not intend to change within the next 6 months. Now, please look again at the last two of the four assumptions shown previously for the PAPM. It should be apparent that the TMC precontemplation stage now clearly violates the third PAPM assumption, as the barriers to change may be based on: (1) not being aware, (2) not being personally engaged, or (3) a rejection of the behavior after failing at an attempt to change or simply after rethinking the issue. So, the PAPM is attempting to include variables that the TMC would assess with additional constructs (pros, cons, efficacy, and processes) within the stage construct.

In the PAPM, the issue of how to handle the person who attempts and then rejects change is resolved by a stage labeled "decides not to act." From an intervention perspective, this is an important stage because it represents a relatively formidable challenge to the health-promotion professional: how does one change behavior among people who have actively rejected the health-protective behavior, perhaps even after making a change attempt? Clearly, these people are qualitatively different from those who are true precontemplators and thus the intervention approach may also be different. Indeed, in any given population (for any given health behavior) a substantial number of people may be identified and classified as "rejectors."

Another important difference between the TMC and the PAPM is that the PAPM does not prescribe change processes. Instead, the PAPM posits that successful movement from any one stage to a succeeding stage may result from any number of intervention techniques, and these techniques will naturally vary as a function of the population and the health behavior in question. This may make the PAPM more compatible with the use of other theories described in this volume, as they may provide valuable insight into creating movement through stages of the PAPM. The concept of stage-targeting or stage-matching is very much a part of the PAPM; the difference is simply the lack of prescribed change processes. Examples of techniques to move people forward are provided in **TABLE 6-6**.

An excellent applied example of the PAPM can be found in an article describing its application to the public health issue of home radon testing (Weinstein, Lyon, Sandman, & Cuite, 1998). These researchers sought to move people from stage 3 (undecided) to stage 5 (decided), and they also sought to move people already in stage 5 to stage 6 (action). Their experiment was eloquently simple. They began by selecting a city with high radon levels: Columbus, Ohio. They mailed out a radon information video and questionnaire to over 4000 residents. The questionnaire assessed stage relative to home radon testing and it was determined that 1897 respondents were either in stage 3 (28.8%) or in stage 5 (71.2%). These respondents were randomly assigned differing interventions: (1) to receive no further intervention (control), (2) a video designed to increase perceived susceptibility to radon (high likelihood), (3) a video designed to show people how easy it is to test their home for radon (low effort), or (4) an intervention that combined the high likelihood video with the low effort video. Consistent with the tenets of the theory, the high likelihood video produced the greatest movement from stage 3 to stage 5 and the low effort video produced the greatest movement from stage 5 to stage 6. The researchers also found that 32.5% of the respondents in stage 5 who viewed the low effort video subsequently ordered radon test kits, as opposed to 10.4% who viewed the high likelihood video and 8.0% of those in the control condition. Of the respondents in stage 5, viewing both videos (high likelihood and low

> *Movement from any one stage to a succeeding stage may result from any number of intervention techniques, and these techniques will naturally vary as a function of the population and the health behavior.*

TABLE 6-6 Progressing through the Stages of the Precaution Adoption Process Model	
Stage Transitions	**Intervention Strategies**
Stage 1 → Stage 2	Increase awareness of the health risk by enhancing exposure to information through media and other messages.
Stage 2 → Stage 3	Media messages about the risk behavior, communication from significant others (e.g., close friends or relatives), personal experience with the health-risk behavior, or having experienced risk behavior–associated adverse outcomes.
Stage 3 → Stage 4 or Stage 5	Enhance perceived susceptibility to the consequences associated with adverse outcomes of health-risk behavior, perceived severity of the consequences associated with the health-risk behavior, perceived efficacy to perform the health-protective behavior, and social norms supportive of action to reduce the health-risk behavior, as well as reduce perceived barriers to adopting the health-protective behavior. Fear and worry will affect likelihood of protective behavior adoption. In addition, beliefs about the difficulty of adopting and performing the protective behavior and the effectiveness of the protective behavior will influence adoption. Recommendations from others are also critical influences affecting the likelihood of adopting protective behaviors.
Stage 5 → Stage 6	Time, effort, and resources; detailed "how-to" information; reminders and cues to action; assistance from significant other (e.g., similar to helping relationships in the TMC) in changing behavior.

effort), 35.8% subsequently ordered a home test kit. The example illustrates the value of stage-matched interventions and suggests that a key aspect of any behavioral intervention is to "begin where the people are" relative to their progression toward adopting health-protective behaviors.

Stage models of behavior change can be valuable theoretical frameworks guiding the development, implementation, and evaluation of health-promotion programs across a diverse range of health behaviors. Further research is needed to determine the relative efficacy, impact, and cost-effectiveness of programs based on stage models relative to programs based on nonstage models. Moreover, research investigating whether these models can be applied beyond the individual level is imperative; specifically, can communities be "staged" (Bowen, Kinne, & Urban, 1997; Prochaska, J. M., Prochaska, J. O., & Levesque et al., 2001) and can appropriate processes of change be applied to

promote community-level change? This is a question of emerging importance given the advent of community-level and social marketing interventions that are specifically designed to target entire communities rather than individuals. Recently, theorists have integrated the TMC and community psychology theories to develop community readiness models (Edwards, Jumper-Thurman, Plested, Oetting, & Swanson, 2000; Oetting et al., 1995; Plested, Thurman, Edwards, & Oetting, 1998). Also, what is the relative efficacy of stage-matched interventions for chronic behaviors (e.g., diet) as opposed to infrequent or episodic health behaviors (e.g., vaccination, mammogram, and colonoscopy)? Further research is needed to understand and quantify the applicability of stage models for the aforementioned behaviors/situations. These models, as is true for all models of behavior change, are dynamic and continue to evolve as new empirical data are discovered and integrated into the models. As these models

A key aspect of any behavioral intervention is to "begin where the people are" relative to their progression toward adopting health-protective behaviors.

continue to gain traction within the field of health-promotion research and practice, a growing body of empirical evidence will be available to evaluate the models' applicability for newer health behaviors, to determine how best to utilize these models to understand and predict human behavior, to develop effective interventions, and to better understand their limitations.

▸ An Applied Example

A computer-delivered TMC-tailored feedback system was designed and developed to promote contraceptive and condom use (dual method use) for at-risk young women who were not planning to become pregnant in the next two years. Project PROTECT was a randomized trial that screened, recruited, and randomized women at baseline into an enhanced standard care group or a TMC intervention group (Peipert et al., 2007, 2008), with a nearly 60% participation rate. All participants ($n = 542$) received a medical exam at baseline to ensure that they did not have a sexually transmitted infection (STI). Incident STIs and pregnancies were then tracked throughout the next 24 months of the study. Women randomized to the enhanced standard care condition received a medical evaluation, treatment, and one computer-delivered session of generic information and advice to use contraception and condoms. Women randomized to the TMC treatment group received a medical evaluation, treatment, and up to three sessions (1 month apart) of computer-delivered feedback that was tailored to their readiness to use contraception and readiness to use condoms.

The TMC intervention was delivered by a computer and took approximately 30 minutes and included sections on both contraceptive and condom use within each session. Pilot testing of

parts of the intervention supported its acceptability (Brown-Peterside, Redding, Ren, & Koblin, 2000; Redding, Brown-Peterside, Noar, Rossi, & Koblin, 2011). The tailored feedback on stages of contraceptive use, pros and cons of contraceptive use, and efficacy for contraceptive use started the intervention session. The TMC condom-use section came next and was more inclusive, targeting stages of condom use in general, stages of condom use for main partner(s), stages of condom use for other partner(s), pros and cons of condom use, efficacy for condom use, and processes of condom use (Redding, Morokoff, Rossi, & Meier, 2008). Data were gathered to inform the tailoring process and to decide which processes of change to provide feedback for in each stage of condom use. The TMC treatment group showed a marked difference in dual method use at the end of the study. In fact, they were 70% more likely to use dual methods; however, even with this magnitude of behavior change, no differences were observed on incident STIs or unintended pregnancies (Peipert et al., 2008).

▸ Take Home Messages

- Stage theories are useful for designing stage-targeted and stage-matched interventions based on people's readiness to change their behavior.
- Stage theories allow more precise targeting of interventions relative to nonstage models for planning, implementing, and evaluating health-promotion interventions.
- The TMC has five stages that describe people's intention to change behavior, along with the processes of change that facilitate progression through the stages and, ultimately, to behavior change.
- Individuals' progress through the stages of change is rarely linear; people often relapse and/or re-cycle through earlier stages.
- Processes of change are the essential components of the TMC and are associated with various techniques to achieve stage progression.
- The PAPM has similar stages to the TMC; however, it adds additional stages and precision.

▶ References

Bandura, A. (1986). *Social foundations of thought & action: A social cognitive theory.* Upper Saddle River, NJ: Prentice Hall.

Bernard, P., Romain, A., Trouillet, R., Gernigon, C., Nigg, C., & Ninot, G. (2014). Validation of the TTM processes of change measure for physical activity in an adult French sample. *International Journal of Behavioral Medicine, 21*(2), 402–410.

Blissmer, B., Prochaska, J. O., Velicer, W. F., Redding, C. A., Rossi, J. S., Greene, G. W., & Robbins, M. (2010). Common factors predicting long-term changes in multiple health behaviors. *Journal of Health Psychology, 15*(2), 205–214.

Bowen, D. J., Kinne, S., & Urban, N. (1997). Analyzing communities for readiness to change. *American Journal of Health Behavior, 21*(4), 289–298.

Brown-Peterside, P., Redding, C. A., Ren, L., & Koblin, B. A. (2000). Acceptability of a stagematched expert system intervention to increase condom use among women at high risk of HIV infection in New York City. *AIDS Education and Prevention, 12*(2), 171–181.

Cabral, R. J., Galavotti, C., Gargiullo, P. M., Armstrong, K., Cohen, A., Geilen, A. C., & Watkinson, L. (1996). Paraprofessional delivery of a theory-based HIV prevention counseling intervention for women. *Public Health Reports, 3*(Suppl. 1), 75–82.

Campbell, S., Bohanna, I., Swinbourne, A., Cadet-James, Y., McKeown, D., & McDermott, R. (2013). Stages of change, smoking behaviour and readiness to quit in a large sample of indigenous Australians living in eight remote North Queensland communities. *International Journal of Environmental Research and Public Health, 10*(4), 1562–1571.

DiClemente, C. C., & Prochaska, J. O. (1982). Self-change and therapy change of smoking behavior: A comparison of processes of change in cessation and maintenance. *Addictive Behavior, 7*(2), 133–142.

DiClemente, C. C., Prochaska, J. O., Fairhurst, S., Velicer, W. F., Velasquez, M., & Rossi, J. S. (1991). The process of smoking cessation: An analysis of precontemplation, contemplation and preparation stages of change. *Journal of Consulting and Clinical Psychology, 59*, 295–304.

DiClemente, C. C., & Velasquez, M. W. (2002). Motivational interviewing and the stages of change. In W. R. Miller and S. Rollnick (Eds.), *Motivational interviewing: Preparing people for change* (2nd ed., pp. 217–250). New York, NY: Guilford Press.

Edwards, R. W., Jumper-Thurman, P., Plested, B. A., Oetting, E. R., & Swanson, L. (2000). Community readiness: Research to practice. *Journal of Community Psychology, 28*(3), 291–307.

Ergul, S., & Temel, A. B. (2009). The effects of a nursing smoking cessation intervention on military students in Turkey. *International Nursing Review, 56*, 102–108.

Evers, K. E., Harlow, L. L., Redding, C. A., & LaForge, R. G. (1998). Longitudinal changes in stages of change for condom use in women. *American Journal of Health Promotion, 13*(1), 19–25.

Hall, K. L., & Rossi, J. S. (2008). Meta-analytic examination of the strong and weak principles across 48 health behaviors. *Preventive Medicine, 46*, 266–274.

Huang, C., Guo, J., Wu, H., & Chien, L. (2011). Stage of adoption for preventive behaviour against passive smoking among pregnant women and women with young children in Taiwan. *Journal of Clinical Nursing, 20*(23–24), 3331–3338.

Janis, I. L., & Mann, L. (1977). *Decision making: A psychological analysis of conflict, choice and commitment.* New York, NY: The Free Press.

Miller, W. R., & Rollnick, S. (2002). *Motivational interviewing: Preparing people for change.* New York, NY: Guilford Press.

Noar, S. M., Benac, C., & Harris, M. (2007). Does tailoring matter? Meta-analytic review of tailored print health behavior change interventions. *Psychological Bulletin, 133*(4), 673–693.

Oetting, E. R., Donnermeyer, J. F., Plested, B. A., Edwards, R. W., Kelly, K., & Beauvais, F. (1995). Assessing community readiness for prevention. *The International Journal of the Addictions, 30*(6), 659–683.

Peipert, J. F., Redding, C. A., Blume, J., Allsworth, J., Ianuccillo, K., Lozowski, F., ... Rossi, J. S. (2007). Design of a stage-matched intervention trial to increase dual method contraceptive use (Project PROTECT). *Contemporary Clinical Trials, 28*, 626–637.

Peipert, J. F., Redding, C. A., Blume, J., Allsworth, J., Matteson, K., Lozowski, F., ... Rossi, J. S. (2008). Tailored intervention trial to increase dual methods: A randomized trial to reduce unintended pregnancies and sexually transmitted infections. *American Journal of Obstetrics & Gynecology, 198*(6), 630.e1–630.e8.

Plested, B. A., Thurman, P. J., Edwards, R. W., & Oetting, E. R. (1998). Community readiness: A tool for effective community-based prevention. *Prevention Researcher, 5*(2), 5–7.

Prochaska, J. M., Prochaska, J. O., & Levesque, D. A. (2001). A transtheoretical approach to changing organizations. *Administration and Policy in Mental Health, 28*(4), 247–261.

Prochaska, J. O. (1979). *Systems of psychotherapy: A transtheoretical analysis.* Homewood, IL: Dorsey Press.

Prochaska, J. O. (1986). Patterns of change in smoking behavior. *Health Psychology, 5*, 97–98.

Prochaska, J. O. (1994). Common principles for progression from precontemplation to action based on twelve problem behaviors. *Health Psychology, 13*, 47–51.

Prochaska, J. O., & DiClemente, C. C. (1983). Stages and processes of self-change in smoking: Towards an integrative model of change. *Journal of Consulting and Clinical Psychology, 51*, 390–395.

Prochaska, J. O., DiClemente, C. C., & Norcross, J. C. (1992). In search of how people change: Applications to the addictive behaviors. *American Psychologist, 47*, 1102–1114.

Prochaska, J. O., Redding, C. A., & Evers, K. (2008). The transtheoretical model and stages of change. In K. Glanz, B. K. Rimer, & K. V. Viswanath (Eds.), *Health behavior and health education: Theory, research and practice* (4th ed., pp. 170–222). San Francisco, CA: Jossey-Bass.

Prochaska, J. O., Velicer, W. F., DiClemente, C. C., & Fava, J. (1988). Measuring processes of change: Applications to the cessation of smoking. *Journal of Consulting and Clinical Psychology, 56*, 520–528.

Prochaska, J. O., Velicer, W. F., Guadagnoli, E., Rossi, J. S., & DiClemente, C. C. (1991). Patterns of change: Dynamic typology applied to smoking cessation. *Multivariate Behavioral Research, 26*, 83–107.

Prochaska, J. O., Velicer, W. F., Rossi, J. S., Goldstein, M. G., Marcus, B. H., Rakowski, W., ... Rossi, S. R. (1994). Stages of change and decisional balance for twelve problem behaviors. *Health Psychology, 13*, 39–46.

Pruitt, S. L., McQueen, A., Tiro, J. A., Rakowski, W., DiClemente, C. C., & Vernon, S. W. (2010). Construct validity of a mammography processes of change scale and invariance by stage of change. *Journal of Health Psychology, 15*(1), 64–74.

Rakowski, W., Dube, C. A., & Goldstein, M. G. (1996). Considerations for extending the Transtheoretical model of behavior change to screening mammography. *Health Education Research, 11*(1), 77–96.

Rakowski, W. R., Ehrich, B., Goldstein, M. G., Rimer, B. K., Pearlman, D. N., Clark, M. A., ... Woolverton, H. (1998). Increasing mammography among women aged 40–74 by use of a stage-matched, tailored intervention. *Preventive Medicine, 27*, 748–756.

Redding, C. A., Brown-Peterside, P., Noar, S. M., Rossi, J. S., & Koblin, B. A. (2011). One session of TTM-tailored condom use feedback: A pilot study among at risk women in the Bronx. *AIDS Care, 23*(1), 10–15.

Redding, C. A., Morokoff, P. J., Rossi, J. S., & Meier, K. S. (2008). A TTM-tailored condom use intervention for at-risk women and men. In T. Edgar, S. Noar, & V. Friemuth (Eds.), *Communication perspectives on HIV/AIDS for the 21st century* (pp. 423–428). Mahwah, NJ: Lawrence Erlbaum Associates.

Redding, C. A., Prochaska, J. O., Pallonen, U. E., Rossi, J. S., Velicer, W. F., Rossi, S. R., ... Maddock, J. E. (1999). Transtheoretical individualized multimedia expert systems targeting adolescents' health behaviors. *Cognitive & Behavioral Practice, 6*(2), 144–153.

U.S. Department of Health and Human Services (USDHHS). (1990). *The health benefits of smoking cessation: A report of the Surgeon General (DHHS Publication # CDC 90-8416)*. Washington, DC: U.S. Government Printing Office.

Velicer, W. F., DiClemente, C. C., Rossi, J. S., & Prochaska, J. O. (1990). Relapse situations and self-efficacy: An integrative model. *Addictive Behaviors, 15*, 271–283.

Velicer, W. F., Prochaska, J. O., Bellis, J. M., DiClemente, C. C., Rossi, J. S., Fava, J. L., & Steiger, J. H. (1993). An expert system intervention for smoking cessation. *Addictive Behaviors, 18*, 269–290.

Velicer, W. F., Redding, C. A., Sun, X., & Prochaska, J. O. (2007). Demographic variables, smoking variables, and outcome across five studies. *Health Psychology, 26*(3), 278–287.

Weinstein, N. D. (1989). Optimistic biases about personal risks. *Science, 246*(4935), 1232–1233.

Weinstein, N. D., Lyon, J. E., Sandman, P. M., & Cuite, C. L. (1998). Experimental evidence for stages of health behavior change: The precaution adoption process model applied to home radon testing. *Health Psychology, 17*, 445–453.

Weinstein, N. D., & Sandman, P. M. (2002). The precaution adoption process model and its application. In R. J. DiClemente, R. A. Crosby, & M. C. Kegler (Eds.), *Emerging theories in health promotion research and practice* (pp. 16–39). San Francisco, CA: Jossey-Bass.

Chapter Opener: © Henrik Sorensen/Getty Images; © MeskPhotography/Shutterstock; © Hero Images/Getty Images; © lzf/Shutterstock

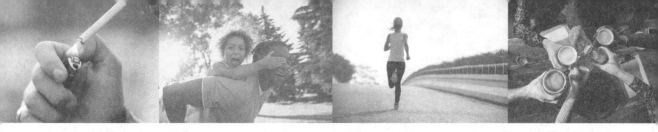

CHAPTER 7

Social Cognitive Theory Applied to Health Behavior

Richard A. Crosby, Laura F. Salazar, and Ralph J. DiClemente

We've learned that stigma and silence don't just fuel ignorance, they foster transmission and give life to a plague.

—**President Barack Obama**, speaking about the 35th anniversary of HIV/AIDS

PREVIEW

An individual's decision to adopt health behaviors is influenced by socially ingrained distal and proximal environmental influences as well as their personal characteristics. As is evident in this quote from former President Obama, these environmental influences may be strongly embedded social factors that have profound impact on health behavior and thus disease. Social cognitive theory contends that the triad of behavior, the environment (social, physical, economic, legal/policy), and the individual form a reciprocal web of causation that, when understood, can be used to construct changes and intervention programs that will ultimately lead to improved public health.

OBJECTIVES

1. Understand the five key constructs of social cognitive theory and be able to apply each one in the context of a health-promotion program.
2. Explain reciprocal triadic causation and describe the implications of this to health-promotion practice.
3. Describe the threefold stepwise implementation model and explain how key social.
4. Cognitive principles would be employed in each of the three levels.

▶ Introduction

Thus far in this text, you have been introduced to highly structured theories with well-articulated constructs and well-specified interrelationships. In contrast, social cognitive theory (SCT), one of the most valuable assets in the field of health behavior, asserts in general terms that the environment (social, physical, economic, legal/policy) and the personal characteristics of the individual interact with behavior in a reciprocal fashion. This interaction, while ostensibly straightforward, can be complex; however, this is a key strength of SCT.

Historically, it is important to note that SCT evolved from Albert Bandura's social learning theory. Albert Bandura, a highly acclaimed psychologist whose career has spanned seven decades and who initially pioneered innovative research examining the foundations of human learning, first developed social learning theory to explain the basic process of learning. He suggested that learning occurs within a social context and involves observing the behaviors of others, modeling those behaviors, being reinforced for performing these behaviors, and basic cognition pertaining to the behaviors. In essence, social learning theory suggests that people learn new behaviors through observing others, imitating their behavior, and then being reinforced by the observed outcomes of the behavior. For example, a robust research literature has shown that adolescents who are exposed to televised violence are more likely to engage in aggressive behavior and commit violent acts. This occurs as a consequence of observation, modeling and reinforcement.

Bandura later expanded social learning theory to suggest that the social context, the larger environmental factors, the individual, and the individual's behavior are intertwined—this expansion was termed social cognitive theory. SCT was not developed specifically to explain health behaviors per se, although it has been applied effectively to a range of health behaviors. The elegance of SCT in the context of the new public health (see Chapter 1) lies in its inherent assumption that nearly all human behavior is influenced by the immediate social environment in which the behavior occurs. In the words of Bandura (2004, p. 143), "Human health is a social matter, not just an individual one. A comprehensive approach to health promotion also requires changing the practices of social systems that have widespread effects on human health." These social systems may be extremely influential, especially for those health behaviors that occur on daily basis. **BOX 7-1** provides an example relative to obesity.

BOX 7-1 Obesity as a Socially Generated Form of Disease

An eloquent longitudinal study, spanning a period of 32 years and including several thousand people, found incredibly strong evidence suggesting that obesity "spreads" from person-to-person as a function of social ties. This evidence came from a social network analysis, using study volunteers as the "ego" (middle of their own social network) and their friends, siblings, spouses as "alters" (people connected to the ego in a social manner). The impetus for this research was the basic observation that obesity occurs among people of all socioeconomic levels and its spread cannot be explained by genetics. The basic hypothesis set forth by the researchers was that "diverse phenomena can spread within social networks." They further suggested that "evident appearance and behavior of those around them" is likely to be a strong factor in explaining how obesity may spread based on social ties. Their results were compelling. For instance, friendship alters of obese egos had a 57% greater chance of also being obese. If the friendship alter was the same sex, these odds increased to 71%. If the friends were both males, the odds increased to 100%. After investigating two alternative explanations (smoking behaviors and geographic distance between egos and alters), the strength of social ties in explaining the spread of obesity remained unchanged.

Christakis, N. A., Fowler, J. H. (2007). The spread of obesity in a large social network over 32 years. *New Egland Journal of Medicine, 357*, 370–379.

This chapter will provide you with a practical introduction to SCT—one that will enable you to apply key principles of the theory to complex health behaviors, such as obesity. First, we describe the five key constructs of SCT. Next, we explain how these constructs are related to the interaction among person, environment, and behavior. Finally, the chapter concludes by describing a process for implementing SCT in the context of changing people's dietary behaviors. Throughout this chapter, we will emphasize the point that social cognitive approaches to health promotion rely on a multilevel intervention strategy that targets both the person and his/her immediate social environment. Achieving this multilevel intervention approach is perhaps one of the most important challenges in the new public health.

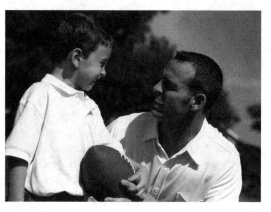

FIGURE 7-1 Parental influence on children
© LiquidLibrary.

▶ Key Concepts

Five Key Constructs of Social Cognitive Theory

Social cognitive theory was developed and has been refined to apply to health behavior by Albert Bandura (1986, 2004). As stated previously, SCT has its origins in social learning theory (a theory used in education and psychology), but the two theories are not the same. The key difference is that SCT is predicated on the concept that the social environment is a central influence on behavior, making personal characteristics alone an inadequate explanation of health behaviors. For example, a central learning environment for children is the home, where the family exerts a strong influence on many behaviors, including what children wear (see **FIGURE 7-1**).

SCT is broad in scope and entire textbooks have been devoted to this theory. Scholars in the social and behavioral sciences would, no doubt, debate whether SCT could be conceptualized by understanding only five constructs. However, it is important to know that these five constructs stem from a landmark article authored by Bandura (2004), which specifically examined SCT in the context of health promotion.

The five key constructs are:

- Knowledge
- Perceived self-efficacy
- Outcome expectations
- Goal formation
- Sociostructural factors

Knowledge

According to Bandura, **knowledge** is a precondition for behavior change. This is a relatively simple idea and one that is quite easy to accept. For example, people who become aware that certain foods and food additives may cause cancer (e.g., artificial sweeteners, nitrosamines, foods high in saturated fats) clearly have a foundation for behavior change. Whether these same people will actually avoid eating some of these foods is, of course, a whole different question. Thus, like the construct of information in the information–motivation–behavioral skills (IMB) model (see Chapter 4), knowledge is viewed as a "gateway" that must be passed before more complex personal and social issues come into play. Indeed, an old adage in health behavior is that "knowledge is a necessary, but not sufficient, basis for

An old adage in health behavior is that "knowledge is a necessary, but not sufficient, basis for behavior change."

behavior change." It is worth bearing in mind that massive public efforts are devoted to this task. Countless media campaigns, billboards, pamphlets/ brochures, and posters have been designed specifically to enhance the public's knowledge about the risk and protective factors relevant to chronic and infectious disease prevention (see **FIGURE 7-2**).

One good way of thinking about knowledge acquisition is as a fundamental starting point for all health-promotion programs.

Bandura (1986) also distinguishes different types of knowledge. In the context of health promotion, **content knowledge** involves understanding the advantages and drawbacks of a given health behavior, though this represents a minimal awareness only. The more advanced type of knowledge, **procedural knowledge**, involves understanding how to engage in a given health behavior.

A good example of procedural knowledge is learning how to recognize the food additives (shown in the required listing of ingredients) that are implicated in cancer development. Learning how to prepare meals that are both low in saturated or trans fats and delicious would be another example of procedural knowledge relevant to cancer prevention. Again, however, knowing how to do something and actually doing it (especially on a regular basis) are two very different things. Procedural knowledge is, nonetheless, a critical point to consider in health-promotion programs (see also

Chapter 11 regarding diffusion of innovations theory). Thinking sequentially, a health-promotion program using SCT as a guide would begin by creating awareness of the health behavior and proceed to building levels of procedural knowledge.

Perceived Self-Efficacy

The next step is to provide people with the confidence and ability they need to actually adopt the health-protective behavior, known as **perceived self-efficacy**. Perceived self-efficacy is perhaps the most widely known theoretical construct in the field of health behavior. Perceived self-efficacy is a person's perception of his or her ability to perform a specific behavior. Procedural knowledge of how to perform a specific behavior, especially when the behavior is moderately to extremely complex, can set the stage for increased perceived self-efficacy.

It is vital to understand that self-efficacy is **task-specific**. This means, for example, that one person may have a strong sense of self-efficacy for a given health behavior such as exercising, but may have a very weak sense of self-efficacy when it comes to eating healthy foods. Consider the case of an overweight woman who wants to lose weight. She may love cooking and may devote quite a lot of time and effort to preparing food, so when presented with the content knowledge that eating a vegetable-rich diet may be a highly effective method of weight loss, she could quickly and easily acquire the procedural knowledge (i.e., various recipes that show how to cook vegetarian meals) needed to enhance her sense of self-efficacy to prepare healthy, vegetable-rich meals. Alternatively, when presented with content knowledge about the weight-loss benefits of aerobic exercise without adequate procedural knowledge, she may fail to perceive an ability to begin a program of regular workouts; this low level of self-efficacy effectively precludes any further progression on her part toward this second method of weight control.

> *Perceived self-efficacy is a person's perception of his or her ability to perform a specific behavior.*

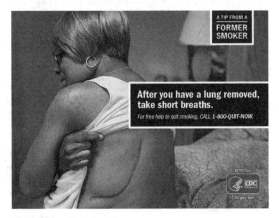

FIGURE 7-2 Media campaign to raise awareness of tobacco risks

Reproduced from CDC.

It is also worth noting that self-efficacy is indeed a **perception**. As you can imagine, perceptions that people hold may or may not mirror reality. A person, for example, may perceive low self-efficacy for the protective behavior of being vaccinated against influenza. This person may have low literacy and fear that he/she cannot fill out the required forms to receive the vaccine, when in reality, the few questions presented on the form may be asked orally and literacy issues can be circumvented when receiving the vaccine. However, in the absence of sufficient self-efficacy, this person may never present himself/herself for the flu vaccine, making the perception the more important factor from a health-promotion viewpoint.

A vignette may be useful to understanding the vital role of perceived self-efficacy. Consider the use of natural family planning (a method of birth control). This method is somewhat complicated to use as it involves charting (on a calendar) a woman's menstrual cycle and using these dates to estimate the likely day of ovulation. Once an ovulation date is estimated, the couple can use that date to plan "safe" days for coital activity. The method can also involve the tactile inspection of the woman's cervical mucus, with a thinning of this mucus being a sign of pending ovulation. Other signs of ovulation, such as changes in body temperature, can also be used as part of this birth control method.

One common problem in the promotion of natural family planning is that women may not have faith in their ability to accurately pinpoint their ovulation dates, and they may further lack the belief that they and/or their male sex partners can reliably abstain from intercourse during "high-risk" days. Until this belief is effectively reversed and women can feel they do indeed have the ability to track their menstrual cycles and control coition on risky days, they are quite unlikely to pursue this behavior. From an SCT viewpoint, the health-promotion challenge in this example is to provide women (and perhaps their male sex partners) with the confidence and ability needed to create a level of perceived self-efficacy that is sufficiently high enough to prompt women to adopt this birth control method.

From an SCT perspective, low self-efficacy generates fleeting or no efforts to perform a given behavior. In the preceding vignette, you can easily imagine that a couple may adopt the use of natural family planning only to abandon the method entirely after a few months. Like all behaviors, the initial period of adoption is unlikely to be smooth or seamless, and the consequent frustration is likely to trigger the abandonment. This is precisely why your health-promotion program should vigorously strive to instill lasting perceived self-efficacy in the people in your target population.

It is important for health-promotion programs to accommodate differences in self-efficacy levels because the range in a population is likely to be broad. For example, there might be a great deal of variance in levels of self-efficacy to abstain from alcohol during a keg party on a college campus. In this case, it is easy to imagine that low self-efficacy, at best, would translate into relatively meager attempts at not drinking. For many students, this low self-efficacy may translate into a complete lack of attempt to abstain from alcohol.

As you can see, the construct of perceived self-efficacy is extremely relevant to the adoption and maintenance of health behaviors that may not always be easy to perform. In essence, strong self-efficacy is a belief that an individual can perform a health-protective behavior even under adverse circumstances. Sometimes referred to as **resilient self-efficacy**, the concept of perseverance even when conditions are not ideal is vital simply because so many health-protective behaviors occur under difficult circumstances. A common example is healthy eating. While most of the time eating a healthy diet may be relatively easy to accomplish, during holidays, business travel, or eating out with friends, it may be extremely challenging. Here are several other examples of health behaviors that

> *The concept of perseverance even when conditions are not ideal is vital simply because so many health-protective behaviors occur under difficult circumstances.*

may be difficult to maintain under certain challenging circumstances:

- Consuming a low-sodium diet
- Consuming a diet low in refined sugars
- Consuming a diet low in saturated fats
- Smoking cessation
- Reduced consumption of alcohol
- Engaging in regular aerobic exercise routines
- Eating a high-fiber diet to prevent colorectal cancer
- Avoiding food additives that may cause cancer
- Using nonhormonal contraceptives

Upon careful and critical reflection of these examples, you may conclude that this list is incomplete. For example, you might ask, "How do these concepts apply to something as simple as hand-washing, but in the context of a place where clean water is not readily available?" Indeed, the potential for challenging circumstances surrounding any given health-protective practice is often a function of the supporting environment. The environmental context may even be financial. Having a Pap test, for example, may be a relatively simple health-protective behavior among women with health insurance; however, for uninsured women, this simple behavior becomes fraught with adversity. The same might be true for women living in highly isolated rural areas who have limited ability to travel to a city that has a gynecological clinic. Medication compliance is yet another example. People who lead relatively stable lives may be able to take a given drug at regular intervals during the day, but people living more chaotic lives (homeless people, for example) may find that such compliance poses overwhelming challenges.

Before we proceed with this discussion of perceived self-efficacy, it is critical to note that any given health behavior may require several distinct skills, and thus perceived self-efficacy may not be uniform across these various skill requirements. Using the vignette as an example, you can see that natural family planning involves multiple skills that are quite distinct: (1) charting the menstrual cycle, (2) using math to pinpoint the day of ovulation, (3) feeling the viscosity of the cervical mucus, (4) reliably measuring and recording daily body temperatures, (5) abstaining from coitus on risky days, and (6) communicating or negotiating with one's sex partner about when to have sex. Thus, when measuring and promoting perceived self-efficacy for the adoption of this birth control method, you can readily see that overall self-efficacy actually breaks down into finer gradients of behavior.

The utility of self-efficacy as SCT construct is that it is very amenable to intervention efforts. According to SCT, people can and do increase their perceptions of self-efficacy based on four methods of learning; **FIGURE 7-3** illustrates these four methods. As shown, the first method refers to one's physiological state. Learning to diminish fear and other negative emotions that may be associated with performing a given health-protective behavior is the goal. For many people, a good example is going to the dentist. The fear of pain alone may preclude people from having strong self-efficacy for something as seemingly benign as a cleaning and checkup. Overcoming these fears and learning to control one's corresponding somatic reactions (e.g., increased blood pressure, pulse, sweating) can be viewed as a basic method in building self-efficacy for receiving dental care.

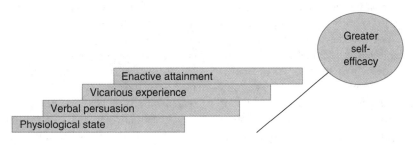

FIGURE 7-3 Four methods of learning

Verbal persuasion is a second method of building self-efficacy. As the label implies, the intent here is to convince people that they can indeed perform a given health-protective behavior. Bandura (1986, p. 400) suggests that these efforts will have their "greatest impact on people who have some reason to believe that they can produce effects through their actions," meaning that verbal persuasion will be more effective when a person can easily modify self-efficacy. Bandura also warns that verbal persuasion beyond a person's actual ability will quite likely be counterproductive.

Applied to health promotion, you can probably imagine settings where verbal persuasion is used and is appropriate. For instance, group-based interventions, such as those used in teen pregnancy prevention programs or in organized weight loss programs (e.g., Weight Watchers), may include activities that will verbally persuade participants that they can talk with their mom about contraception or they can resist the temptations to consume high-calorie foods.

The next method shown in Figure 7-3 is **vicarious experience**. Stated simply, people learn by watching others perform a given behavior; if the given behavior is performed successfully, feedback to the observer may inform their self-efficacy perceptions. Vicarious learning is especially influential on self-efficacy perceptions when people are unsure about their ability (**FIGURE 7-4**). This form of learning is maximized when people observe someone quite similar to themselves successfully performing (or not successfully performing) a given health-protective behavior. Indeed, this theoretical premise is the basis for the use of peer-to-peer teaching models in health-promotion efforts and also health-promotion interventions utilizing media (Romer et al., 2009). The behavior of forcefully taking away a would-be drunk driver's keys is a cornerstone of preventing alcohol-induced auto fatalities. This action is widely advocated to college students, but the behavior is fraught with complications; thus, students may or may not attempt it depending on their perceived self-efficacy (and their level of persistence will vary as a function of self-efficacy). Although verbal persuasion from a campus alcohol prevention program may be somewhat effective at promoting this behavior, that

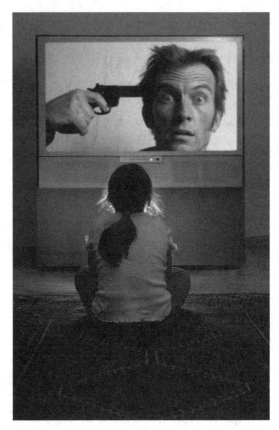

FIGURE 7-4 Vicarious learning in children
© Maica/Vetta/Getty Images

same program might be more effective by showing students a video that portrays a person successfully getting the car keys away from a drunken friend.

Another effective approach, if possible, would be to have a student who successfully performed this delicate behavior describe the experience to the other students (a form of peer teaching). The identification that students have with the student in the video or the speaker (the peer teacher) creates a compelling reason to believe something like, "If he can do it, then so can I." The direct observation of another person performing the behavior is, of course, the most powerful way to learn vicariously. Unfortunately, this is often not possible in connection with so many health-protective behaviors (e.g., condom application, sexual negotiations).

The final and most effective method shown in Figure 7-3 is **enactive attainment**. Enactive attainment is physically guiding or coaching someone through the behavior. We (the authors) have used this method of coaching behavior to affect self-efficacy in many of our interventions designed to increase condom use. Using a penile model, we instruct young people how to correctly apply a condom, then we talk them through the process as they physically perform the behavior, giving them feedback on their mistakes and success as they go. Without enactive attainment, even motivated people may become frustrated and cease trying to use condoms.

People's self-efficacy perceptions are naturally shaped by their experience of effort followed by success or effort followed by failure. Here, however, it is important to note that success and failure are also perceptions. Moreover, it may not always be readily apparent to people whether their efforts succeeded. This is particularly true with health behaviors. For example, a man on the edge of developing hypertension may diligently consume what he believes to be a low-sodium diet (on a daily basis for several weeks), but he may or may not see a corresponding drop in his blood pressure; this makes it quite difficult for this man to objectively know if he has been consuming a low-sodium diet (as so many food products have hidden sodium).

The practical implication in this regard is that health-promotion efforts should structure success experiences for people adopting new behaviors, and these structures should attempt to objectify "winning." Bandura (1986, p. 399) noted that failure experiences early in the process of adopting a behavior are especially damaging to self-efficacy. Again, a clear implication for health promotion in this regard is to provide structured success experiences (i.e., enactive attainment), for people who are initially making efforts to adopt a behavior. Indeed, the initial adoption effort may best be viewed as a fragile period that can benefit greatly from intervention attempts. For instance, La Leche League, an international organization, is dedicated to the promotion of breastfeeding. One of their services is to have a volunteer physically assist new mothers during their first attempts to nurse their newborns. These efforts are quite consistent with enactive attainment, as the intervention occurs at a critical point in mothers' shaping of their self-efficacy perceptions regarding breastfeeding (**FIGURE 7-5**).

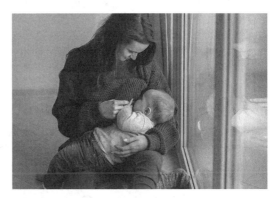

FIGURE 7-5 Building self-efficacy for seemingly simple health behaviors is vital to public health
© Romanova Anna/Shutterstock

A final point about self-efficacy is warranted. **Behavioral capacity** is the actual ability a person has to perform a given behavior. Self-efficacy and a person's actual behavioral capacity may often be misaligned, meaning that self-efficacy may sometimes be higher than actual ability. In this scenario, performance of the behavior is limited by behavioral capacity rather than self-efficacy, and the important implication for health behavior is that intervention efforts must focus on increasing both self-efficacy and behavioral capacity. This is precisely why teaching people the requisite skills to perform a given health behavior is so vital to the success of health-promotion programs (see **FIGURE 7-6**).

> *A clear implication for health promotion in this regard is to provide structured success experiences.*

Outcome Expectations

If you think about self-efficacy as one of the engines on a figurative jet moving toward long-term adoption of health-protective behavior, the engine propelling the other side of the jet would be **outcome expectations**. Favorable perceived self-efficacy is only half of the behavior change equation, and it may not be sufficient for a person to change or adopt a health behavior. Before behavior change occurs, there must be a sufficiently strong belief that

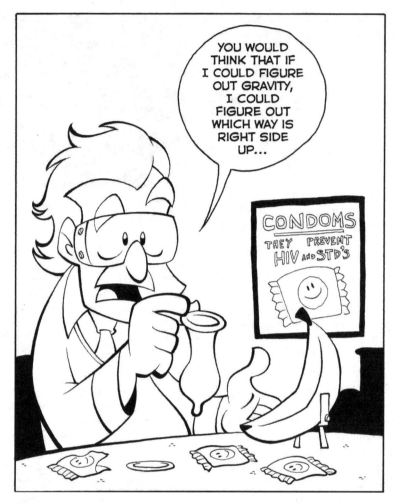

FIGURE 7-6 Even seemingly simple health behaviors may be complex to members of the target audience
Copyright 2011 by Justin Wagner; reprinted with permission.

the health behavior will "pay off" in either the short term or long term. Outcome expectations are the anticipated positive outcomes that stem from engaging in the behavior; in other words, the belief that if I do X, then Y will happen. One example would be, "If I use a condom, then I will avoid getting HIV."

Although self-efficacy must be strong, outcome expectations must also be favorable enough to help propel the person into action. For some health behaviors, the outcome expectation is linked to perceived self-efficacy level, meaning that the perceived anticipated outcome is a function of how adequately the health behavior can be performed.

For example, with the belief that, "If I can use a condom correctly, then I will avoid getting HIV," a successful outcome relies heavily on correctly performing a behavior. Of note, both self-efficacy and outcome expectations are based on perceptions; thus, each is amenable to intervention.

Perceptions of outcome expectations can be influenced by vicarious learning. Just as self-efficacy can be improved through vicarious learning, the same is true regarding one's beliefs in a positive outcome following the behavior. For example, suppose a young woman who frequently smokes cigarettes, observes that her close friend recently quit smoking, and in doing so dramatically improved her smile (the yellow stains subsided). The outcome expectation (quitting will lead to a sexier smile) in this case was learned vicariously. Notice, however, that this example was not based on the well-established physiological benefits of smoking cessation (e.g., less LDL cholesterol production, improved oxygenation of red blood cells, less blood platelet adherence to artery walls) because these outcomes are not readily or easily observable. Indeed, when applying SCT to health behaviors, one of the greatest challenges lies in helping people develop positive outcome expectations for behaviors that produce long-term, rather than short-term, benefits.

For many health behaviors, there is no need to rely on vicarious learning to acquire positive outcome expectations simply because the positive outcome can be experienced as a direct and immediate consequence of the behavior. The endorphin "high" that runners experience during and immediately after a good run sets up a positive outcome expectation for the next run. The sense of satisfaction and self-control that a person experiences when turning down offers of high-calorie foods sets up a positive outcome expectation for the next opportunity to forego this oral pleasure in favor of feeling good about oneself. Again, the intervention implications suggest that outcome expectations can be structured in health-education/health-promotion programs so that people perceive a worthwhile reason for expending their effort. This is similar to expected net gain—that is weighing pros and cons—in the health belief model (see Chapter 5).

As you might imagine, the social environment is also important in shaping perceived outcome expectations. Although altering people's perceptions about personal outcomes is a worthy endeavor, outcomes that are social in nature may be perceived as more meaningful. Consider that an individual may perceive that engaging in the health behavior of altering their diet and exercising will have the anticipated outcome of lowering their blood serum cholesterol levels. However, in the past few decades, the positive outcomes of these health behaviors have been socially expanded, and now people who are watching their cholesterol are considered healthy and responsible, and people who are runners are viewed as role models for others. Additionally, health and life insurance companies give better rates to people testing lower for LDL cholesterol and with better overall cholesterol levels. All of these outcomes are quite likely to have sufficient strength to drive continued diet and exercise behaviors; however, it is worth noting that these outcomes were socially engineered. While a medical doctor, for instance, may congratulate a patient for lowering his or her cholesterol level by 10 points, the clinical significance of this outcome may be quite small in the larger picture of risk for heart disease and stroke. Herein lies the ultimate paradox in prevention: it is difficult to convince people their actions are paying off because seemingly nothing (as in no heart attack or stroke) is happening. Thus, health-promotion efforts have created shorter-term, highly observable surrogates to the longer-term and more elusive outcome expectations that may actually be of physical value.

A streamlined method of thinking about outcome expectations is shown in **FIGURE 7-7**.

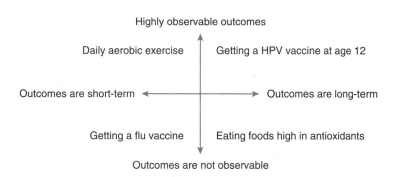

FIGURE 7-7 A matrix of outcome expectations

The figure depicts two bipolar continuums shown in a perpendicular fashion. The vertical continuum in the figure is the level of observability; in this case, observability means the ability to learn through watching outcomes happening to others (vicarious learning), as well as learning directly through personal experience. The horizontal continuum is the level of immediacy (short-term vs. long-term). Simply stated, outcome expectations may be highly observable and immediate (ideal circumstances for behavior change) or not observable and long-term (extremely challenging circumstances for behavior change). It could be argued that relatively long-term outcomes that are nonetheless observable may be only modestly challenging for health-promotion efforts, because surrogate short-term outcomes (as was exemplified by the cholesterol example) may be socially structured. In this situation, vicarious learning that demonstrates the long-term outcome may also occur.

Figure 7-7 can be used to gauge the difficulty of changing a given health behavior. The most challenging behaviors will be those found in the lower-right quadrant. Consider the daily behavior of eating foods that are high in antioxidants (properties of foods that may prevent cancer). There is no observable benefit to this daily health behavior and the outcomes are extremely long term, so reinforcement through a tangible physical benefit for the behavior is entirely lacking. Conversely, behaviors located in the upper-left corner are relatively easy to change because their benefits are quickly observable. For example, for most people only a few weeks of regular aerobic exercise will produce a noticeable increase in daily energy and alertness, and these readily noticeable effects may even include desired weight loss. This figure is important to consider when planning a health-promotion program, in that the targeted behaviors may have long-term, but not readily observable, outcomes; thus, they may or may not be readily amenable to change. For those behaviors characterized by the lower-right quadrant (e.g., reduced saturated fat intake to avoid heart disease and stroke, increased vegetable consumption to protect against colorectal cancer, calcium

supplements to avoid osteoporosis), more intensive interventions efforts will be required.

Outcome expectations can also include negative perceptions. Globally, it is not uncommon for women attempting to negotiate condom use with a resistant male partner to be physically abused for doing so. People who smoke have probably observed the weight gain that most often occurs for people who have recently quit. The Internet has created a media environment that magnifies the extremely small number of adverse vaccine-related events and, as a consequence, people may perceive that flu vaccines, HPV vaccines, or other vaccines can be painful, debilitating, or even deadly. The prospect of developing chronic joint pain as a consequence of high impact aerobic exercise (e.g., running on pavement, tennis, contact sports) is a realistic perception of "cost" for people considering the outcome expectations of this repeated form of exercise. Addressing and minimizing negative expectations, as you might imagine, is therefore a primary obligation of any health-promotion program. **BOX 7-2** provides an example related to negative perceptions about the HPV vaccine, held by parents of adolescent females.

At this point in discussing SCT, we want introduce the concept of **expectancies** and how *expectancies* differ from *expectations* in SCT. Expectancies entail the expectation that Y will occur following X and a positive or negative value attached to Y.

Some people may value an outcome more than others. In our experience of teaching SCT to students, we typically find that confusion between the two terms is commonplace—understandably so, considering how similar the two terms are. One strategy that may help is to think about the last several letters in the term expectancies ("ncies") and try to find the word "nices." If something is considered "nice," then there is a value attached. Stated differently, expectancies include the personal evaluation of anticipated outcome.

The concept of expectancies' "nices" is relevant to the concept of **reinforcement**. Reinforcement is the final aspect of outcome expectations

BOX 7-2 Are Negative Outcome Expectations a Factor for Parents in Having Daughters Vaccinated Against Human Papillomavirus?

A study of parents with adolescent daughters found that negative expectations regarding the vaccine against human Papillomavirus (HPV) were the strongest predictor of whether their daughters had begun the vaccine series or parents intended for them to do so. Negative expectations included medical side effects of the vaccine itself and the notion that girls having the vaccine would be more likely to engage in sex. The path coefficient (this is just a value between 0.00 and 1.00, with larger numbers meaning a greater level of association) for the association between having negative expectations and uptake/intent was 0.39 while the coefficient between perceived vaccine effectiveness and uptake/intent was only 0.23. The 0.39 coefficient was inverse, meaning that as the level of negative expectations increased, the odds of uptake/intent decreased. Negative expectations rivaled the strength of association between provider recommendation (traditionally an exceedingly strong predictor of HPV vaccine uptake/intent) and uptake/intent. The study provided clear and compelling evidence that HPV vaccine promotion efforts directed towards parents of adolescent daughter must begin by addressing and rectifying their negative expectations about having their daughters received the HPV vaccine.

Dayal, K., Robinson, S., Schoening, J., Smith, M. C., & Kim, S. C. (2017). Predictors of human Papillomavirus vaccine uptake or intention among parents of preadolescents and adolescents. *Journal of Nursing Education and Practice, 7*(6), 35–42.

that we will address in this chapter; it can take the form of adding something good (**positive**) or subtracting something bad (**negative**) and always involves an increase in the behavior. Regardless of whether the reinforcement is positive or negative, reinforcement usually takes the form of experiencing tangible and immediate benefits for performing a behavior.

Positive reinforcement generally involves a perceived reward following the behavior; thus, the behavior will be repeated in the future. These rewards may be socially constructed; examples include organizations that reward weight loss with applause (social approval), insurance companies that reward smoking cessation with a policy discount, and employers who reward "perfect health" (absence of sick days) with financial bonuses. When positive reinforcements are socially structured, they are termed **extrinsic**. Conversely, positive reinforcements may be **intrinsic**, meaning they are not socially structured. Examples include the previously mentioned "runner's high," as well personal rewards experienced for outcomes such as losing weight (increased satisfaction with body image) or controlling hypertension through diet (less reliance on hypertension medication).

Negative reinforcement takes the form of removing something that people classify as undesirable. A good example is using contraception. For many people of reproductive age, one immediate outcome of using highly reliable contraceptive methods is substantially less concern during sex about becoming pregnant or causing a pregnancy. The reinforcing effect of the outcome is the removal (hence, negative) of something that is not wanted, and so the overall consequence is considered good. Bandura suggested that health-promotion programs use extrinsic reinforcement (positive or negative) only as an initial method of structuring valued outcome expectancies in people, as a drawback of long-term reliance on extrinsic reinforcements is that they may disappear (as would be the case if insurance companies stopped providing discounts to people for smoking cessation). Structuring health-promotion programs to set up intrinsically reinforced behavior patterns should also be utilized as a promising strategy for lasting behavior change.

Before introducing you to the next construct, we would like you to take a look back at the constructs of self-efficacy and outcome expectations in a combined fashion. Remember our dual jet

The reinforcing effect of the outcome is the removal (hence, negative) of something that is not wanted, and so the overall consequence is considered good.

engine analogy? Two jet engines working together determine the speed of the jet. In SCT, these two constructs work together to determine the **level of motivation** a person may experience relative to the potential adoption of a health-protective behavior. Think about this in relation to adopting a low-sodium diet in hopes of controlling borderline hypertension (in lieu of using medication). Once a person has a sufficient level of knowledge about the health condition (hypertension) and procedural knowledge about the health-protective behavior (consuming a low-sodium diet), he or she may still be a long way from making the dietary changes needed to achieve a clinically significant drop in dietary sodium. Clearly, the next step is acquiring a sense of motivation. SCT contends that motivation is the product of expectancies and self-efficacy and involves a person's answer to two questions: (1) "Will adopting the health-protective behavior reliably lead to a valued outcome?" and (2) "Can I realistically perform the necessary behaviors?" People with doubts about an affirmative answer to either question are not likely to attempt adopting the behavior. This makes sense, in that people simply see no reason to invest in change without a payoff and they see no reason to make a reasonable attempt at change if they have a low level of perceived self-efficacy for that behavior. As such, the person must be convinced that controlling hypertension though a low-sodium diet will work, is valuable, and that he/she has the ability to achieve and maintain the low-sodium diet. Once this level of motivation is experienced, the person is ready to formulate goals.

Goal Formation

According to the principles of SCT, behavior change is best achieved by breaking goals down into a progressive series of subgoals (Bandura, 1986). Applied to health, this principle typically implies that well-defined and easy-to-measure behaviors should be the subgoals that lead to a grander (but perhaps elusive) behavioral change goal. The control of diabetes serves as a good example of the difference between goals and subgoals. For a diabetic, a diet-induced, clinically significant decline in otherwise elevated blood sugar levels represents an admirable goal. This diet-induced overall decline in blood sugar, however, is a product of a daily battle of willpower versus an overwhelming selection of tempting foods that are high in refined sugar. The goal may be beyond someone's capacity to envision, thereby not sufficient to create behavior change. Guiding the efforts of the diabetic, a health educator may help this person formulate daily subgoals that are defined by measurable behaviors rather than the outcome of glucose test. Daily subgoals may include eating less than two servings of carbohydrates, not consuming any food classified as a dessert, and consuming at least 50% of their daily calories in the form of protein. Each day, this person can measure achievement of the three subgoals, and so each day the person has a potential to reach their overarching goals. In this scenario, self-efficacy perceptions are likely to increase and the experience of positive outcomes sets up subsequent behavioral efforts for the next day. The subgoals may not have a clinical benefit per se; however, they serve to enhance a person's self-efficacy and expectancies, thereby motivating the continued behavior that will eventually lead to clinically meaningful outcomes.

The subgoals may not have a clinical benefit per se; however, they serve to enhance a person's self-efficacy and expectancies, thereby motivating the continued behavior that will eventually lead to clinically meaningful outcomes.

Sociostructural Factors

Goal attainment through motivated behavior (positive outcome expectancies combined with sufficient levels of perceived self-efficacy) is a function of the supporting factors, as well as the impeding factors, of a person's environment. Stated another way, the world people live in enables and limits their ability to effectively engage in goal-directed behavior. Again, a vignette may be helpful.

Imagine a relatively poor region of rural America where people have traditionally consumed diets high in fat and refined carbo-hydrates (soda, white bread, cakes, biscuits, etc.). Imagine also that the relative geographic isolation from urbanized centers necessitates a small string of grocery stores scattered through-out the area. Each of these small grocery stores serves relatively few people, thereby causing a high risk of financial loss to the owners who opt to stock foods with a short shelf life, such as fresh produce. People in this area commonly develop diabetes, heart disease, and colorectal can-cer (three likely outcomes of a high-fat, highly refined diet). Although they may be exposed to public health campaigns (e.g., the Centers for Disease Control and Prevention's *5-A-Day* campaign) and as a result feel a need to change their diet to protect their health, the challenges imposed by the cultural and physical environ-ment make it difficult. The self-efficacy equa-tion is much different for these rural residents as compared to people living in a suburban Cal-ifornia town where local norms support healthy eating and fresh foods are widely available and largely affordable. Enhancing self-efficacy in a rural area would have to include altering the perception and suggesting that a person can defy long-standing customs by not eating fat-laden, and sugar-laden meals at least twice each day. It would also include altering perceptions of being able to find and obtain fresh produce during months of the year when local gardens are not producing food. In the absence of a critical mass of like-minded healthy eaters, the rural person may even find that obtaining procedural knowl-edge about preparing healthy foods is a difficult task. Moreover, socially structured reinforce-ment for eating low-fat protein alternatives and consuming nonprocessed foods that are high in fiber may be entirely absent. As you can quickly see in this brief example, motivated behavior change among people in a rural area may not be well supported.

At this point you have observed several parallels between these five key constructs of SCT and other theoretical constructs. This fifth construct (sociostructural factors) is parallel to the concept of perceived behavioral control in the theory of planned behavior (see Chap-ter 4). Furthermore, you should be able to see clear evidence of a value–expectancy approach in the part of this chapter that introduced the construct of outcome expectations. Outcome expectancies ("nices," or the expectation plus the person's evaluation of "good versus bad") in SCT parlance are similar to the attitudes construct in the theory of reasoned action/theory of planned behavior.

Reciprocal Triadic Causation

Reciprocal triadic causation is perhaps the single most important aspect of SCT as applied to health promotion. The concept (see **FIGURE 7-8**) is seem-ingly simple but becomes a bit complicated upon further exploration. As shown in Figure 7-8, the triad consists of the environment, the person, and the behavior.

In reviewing this figure, let's start with the environment. Specifically, let's consider the line extending from the environment to behavior. The environment represents any social, eco-nomic, policy, legal, or physical influence that can act on behavior. The strength of this influ-ence is not difficult to understand, as shown by the multiple examples that have already been provided in this chapter and throughout this text, though some additional examples include

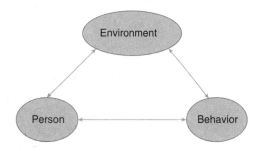

FIGURE 7-8 Reciprocal triadic causation

state programs that provide free vaccines to children; local, state, and federal laws that prohibit smoking in public places; cultural norms that shape eating behaviors; taxes on alcohol to curb drinking; and redesigning public streets and sidewalks to make walking more accessible and safer. So, at this point, your logical questions should be, "Why is the arrow bidirectional, indicating that behavior influences environment?" The forthcoming answer is your introduction to the concept of reciprocality. At both an individual level and a collective level, people do indeed shape their environments. The most obvious example is when a person selects his or her environment. Consider, for instance, a person who moves to a city to (in part) enjoy the health benefits they perceive to be abundant there. U.S. cities like San Diego, CA, Seattle, WA, and Burlington, VT are well known for their built environments relative to fitness and their cultural and physical supports for alternative foods that constitute a heart-healthy diet. In this case, the person's influence on the new environment is that he or she joins an existing group of people, thereby magnifying and supporting these fitness- and diet-enabling macrostructures. At the collective level, SCT suggests that people shape the environment, which in turn shapes the people. (At this point you can see why the term "reciprocal" is used in SCT.) Consider a scenario that has been and is currently being played out in many U.S. cities: the creation and passage of environmental tobacco smoke (ETS) laws. These laws are often opposed by avid smokers and by those who profit tremendously from the sale of tobacco. Given these factors, a rather large number of citizens are needed to effectively lobby for passage of ETS laws. Bandura has termed a community's perceived ability to shape the environment **collective self-efficacy** (1998). Even with these barriers, through lobbying efforts and advocacy, ETS laws have been passed successfully in many states and counties across the United States. As a result, fewer teens and young adults have started to smoke and there is less prevalence of smoking. With their passage and implementation, these ETS laws illustrate the

reciprocal action between individuals and their effect on the environment.

Next, let's consider the line from the environment to the person. Here, it is important to define what constitutes the "person" in Bandura's model of reciprocal triadic causation. The person in this model represents the sum of all cognitive attributes, many of which you know about already (e.g., self-efficacy, outcome expectations, outcome expectancies). A good example of environment-to-person influence would be an environmental factor such as a policy or law having an effect on a teen female's level of self-efficacy to obtain birth control pills. In a nation such as the Netherlands, the applicable policy and social environments largely support this behavior, making it relatively simple; this is in contrast to the United States, where these types of supports are lacking.

Another example would be the behavior of people beginning to eat a low-fat diet to prevent heart disease. In some social settings, positive extrinsic reinforcement, such as social recognition and praise, for eating a vegetarian diet would be abundant, whereas other social settings might lack any social reinforcement of this behavior, and still others may actually view the behavior as odd or deviant. Thus, depending on the context, the environment can either promote healthy eating through availability and social norms or it could hamper such efforts.

The environment can also have a tremendous influence on outcome expectancies. For example, the outcome expectation of being overweight as a consequence of not eating healthy food may be valued very differently by men versus women or by urban versus rural populations. For men, being overweight might not matter as much, but for women it may matter a great deal, mainly due to gender stereotypes. In an urban area where socioeconomic status is reflected by how thin you are, not being overweight may be of greater importance than in a rural area where there is more homogeneity and being overweight is the norm.

Next, consider the arrow extending from the person to the environment. In this case, the arrow can only be understood by thinking about people (collectively) rather than a person (individually). In essence, the collective cognitions of a community or society define the sociocultural environment. For example, when a community of young gay men all begin to view HIV/AIDS as a medically manageable disease (much like diabetes), that view creates a sociocultural environment. In turn, that environment may influence outcome expectancies among community members relative to behaviors such as condom use. Please recall that outcome expectations are value-free and outcome expectancies ("nices") are value-laden. Stated differently, only the expectancy takes into account how people feel about the outcome. In this example, people who feel that getting HIV is less threatening will have less compelling outcome expectancies, compared to those who view HIV in a more devastating manner.

Let's look at the bidirectional arrow shown across the bottom of Figure 7-8. First, consider the arrow extending from the person to the behavior. This pathway represents classic psychological theory, in that people's cognitions will dictate their behavior. You may recall that we previously stated that the person represents the sum of all cognitive attributes (e.g., self-efficacy, outcome expectations, and outcome expectancies). A large number of health-promotion efforts have focused solely on altering cognitions to foster behavioral change. However, SCT posits that this single pathway is embedded within the larger context of reciprocal triadic causation and the environment also plays a critical role. An example of how the environment may shape cognition can be found in the concept of "defensible space." Defensible space, a sociological concept, implies that a bounded geographic area can become a type of personalized territory for a social community. Applied to otherwise public urban environments, an example of defensible space is city-owned vacant piece of land. As neighbors to this land begin to "claim" it for their recreation needs, for example, the area becomes branded as a place to play sports, walk, or just be outside on a nice day. In the absence of this

branding, the vacant space may well become a place for the sale/exchange of drugs or sex, with the corresponding levels of people who may be living outside of the law, and perhaps capable of violence. Evidence accumulated since the 1970s in the United States suggests that space that is not defended and branded by an established segment of the law-abiding community will become a place for the perpetration of violence and other crimes (Perkins, Wandersman, Rich, & Taylor, 1993). This concept of the physical environment shaping the perceptions/cognitions/behaviors of people is so powerful that it has been used by urban planners as a method or preventing crime through environmental design.

Next, consider the reciprocal pathway extending from the behavior back to the person—this is somewhat more perplexing. In this pathway, a behavior is posited to influence cognition. This pathway is actually quite common. Think about a time when you engaged in a health behavior with a given outcome expectation in mind and that outcome did not occur. This was most likely a disappointment to you and you may have said to yourself something like, "Why should I do X if Y doesn't happen?" Think about a person who switches to a low-fat diet to lose weight (i.e., the "person" is represented by the outcome expectation). The person may eat a low-fat diet, thus performing the behavior perfectly. But, perhaps as a consequence of their basic physiology, the outcome of the effort does not happen—in other words, they may be cursed with a slow metabolism and therefore did not lose any weight. Consequently, they altered their outcome expectation as a result of engaging in the behavior.

Finally, it is important to understand that reciprocal triadic causation involves all three pathways collectively. For instance, our cursed dieter lives in a nonsupportive environment where high-fat foods are emphasized (see **FIGURE 7-9**) and outcome expectations, in the form of extrinsic positive reinforcement such as social praise from family and friends, may be lacking. Without these outcomes being realized, the person may easily lose interest in repeating

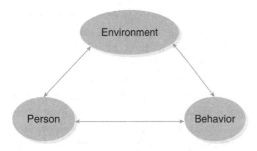

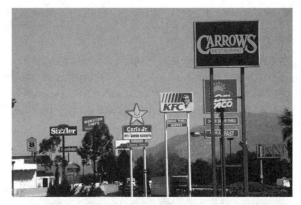

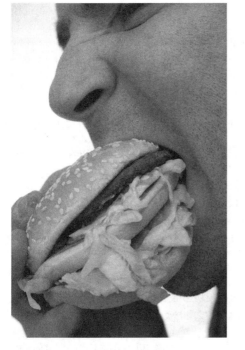

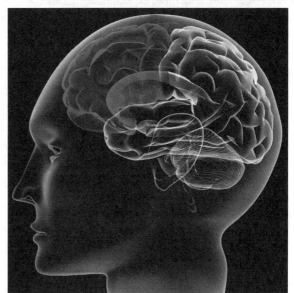

FIGURE 7-9 Example of reciprocal triadic causation

Photos clockwise from top, © Davis Barber/PhotoEdit, Inc., © Wallenrock/Shutterstock, © YAKOBCHUK VASYL/Shutterstock

the behavior day after day and may succumb to eating unhealthy foods. Thus, it is the behavior that led the person to change his or her outcome expectation (a cognition). However, this altering of outcome expectations is less likely to occur in a supportive environment, which provides extrinsic positive reinforcement for the dieting behavior. The triangle, in essence, operates as a whole, never as independent parts. The intervention implications for reciprocal triadic causation are rich, as they include potential changes to the social, political, and economic environment as well as the more traditional cognitive approaches.

Threefold Stepwise Implementation Model

Bandura (2004) distinguished three levels of readiness to adopt a given health behavior. These levels of readiness are quite distinct from the levels that constitute the stage models you learned about in Chapter 6. The primary difference is that Bandura's levels are centered upon self-efficacy and outcome expectations. The utility of the three levels is that they collectively provide guidance into the often overwhelming question of how best to tailor health behavior interventions to a broad range of very different people.

Level One: High Self-Efficacy and Strong Outcome Expectations

People at this level require very little, if any, intervention before they adopt the health behavior that corresponds with their high level of self-efficacy and their strong outcome expectation. Thus, relatively low-intensity intervention efforts may be sufficient to promote the adoption of a given health behavior among people who are already at this advanced level of readiness. Keep in mind, however, that self-efficacy and outcome expectations are very specific constructs—they are far from universal across health behaviors. This means that readiness is a concept that applies to very narrowly defined health behaviors, such as eating a low-sodium diet to prevent or control hypertension, exercising to increase cardiovascular fitness, or eating a low-sugar diet to prevent diabetes. In the context of very specific health-promotion programs (those targeting a single health behavior), relatively simple media messages may be sufficient to move "level one" people from readiness to action. Whether the initial action of these people evolves into long-term maintenance is a question that is most likely dependent on environmental supports for the behavior.

Level Two: Doubts About Self-Efficacy and Weak Outcome Expectations

People at this level are quite obviously distinct from people at the first level and thus their intervention needs are far more intense. For "level two" people, multiple intervention points will be required to move them to level one so that they can then progress to behavior change. Intervention points can be conceived by thinking about reciprocal triadic causation (see Figure 7-6). Intervention at the person level may include efforts to enhance skills and build self-efficacy using the methods shown in Figure 7-3. Intervention at the environmental level (top of Figure 7-6) may include the social creation of surrogate outcomes that can be more quickly realized compared to the long-term physical outcomes that may have initially been the motivation for behavior change.

Level Three: Belief That Personal Control over Behavior Is Lacking

People at this level require intensive intervention before they can progress to level two and eventually to level one. Unlike people at levels one and two, people at this level may hold a universal perception that they are unable to change their health behaviors. The goal here involves **personal agency**. Personal agency is similar to the concept of volitionality as described in Chapter 2 and refers to the larger perception of having any control in performing the behavior. If people do not have a sense of personal agency to perform a behavior, then they will not even try. Personal agency must be established before attempts to enhance self-efficacy and/or outcome expectations can effectively occur. At this point, you should be able to see that the lack of agency is deeply connected to the tenets of triadic reciprocal causation.

Putting It All Together

An all-too-common abuse of SCT is that researchers use isolated parts and pieces of the theory and then claim to have "used SCT." We ask you not to make this mistake in scholarship. Instead, think of SCT as a set

> *If people do not have a sense of personal agency to perform a behavior, then they will not even try.*

of principles that can be used (in varied combinations) to design a health-promotion program for optimal effectiveness. Always think first about planning a program that will use the five key constructs to achieve the adoption of a very specific health behavior. Keep in mind that SCT is not designed for broadly defined behaviors such as avoiding heart disease. Your health-promotion program should always include plans to build self-efficacy and address outcome expectations for those "level two" and "level three" people described in the previous section. Never ignore knowledge (especially procedural knowledge), despite its lack of glamour in the world of health promotion and remember the principles associated with goal attainment. Perhaps most importantly, full consideration of the fifth construct (supporting and impeding factors) invariably leads you to think about the environment and how it is influencing unhealthy behavior, as well as how it can be altered to influence the adoption of health-protective behaviors. When you begin to seriously contemplate these environmental influences, you have made a leap into the realm of reciprocal triadic causation. Making this leap is important and it also carries a tremendously large ethical responsibility. In short, providing people with the awareness of a health threat and the recommendation of a corresponding protective behavior is never enough. Your program must also diagnose and alter the key intervention points in Figure 7-8. If your program promotes mammography among low-income women without creating policy and an economic mechanism that will pay for the mammography, then your program will be not only less than optimally effective, but also unethical from a practice viewpoint. Diagnosing a problem in health behavior is not unlike a physician diagnosing a physical pathology in a medical patient: once you make the diagnosis, you have an obligation to do all that is possible to intervene.

▶ An Applied Example

Mammography serves as an excellent example of how SCT might be applied to prevent morbidity and mortality. One chronic challenge in the early diagnosis of breast cancer is reaching low-income Hispanic women, especially those who lack adequate health insurance. SCT can be used as a guide to develop effective approaches to the promotion of mammography, even in this challenging scenario.

The health-promotion program may begin by mounting a media campaign designed to raise awareness of breast cancer and the incredible advantage of early diagnosis. This part is "bread and butter" health promotion and is not at all unique to SCT. However, SCT would suggest that women most in need of a mammogram (e.g., women over 40 who have never had one) probably lack self-efficacy and/or a sufficient belief in the health-protective value of having a mammogram.

Addressing the self-efficacy issue is, of course, potentially quite difficult. Building self-efficacy may indeed require personal-level intervention approaches. One approach that may work is to have lay health advisors (LHAs) perform outreach to underserved women of this population. As the name suggests, LHAs are not health professionals, but rather volunteers from the community who provide education for people who enroll in health-promotion efforts. SCT would suggest that the LHAs should be quite similar to the women in the target population, relative to gender, ethnicity, income, etc. This similarity has the potential to foster improved conditions for vicarious learning. LHAs may find that many women lack self-efficacy for even making an appointment to have a mammogram, let alone the process of completing insurance, medical, and payment-related paperwork. Although the LHAs could complete these tasks on behalf of women, doing so would not address the long-term maintenance of the behavior. Instead, LHAs can and should teach women the requisite skills, thereby building self-efficacy in the population relative to obtaining a mammogram. At the same time, LHAs can promote the strong connection between early detection of breast cancer and greatly heightened odds of cancer survival (thereby increasing outcome expectations). While other theories of health behavior may stop at this point, the SCT concept of reciprocal triadic causation demands that the health-promotion program diagnose and alter aspects of the environment in a way that optimizes the chances of women obtaining mammography services. Clinics that serve this population may require intervention regarding how women make mammography appointments and complete medical paperwork. Clinics that have limited hours, lack user-friendly protocols for completing paperwork, and do not have Spanish-speaking staff are clearly at odds with program goals and these barriers demand substantially higher levels of motivation (self-efficacy plus positive outcome expectations) from women in the target population. Of course, leveraging change in clinic protocols and policies will not be easy to achieve, but expecting women to magically overcome these long-standing barriers is simply not realistic, thereby suggesting the wiser course of program effort should be focused on a systems-level change. (Please be aware that systems-level change is quickly becoming a predominate paradigm in the new public health—see Midgley, 2000).

SCT is perhaps one of your most valuable tools as a health-promotion professional. The theory demands that you pay strict attention to environmental-level, as well as personal-level, variables that may influence health behaviors. More importantly, the theory demands that you understand the reciprocal pathways that occur between the person, the environment, and the behavior in question. Armed with the five key constructs, you should be able to see that behavioral intervention under an SCT framework will be labor intensive, especially with respect to building self-efficacy and bolstering outcome expectations. The step-wise implementation model also suggests that your health-promotion program can never be a "one size fits all" approach— instead, different degrees of intensity will be required depending on the level of readiness to adopt any given health behavior.

▶ Take Home Messages

- A comprehensive approach to health promotion requires recognition that nearly all human behavior is influenced by the immediate social environment in which it occurs.
- Knowledge is the fundamental starting point for most health-promotion programs and encompasses both an awareness of the advantages/disadvantages of a behavior (content knowledge) and an understanding of how to perform the behavior (procedural knowledge).
- To achieve behavior change, individuals must have confidence that they can actually adopt the behavior and maintain it under adverse circumstances. These concepts are known as perceived self-efficacy and resilient self-efficacy, respectively, and are fundamental in social cognitive theory.
- Self-efficacy can be built through diminishing one's fear and negative emotions associated with the behavior and exposing them to others performing the behavior (vicarious learning), as well as through verbal persuasion and coaching (enactive attainment).
- Individuals' anticipated pay-off for performing a behavior, or outcome expectations, can be affected by vicarious learning, direct experiences with the behavior, a supportive social environment, and through reinforcement.
- Behavior change is best achieved through breaking the behavior down into measurable and achievable subgoals; however, it is important to recognize that goal attainment is strongly affected by supporting and impeding factors in one's environment.
- The relationships between individuals' cognitions, behaviors, and environment are each reciprocal. This phenomenon, known as reciprocal triadic causation, is central to social cognitive theory.

▶ References

Bandura, A. (1986). *Social foundations of thought & action: A social cognitive theory.* Upper Saddle River, NJ: Prentice Hall.

Bandura, A. (1998). Health promotion from the perspective of social cognitive theory. *Psychology & Health, 13,* 623–649.

Bandura, A. (2004). Health promotion by social cognitive means. *Health Education & Behavior, 31,* 143–164.

Midgley, G. (2000). *Systemic intervention: Philosophy, methodology, and practice.* New York, NY: Kluwer Academic/Plenum.

Perkins, D. D., Wandersman, A., Rich, R. C., & Taylor, R. B. (1993). The physical environment of street crime: Defensible space, territoriality and incivilities. *Journal of Environmental Design, 1*(1), 29–49.

Romer, D., Sznitman, S., DiClemente, R. J., Salazar, L. F., Vanable, P. A., Carey, M. P., ... Juzang, I. (2009). Mass media as an HIV-prevention strategy: Using culturally sensitive messages to reduce HIV-associated sexual behavior of high-risk African-American youth. *American Journal of Public Health, 99*(131), 2150–2159.

Chapter Opener: © MeskPhotography/Shutterstock; © Hero Images/Getty Images; © lzf/Shutterstock; © Henrik Sorensen/Getty Images

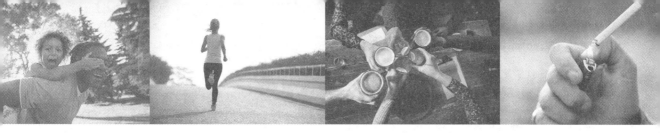

CHAPTER 8

Health Communication: Theory, Social Marketing, and Tailoring

Laura F. Salazar, Richard A. Crosby, Ralph J. DiClemente, Seth M. Noar, and Anne Marie Schipani-McLaughlin

The more elaborate our means of communication, the less we communicate.

—**Joseph Priestly**

PREVIEW

Communication has been conceptualized as both art and science. As such, it takes both talent and knowledge of underlying scientific principles to communicate effectively. Health communication is no different and requires an understanding of theoretical perspectives coupled with some level of creativity to capture the attention of the target audience, convey the message, and ultimately change health behavior.

OBJECTIVES

1. Understand that effective health communication is complex and multidimensional.
2. Understand the importance of attitudes in health communication initiatives.
3. Describe the reception–yielding model, the input communication and output persuasion matrix, and the elaboration likelihood model and explain how the key principles from each would be used effectively in a health communication initiative.
4. Explain social marketing and the difference between an upstream and downstream approach.
5. Understand how the four P's, or the marketing mix, are closely linked.

6. Identify the different behavioral theories that can be used to inform the different aspects of a social marketing campaign.
7. Explain the concept of message tailoring and how it enhances effectiveness in health communication programs.

▶ Introduction

Health-promotion programs are often designed as resource-intensive interventions to achieve large effects. Many of these programs put forth great effort to raise awareness, change attitudes, and teach skills related to engaging in healthy behaviors so that the chances of leveraging substantial and lasting behavior change are strong. Despite the strong appeal of these resource-intensive interventions, one drawback significantly detracts from the overall utility of this approach to improving public health: these types of interventions cannot practically be delivered to entire populations. This is a point that is far from minor when considering that the overall purpose of health promotion is to move the mean level of risk behavior to the left (lowered risk) in any given population (see Figure 1-5 in Chapter 1).

Consequently, the advantage that resource-intensive programs enjoy in terms of effect size (i.e., the magnitude of the intervention's effect on achieving significant mean differences in outcomes) is counterbalanced by a disadvantage in achieving widespread dissemination and adoption. Stated differently, a program that produces big effects will not have a big impact unless it can be delivered to large numbers of people. This simple observation raises the question of whether a less resource-intensive type of intervention that produces smaller effects could potentially be magnified for an overall meaningful contribution through its potential for widespread dissemination. **FIGURE 8-1** illustrates the two paradigms using the analogy of nature to demonstrate.

As suggested by Figure 8-1, programs differ by resource and dissemination levels. As shown, it is no surprise that a low-resource program with low dissemination would result in a "microscopic" net effect. Yet, this microscopic net effect contrasts sharply with the overall impact obtained for a low-resource program that has a *high* degree of dissemination. Thus, we posit that the small effects of a low-resource program can be greatly *amplified* by widespread dissemination throughout large segments of a population, thereby resulting in a colossal, overall public health impact much like that of a hurricane. Conversely, a high-resource program may, in turn, have its large effect *attenuated* due to low dissemination, and so the net effect is somewhat miniscule and may be more like that of a hummingbird. Of course, not surprising, the most desired impact would be to have a high-resource program with a large effect size, but also has the capability to reach a large number of people (high dissemination) resulting in a "cosmic" impact similar to a meteor crashing into Earth.

Because in public health a colossal or cosmic impact is preferable to a microscopic or miniscule one, we need to understand how to best increase dissemination. What mechanisms or modes can we use to amplify rather than attenuate? One such amplification mechanism often used to achieve cosmic results through a broader reach is media, and the discipline most often associated with media-based health promotion is health communication. Health communication, as its name suggests, is the marriage between the fields of communication and health and involves the strategic use of communication to inform, influence, and improve personal and public health (U.S. Department of Health and Human Services, 2000). Health communication can contribute significantly to disease prevention and health promotion. However, before we go any further, it is important to note that health communication is NOT simply a mass media campaign; rather, health communication can be *used* in a media

Resource Level

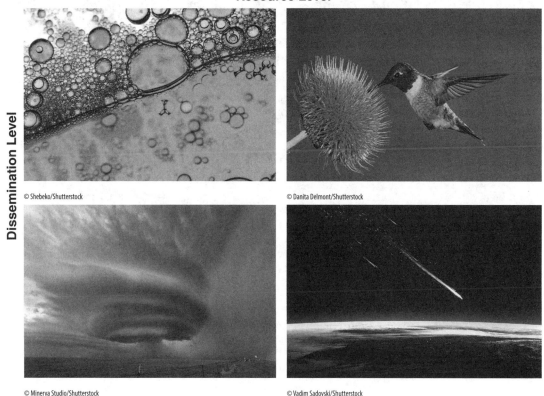

© Shebeko/Shutterstock

© Danita Delmont/Shutterstock

© Minerva Studio/Shutterstock

© Vadim Sadovski/Shutterstock

FIGURE 8-1 Impact of programs as a tradeoff between effects and dissemination

campaign, but is often used in many different contexts, such as:

- Health-professional–patient relations
- Individuals' exposure to, search for, and use of health information
- Individuals' adherence to clinical recommendations and regimens
- The construction of public health messages and campaigns
- The dissemination of individual and population health risk information (risk communication)
- Images of health in the mass media and the culture at large
- The education of consumers about how to gain access to the public health and healthcare systems (U.S. Department of Health and Human Services, 2000, pp. 11–13)

Health communication applied to many of these contexts involves planning and creating different types of communication products, such as writing a brochure on encouraging African American women to get a mammogram, creating a program that teaches physicians and healthcare providers how to communicate with their patients, developing a new website to foster young adults getting tested for STDs and HIV, writing a press release that disseminates a new health risk associated with a food product, or creating a television campaign to raise awareness of type 2 diabetes. Regardless of the context or the nature of the health communication initiative, successful health communication should incorporate several attributes to enhance effectiveness. These attributes are presented in **TABLE 8-1** and suggest that health

> *Health communication must also include scientific principles and research, and be appealing to the target audience.*

TABLE 8-1 Attributes of Effective Health Communication	
Accuracy	The content is valid and without errors of fact, interpretation, or judgment.
Availability	The content (whether targeted message or other information) is delivered or placed where the audience can access it. Placement varies according to audience, message complexity, and purpose, ranging from interpersonal and social networks, to billboards and mass transit signs, to primetime TV or radio, to public kiosks (print or electronic), to the Internet.
Balance	Where appropriate, the content presents the benefits and risks of potential actions or recognizes different and valid perspectives on the issue.
Consistency	The content remains internally consistent over time and is also consistent with information from other sources (the latter is a problem when other widely available content is not accurate or reliable).
Cultural competence	The design, implementation, and evaluation process that accounts for special issues for select population groups (e.g., ethnic, racial, or linguistic) and also educational levels and disability.
Evidence base	Relevant scientific evidence has undergone comprehensive review and rigorous analysis to formulate practice guidelines, performance measures, review criteria, and technology assessments for telehealth applications.
Reach	The content gets to or is available to the largest possible number of people in the target population.
Reliability	The source of the content is credible and the content itself is kept up to date.
Repetition	The delivery of / access to the content is continued or repeated over time, both to reinforce the impact with the target audience and to reach new generations.
Timeliness	The content is presented or available when the audience is most receptive to, or in need of, the specific information.
Understandability	The reading or language level and format (including multimedia) are appropriate for the specific audience.

U.S. Department of Health and Human Services. (2000). *Healthy people 2010: Understanding and improving health* (2nd ed.). Washington, DC: U.S. Government Printing Office.

communication can be very involved. Health communication is not simply telling individuals what they should do to improve their health (e.g., eat less fat) or providing them with basic information (e.g., high cholesterol can lead to heart disease). Health communication must also include scientific principles and research, and be appealing to the target audience.

Health communication in the past decade alone has become even more complex, in that the context in which health communication occurs has changed dramatically. There are evolving communication channels (e.g., social media sites and apps, mHealth, etc.) and health technologies such as bionic implants and medical tricorders in addition to many different health issues vying for attention (e.g., type 2 diabetes, Alzheimer's, cancer, and infectious diseases such as Zika). Thus, to be successful, in addition to incorporating the attributes presented in Table 8-1, health communication should use theory to inform its products, messages, and materials. Moreover, health communication should use research to determine the proper channels and technologies to deliver the various health communication products so that the target audience is reached. Finally, health communication must be creative so that in the midst of countless advertisements and messages, the target audience will pay attention and ultimately use the information in the way it was intended.

This chapter will introduce you to several of the health communication theories and approaches that are used in the creation and design of health communication initiatives: the reception–yielding model, the elaboration likelihood model, and two much broader classes of approaches, known as social marketing and tailored communications.

▶ Key Concepts

The Reception–Yielding Model

Many theories of health behavior (e.g., theory of reasoned action) include the construct of "attitudes" as an important and underlying factor related to behavior. Thus, many times health communication will work through underlying attitudes in order to achieve behavior change. There are a number of ways to change people's attitudes; however, in this chapter we focus primarily on the use of messages that contain information related to the **attitude object** (i.e., the target of judgment, including people, places, and things, that have an attitude or opinion associated with it). This strategy is essentially called **persuasion**.

An early and influential way of thinking about persuasion stemmed from the Yale communication program (Hovland, Janis, & Kelley, 1953), which suggested that attitude change toward a particular issue was likely if people went through a series of cognitions when thinking about the issue: attention, comprehension, learning, acceptance, and retention. This way of thinking was deemed as information processing, because it involved this series of cognitions. McGuire (1968) modified this approach into a more formal model that involved a chain of responses.

The chain of responses begins with the presentation of the message and then progresses through each step: attention to the message, comprehension of the message, yielding to the message, and retention of the message, and concludes with the behavior stemming from the message. Each of these steps (see **FIGURE 8-2**) is linked to the preceding one. McGuire suggested that an individual pass through these stages sequentially if they are to be effectively persuaded (i.e., yield to the message).

These sequential steps represent a model that can be used for designing health communication programs, especially when behavior change is the desired endpoint. "Presentation" is the persuasive message; however, following the presentation of the message, it stands to reason that people must absorb the message before anything else can happen. Attention is a critical aspect of the model, because the persuasive message must capture sufficient mental concentration from people before any effect can be expected to occur. Take a moment and think about the number of messages you are exposed to each day through multiple media channels, then ask yourself, "How many of these messages do I actually pay attention to?" Next, even if people pay attention to the message, they must understand what the message is conveying. Messages should be crafted with the target audience in mind so that they will not only be exposed to the message, but the message will resonate to them, catch their attention, and be understood. According to this model, only then can yielding, or attitude change, occur. Once yielding is achieved, the

Presentation → Attention → Comprehension → Yielding → Retention → Behavior

FIGURE 8-2 Information processing "chain" of responses

level of retention for the newly formed attitude becomes a primary determinant of performing the corresponding behaviors or of taking action. Thus, behavior change is the ultimate goal of this persuasive discourse.

McGuire's model was eventually simplified into a two-step model, the reception–yielding model, where he classified attention and comprehension into the single step of reception and preserved yielding as a single and critical step. The model asserts that the ability of a given health communication message to influence attitude change is a mathematical product of reception probability times yielding probability. There has been much support for this theory in the research literature; however, some research has suggested that reception is not always necessary for yielding, especially when there is another "cue" in the persuasion context, such as the presence of an expert source (Petty, Jarvis, Evans, & Bakker , 1995).

This relatively straightforward model quickly becomes a bit more complex when thinking about variables related to the intended population (the message receivers). For example, in a population experiencing the emotion of fear as a result of a persuasive message, the likelihood of message reception may be diminished, whereas the likelihood of yielding may be elevated. Other research pertaining to the use of fear in health communications has suggested that excessive fear may indeed backfire simply because people may enter a state of defensive denial as a method of coping with the new threat. Consider a health communication message designed to persuade young males to be vaccinated against human papillomavirus (HPV) on the basis of being protected against the acquisition of genital warts. Imagine that the vaccination campaign features photographs of a wart-covered penis (the genital warts caused by this virus can sometimes be quite large and cover a substantial area of the penis). For many young males, viewing such an image may result in a reaction of intense fear associated with being infected by genital warts. An emotional response such as fear may in turn preclude these young men from paying full attention to written or spoken

messages that accompany the image. However, this same image may provoke **yielding**, which in turn could lead to seeking a vaccination. On the other hand, some of the males viewing the penile image may experience such fear arousal that it triggers severe psychological discomfort that can only be resolved by minimizing or discounting the message that inspired the fear in the first place. As was covered in greater detail in Chapter 5, one lesson that has been learned in research pertaining to fear is that messages inspiring this emotion must be "packaged" with messages promoting an effective and easy-to-perform protective response against the threat. Stated differently, fear in the absence of a viable solution is likely to be counterproductive.

The reception–yielding model also produces some intriguing findings in relation to the construct of intelligence. Ironically, high intelligence favors reception, but may work against yielding. This finding may occur because highly intelligent people are able to attend to and comprehend the message (reception), but are less likely to yield because they have greater knowledge of counterarguments. Further, low intelligence favors yielding but works against reception. This relatively robust research finding clearly implies that message development must be based upon a solid foundation of awareness about the target population (i.e., what type of message is most likely to be understood by most people, yet still have a level of sophistication great enough to produce reasonable odds of yielding).

The reception–yielding model has served as the basis for a great deal of research focused upon attitude development and change. Variables that can influence either process are certainly viable targets for intervention via health communication programs. Perceived credibility of the message source, for example, may be critically important to reception. Ultimately, however, it is incumbent on the health-promotion professional to ask the critical question: how can the health communication message optimally ensure that yielding translates

High intelligence favors reception, but may work against yielding.

into an enduring and highly salient attitude that can reliably trigger lasting adoption of health-protective behaviors?

McGuire's Input Communication and Output Persuasion Matrix

McGuire (2013) later conceptualized a more comprehensive communication-persuasion model involving a matrix of communication inputs and persuasive outputs. The model emphasized the importance of different characteristics related to the communication message (i.e., the inputs) and also expanded upon the reception–yielding model's five steps to include 12 steps related to yielding. The matrix is presented in **TABLE 8-2** and shows the input variables used to construct persuasive communications and the meditational output behaviors that must be elicited to achieve behavioral change. The inputs represent characteristics of the persuasion/

communication attempt. Before designing a health communication campaign designed to persuade people to change their health behaviors, formative research is needed on these input variables so that the targeted population can be reached and messages will be more effective. For example, when choosing the source to deliver the communication message, credibility, attractiveness and power have been obvious choices of campaign designers, but they may not always be effective. Thus, formative research is needed to inform each of the input variables and to maximize effectiveness.

A recent study examined the input variables (e.g., sources, message, receiver, channel, context) to inform a Middle East Respiratory Syndrome (MERS) risk communication campaign in Saudi Arabia (Hoda, 2016). The model was used to understand the information-seeking behaviors and preferences among the population of interest. Data were collected from residents of Riyadh via surveys ($N = 658$). Findings indicated that the

TABLE 8-2 McGuire's Communication Persuasion Matrix: Input Communication Variables and Output Mediational Steps of Persuasion

Input Communication Factors	Output Persuasion Steps
1. Source: trustworthiness, attractiveness, credibility of sender, etc. 2. Message: appeal, inclusion or omission, repetitiveness, style, organization, etc. 3. Channel: directness, modality, context, etc. 4. Receiver: person's attitudes, beliefs, prior knowledge, intelligence 5. Context: environmental factors, noise, clutter influencing the message	6. Exposure to communication message 7. Pay attention to message 8. Enjoys and maintains interest in message 9. Learn message contents 10. Generate related cognitions to message 11. Gain relevant skills 12. Agree with communication's position and change attitude 13. Store this new attitude in memory 14. Retrieve new attitude from memory when relevant 15. Decide to act on new position gained through attitude change 16. Act on new attitude 17. Following action, integrate cognition of this behavior 18. Encourage others to adopt new behavior

Modified from McGuire, W. J. (2013). McGuire's classic input-output framework for constructing persuasive messages. In R. E. Rice & C. K. Atkin (Eds.), *Public Communication Campaigns* (4th ed., pp: 133–146). Thousand Oaks, CA: Sage Publications, Inc.

Internet was the most common source of information among participants, as well as the preferred communication channel for a MERS risk communication campaign. The majority of participants (76.9%) reported that physicians and healthcare providers are the most credible information source to deliver a MERS campaign. These results represent the value of examining varying inputs of the Communication Persuasion Matrix during the formative stage to develop more effective health communication campaigns (Hoda, 2016).

In going back to the matrix, we now turn to the outputs, which, similar to the reception–yielding model, also represent a series of sequential, mediating behavioral steps. Persuasive communication messages, if effective, will evoke these series of steps and result in attitude change or adoption of a health behavior. Formative research on how best to affect outputs is critically important. For example, evidence shows that some people are more easily persuaded when they are alone versus being in a group. A public health campaign might have more success using social media to promote health messaging rather than bus advertisements for instance, because, unlike often crowded buses, people are typically alone when they are on social media. By using social media for a health communication campaign, people may be more likely to be exposed (step 1), pay attention (step 2), enjoy the message and maintain interest, and so on and so on all the way to step 13.

McGuire's (2013) input/output model was used to test the health communication inputs of printed health education materials in affecting a comprehensive set of outputs to better understand weight loss (Bull, Holt, Kreuter, Clark, & Scharff, 2001). Researchers examined the effects of printed health education materials on weight loss attitudes, behaviors, and cognitions among a sample of $N = 196$ overweight adults. Participants reviewed one of three health education materials and completed pre- and post-test assessments before and after viewing each of the messages. Different input characteristics were associated with success at each of the output steps. Message attractiveness, encouragement, level of information, and relevance to one's life was associated with the early steps (e.g., attention, liking the message, and understanding) and the mediating steps

(e.g., recalling, keeping materials, and rereading messages). Readiness to change, self-efficacy, and perceived application to one's life were associated with later output steps, including intention to change behavior and showing others the message (Bull et al., 2001). Understanding how input variables affect the output persuasion steps is therefore useful for tailoring public health communication messages to elicit attitude and behavior change.

The Elaboration Likelihood Model

Health communications rely on short but powerful messages that can sometimes be conveyed to massive numbers of people in an effective format. As such, the goals of these communications are quite modest by necessity. Indeed, the goals are typically targeted toward proximal mediators of behavior change. You may recall from Chapter 2 that proximal mediators are directly linked to the behavior, so they exist at the individual level. Attitude toward a given behavior, for example, is perhaps one of the most common proximal mediators of behavior. Thus, changing attitudes toward specified health behaviors is frequently the goal of health communication campaigns. One of the premiere theories used for this purpose is the elaboration likelihood model (ELM) (Petty, Barden, & Wheeler, 2002). The ELM is depicted in **FIGURE 8-3**.

TABLE 8-3 presents the key features of the ELM. As shown, a central tenet of the ELM is that attitude formation occurs through one of two possible cognitive pathways: the **central route** or the **peripheral route**. The central route is cognitive, whereas the peripheral route involves emotion or heuristics (a commonsense rule that people use to make expedient judgments—a mental shortcut to making decisions); an example of a heuristic would be buying a product based on the company's reputation versus doing research about the product itself. Attitudes developed through central route processing are far more likely to be enduring over time than those formed through peripheral routes, and they may have a stronger connection to behavior. Unfortunately, not everyone takes the time to engage in this level of somewhat demanding cognition, so in the peripheral route, people form attitudes about given health behaviors based on

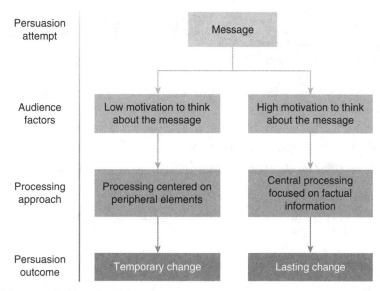

FIGURE 8-3 The elaboration likelihood model

Modified from Kenrick, D. T., Neuberg, S. L., & Cialdini, R. B. (2005). *Social psychology: Unraveling the mystery* (3rd ed.). Boston, MA: Allyn and Bacon.

emotion or mental heuristics. After describing central route processing and peripheral route processing in more detail, examples of ELM applications in health communications will be provided.

Central Route Processing

In essence, the value–expectancy theories described in Chapter 4 each assume a type of mental math that is characteristic of central route processing. Conscious thought pertaining to the behavior in question is the hallmark of central route processing; consequently, health communications aimed at this route typically provide detailed information, thereby allowing people to perform an evaluation. This evaluation then leads to attitude formation. If, for example, a campaign seeks to promote acceptance of the vaccine to prevent infection with HPV, a key aspect of the health communication messaging will be information about the degree of protection the vaccine confers against cancer and genital warts.

Conscious thought pertaining to the behavior in question is the hallmark of central route processing.

The information must also be tailored to the target audience. Men who engage in receptive anal sex, for example, may form a more favorable attitude toward being vaccinated by learning that the vaccine prevents anal cancer, while persons engaging in receptive oral sex may form more favorable attitudes toward HPV vaccination by learning that the vaccine greatly reduces the risk of head, neck, and throat cancers. Information in the campaign relative to the safety of the vaccine and its minimal side effects may also become a valuable aspect of favorable attitude formation. The overall ethic of the campaign should be to provide the target audience with enough information to engage in a "pro vs. con" level of analysis that will culminate in an enduring attitude that has a high probability of being translated into behavior.

Enduring attitudes are resistant to counter-persuasion, meaning that a newly introduced negative idea is unlikely to change the initial decision based on previous comparison. This is important, because modern media can quickly disseminate and magnify faulty information that may unfairly change people's mind about a given health behavior. For example, in a 2010 *Frontline* interview, celebrity Jenny McCarthy spoke out against vaccinations because she believed her son's autism diagnosis started after he received a series of

TABLE 8-3 Key Features of the Elaboration Likelihood Model

- The model is useful in tailoring health communications (i.e., messages) that are widely disseminated to the public.
- The intent is to change a specific attitude, and in turn, the behaviors that correspond to the attitude under consideration.
- Attitude is defined as a relatively enduring evaluation of a person, object, or issue.
- Attitude assessment should be as specific as possible.
- The ELM uses research on persuasion (e.g., studies that determine the role of source attractiveness and credibility, receiver attention and comprehension, message complexity, and the time available to process the message).
- The ELM resolves apparent discrepancies in attitude research by organizing persuasion into two main routes: central and peripheral.
- The central route is very cerebral. Alternatively, the peripheral route is driven largely by emotion. The former produces more enduring (and accessible) attitudes than the latter.
- Increased personal confidence with central route processing may be the mechanism that is associated with more enduring attitudes.
- Central route processing occurs when people are able and motivated (high relevance); the latter can be enhanced through peripheral route processing.
- The peripheral route includes "mental shortcuts" such as "experts are usually right" or "most people prefer." It can also include making associations with valued people, objects, or experiences (advertisers use this often).
- Both routes can function at the same time—each may make a unique contribution to attitude formation.
- The distinction between routes is based on how people process the message rather than the message itself (e.g., understanding that condoms can be effective against HIV if used correctly and consistently vs. condoms must be effective if a famous HIV+ sports figure advocates using them).
- High relevance can be achieved through enhanced personal susceptibility and severity (based on the health belief model, the combination of these factors is known as perceived threat).
- Evidence suggests that enduring attitudes are more resistant to counterpersuasion and have a stronger correlation with behavior.
- People in a positive mood may avoid message processing if they perceive that negative feelings may result (this is a particular challenge for public health).
- A large number of studies have evaluated (and supported) the efficacy of the ELM in relation to changing health behavior.

measles, mumps, and rubella (MMR) vaccinations. McCarthy has authored three books on autism and sparked a controversial movement of parents concerned about the link between vaccines and autism despite the scientific consensus that this link does not exist. A 2014 meta-analysis examining ten studies with over one million children demonstrated that childhood vaccination administration is not linked to autism (Taylor, Swerdfeger, & Eslick, 2014). *Frontline* began reporting on the vaccine debate in "The Vaccine War" starting in 2010 though doctors and public health officials warned that media coverage on the growing skepticism of vaccinations could lead to the return of preventable diseases. Sure enough, the United States has seen spikes in measles, mumps, and whooping cough since 2010. The media attention given to the anti vaccine movement led people to change their minds about vaccination, a trusted health behavior to prevent disease.

Peripheral Route Processing

All too often, people form attitudes based on emotion or feeling. In the business world, advertisers understand this principle well and they use it to instill attitudes that are favorable to their product. One obvious example of this is the use of extremely sexy women in an advertisement for a product such as beer. The resulting emotion for many men is that the beer in question makes them feel good. This is a simple associative process; by pairing the product with sex, the product takes on new meaning and new value.

Peripheral route processing is not intrinsically a bad thing. Realistically, most people are simply not predisposed to engagement in the more demanding central route processing. The obvious downside of peripheral route processing, however, is that the resulting attitudes are not as resistant to counter-persuasion, and so the attitudes formed in this way are far less enduring. With this limitation in mind, it becomes quite reasonable to view health communications aimed at peripheral processing as a method of initially persuading people (through attitude formation) to perform a given health behavior. The continued repetition of this behavior (i.e., maintenance) may then be promoted through subsequent campaigns utilizing communication aimed at central route processing.

Given the value of the peripheral route, this form of health communication can have extreme utility. If, for example, a celebrity figure endorses HPV vaccination, then people listening to or viewing this message may heuristically decide that the vaccine must be a good thing. From a public health perspective, the ability to quickly instill favorable attitudes toward health-related behaviors has great potential to influence population-level health. Historically, this was exactly the intent in 1976 when President Jimmy Carter and First Lady Roslyn Carter were vaccinated against influenza on network

> *It becomes quite reasonable to view health communications aimed at peripheral processing as a method of initially persuading people.*

television. When celebrities like Charlie Sheen announced he was HIV positive, sales of HIV home testing kits dramatically increased. When basketball star Magic Johnson promoted HIV testing, the widespread acceptance of his message among at-risk males made a dramatic impact. This same effect was observed when actress Angelina Jolie announced her double mastectomy and removal of her ovaries and fallopian tubes due to her BRCA1 gene mutation. Following her announcement, research showed that women were more likely to get genetic testing, there were increased genetic testing requests and Internet searches related to BRCA1.

Taking Health Communication to the Next Level: Social Marketing

Although not classified as a theory, we are including a discussion of **social marketing** in this textbook because it is another tool to effectively change and influence behavior. However, it is important to emphasize that social marketing's role does not stop with those individuals whose health behavior is the focus; rather, social marketing can and should target the social and physical determinants of those behaviors (Hastings & Donovan, 2002). Anderson (2006) in his illuminating book, *Social Marketing in the 21st Century*, postulates that social marketing, in order to affect true social change, must switch the focus from the current downstream approach (i.e., targeting the individuals who engage in the behavior) to an upstream approach (i.e., targeting the structures and environmental determinants). Of course, the structures and environmental determinants are not amorphous "things," but individuals who make the decisions, such as the corporate executives, government officials, legislators, media gatekeepers, community activists, lobbyists, and anyone else who plays a role.

Consider for a moment, the major public health problem of childhood obesity. It makes considerable sense to focus resources and efforts toward influencing the school superintendents, as these people decide what meals are served in their school districts and how much time for physical activity is allotted for kids during the school day. Additionally,

Social marketing is yet another tool for public health researchers and practitioners to use as a means to achieve the end of an improved public health.

efforts should be directed toward influencing local government officials who regulate zoning ordinances for new developments (and can ensure walkability) or who can regulate what restaurants can and cannot serve. This upstream approach should be the strategy utilized and is congruent with the new public health, which focuses on environmental factors and how those factors affect individual behavior. Thus, social marketing is yet another tool for public health researchers and practitioners to use as a means to achieve the end of an improved public health.

Social marketing is included in this chapter on health communication because it incorporates principles of health communication in its endeavors. Social marketing has been defined previously as a practice, a discipline, a strategy, and a framework, but it should never be classified as a theory. Social marketing uses principles and techniques borrowed from commercial marketing to sell products. It is important to understand that in this milieu, products are referred to as ideas, behaviors, health programs, and so forth, which are meant to enhance health and alleviate social issues. Social marketing is used to benefit the greater good of the target population, rather than to make a profit for the marketer. Thus, it is consumer-oriented, in that the needs of the consumer are considered rather than the needs of the marketer. Some of the strengths of social marketing interventions include its cost-effectiveness, audience-driven nature, utilization of a wide range of communication channels across a wide range of settings, ability to change social norms and promote an environment of change, ability to change a wide range of health behaviors, and its empowerment of communities. In the last three decades, social marketing has been applied successfully to programs concerned with obesity prevention, smoking cessation and prevention, heart disease prevention, breast cancer screening, family planning, reproductive health, HIV/AIDS, and violence prevention.

However, we encourage future social marketers to heed the call to take social marketing into the 21st century by targeting the decisionmakers and policymakers located upstream to achieve bigger and better results.

At this point, you are most likely wondering, "But what exactly is social marketing?" Social marketing involves a mix of elements that must integrate and work collectively toward achieving the desired outcome—influencing individual behavior—and should coordinate with each other to be effective (Winett, 1995). These elements include the four P's from classical marketing: product, price, place, and promotion. Another "P" (positioning) is also included at times; however, we won't articulate this "P" in this chapter, as it refers to a product filling a special niche. As we stated earlier, social marketing is not considered a theory, but each of these elements constituting social marketing can be informed by many of the behavioral theories described in this textbook (Winett, 1995). These elements are described in the next sections.

Product

In social marketing, the **product** can be something tangible such as an actual product (e.g., dental floss, condoms), program (e.g., an HIV prevention program, a smoking cessation program), or service (e.g., mammogram, colonoscopy, STD screening, HPV vaccine), or an intangible one such as behavioral practices (e.g., exercising, breastfeeding, good nutrition) or a change in attitudes, beliefs, or ideas. When designing the product, social marketers must be informed by research and can greatly enhance their efforts by using theory. First, it is extremely important to know the perceptions of the target audience regarding the problem being addressed and also whether the product might be an adequate solution to the problem. Formative

When designing the product, social marketers must be informed by research and can greatly enhance their efforts by using theory.

research at this stage is critical and it supports social marketing's consumer-oriented approach. Focus groups, elicitation interviews, and surveys with the target population and with others such as decisionmakers and policymakers will help understand perceptions to design a better product.

Winett (1995) delineated the different theoretical models that are relevant to each of the five marketing elements. These are presented in **TABLE 8-4** and provide a guide for social marketers to select a theory that can inform each element. This is not to say that there are no other equally valid theories, but it is a good starting point. As the table shows, he suggested two theories might be helpful for product design: diffusion theory (see Chapter 10) and stages of change (see Chapter 6).

Diffusion theory (see Chapter 11) suggests that when designing a new product the marketer should consider characteristics such as trialability (i.e., the minimal cost or commitment to try it), compatibility (i.e., suitability for existing cultural values and norms), and relative advantage (i.e., perception as an improvement over what is currently being used or done). From the stages of change model (see Chapter 6), the marketer must consider how to match product characteristics to the different stages of the target audience. For example, audience members who are in the precontemplation or the contemplation stage will view the product characteristics differently than a member who is in the action stage. Also, many of the value–expectancy theories (see Chapter 4) can be used to inform marketers how to design products that will be more readily adoptable. For example, from the theory of reasoned action (see Chapter 4), attitudes toward a behavior are based on an individual's underlying beliefs regarding negative and positive outcomes associated with the behavior. Thus, when designing a "behavior" product, the social marketer should be informed of what the target audience's attitudes are toward that behavior. Then, the reception–yielding model and/or the ELM would be instrumental in helping the social marketer craft the relevant communication message to persuade the target audience to adopt the product (i.e., engage in the behavior).

TABLE 8-4 Interactive Marketing Variables, Relevant Theories or Models, Principles, and Procedures

Variable	Theory or Model	Principles	Procedures
Product	Diffusion theory	Product design	Trialable Fit Relative advantage Simple Observable Reinvention
	Stages of change	Matching	Precontemplation Action Contemplation Maintenance Preparation
Price	Behavior analysis Social cognitive theory	Reinforcement	Contingency management Shaping and successive approximation Feedback and goal setting

(continues)

TABLE 8-4 Interactive Marketing Variables, Relevant Theories or Models, Principles, and Procedures *(continued)*			
Variable	**Theory or Model**	**Principles**	**Procedures**
Promotion	Theory of reasoned action Health belief model Protection motivation theory Social cognitive theory Behavior analysis	Cognition ↔ Behavior (reciprocal influence, spiraling)	Information framing Tailoring Saliency Vulnerability Fear arousal Two-sided messages Benefits–cost ratio Modeling Coping Reinforcement Cues to action Prompts Discriminative stimulus
Place	Public health Ecological	Environmental design	Passive intervention
Positioning	Stages of change Developmental	Matching	Segmentation

Reproduced from Winett, R. A. (1995). A framework for health promotion and disease prevention programs. *American Psychologist, 50*(5), 341–350.

Price

The **price** of the product can be a monetary cost in some instances, such as the cost of getting a mammogram or the cost of buying condoms, but price can also refer to psychological or social costs; in other words, price is what the members of the target audience must go through in order to get the product. Some products may entail experiencing embarrassment (e.g., an overweight individual who exercises in public or a young man going into an STD clinic), fear (e.g., a young woman who tries to negotiate condoms with her older sex partner), physical exertion and sweating (e.g., exercise), loss of time (e.g., making an appointment for a mammogram and going to the appointment), or even being ostracized (e.g., a smoker who tries to quit while all his friends continue to smoke). These are all considered as costs,

and marketers must consider that product design influences costs; thus, marketers should try to figure out how to minimize costs and maximize benefits when they are designing the product. When deciding to buy or adopt the product, individuals will typically do a cost–benefit analysis to determine if the benefits outweigh the costs.

Again, for this element, research is needed to help determine the perceptions of the target audience regarding the costs and benefits of the product. Referring back to Table 8-4, we can also consider using social

When deciding to buy or adopt the product, individuals will typically do a cost–benefit analysis to determine if the benefits outweigh the costs.

cognitive theory (see Chapter 8) to inform price. One central tenet of social cognitive theory is reinforcement. Designing a product that will essentially reinforce its use will result in a better cost–benefit ratio. Also, instead of having the ultimate goal behavior (e.g., running a 10K) as the product, breaking the behavior down into smaller, successive behaviors (e.g., walking a mile, then three miles, then running three miles, etc.) will increase adoption of the product because the behavior is reinforced and costs are reduced with each successful goal obtainment. This concept is known as **shaping** and **successive approximation**. Self-efficacy also needs to be considered when addressing price, because if members of the target audience perceive low confidence in performing the behavior or adopting the product, this will result in a higher cost response. Expectancies also play a role, in that if targeted audience members place a low value on the consequences of adopting the product, then the perceived benefits might not overcome perceived costs. Although not highlighted in Table 8-4, another theory that could inform price is the health belief model (HBM) (see Chapter 5). The HBM component of barriers and benefits is directly relevant to how social marketers must balance costs and benefits when addressing price (Lefebvre, 2001). The other value–expectancy theories also are relevant in that they can help the marketer understand the mental math the target audience might go through when deciding to adopt the product.

Place

Place refers to the point of contact with the target audience. Think of place as the different channels used to get the product to the target audience. Place can be a physical location (e.g., health clinic, retail store, school, mall) or for an intangible product, place can be the media channel that gets the product delivered to the audience (e.g., television or radio ad). Thus, the possibilities are almost limitless. Accessibility is a critical component that the marketer needs to consider, as this is the function of the product (Lefebvre, 1992). Research to inform decisions regarding place should be focused on determining the activities and habits of the target audience, as well as their experience

and satisfaction with the existing delivery system (Weinreich, 2006).

At this point, you can begin to see that each element of the marketing mix is interconnected. For example, when addressing place, if it is not convenient or access is difficult, then price goes up. Also, environmental characteristics of place other than geographic location can also affect adoption. If, for example, a social marketer wants to increase the percentage of women over 40 who get annual mammograms in a local community, and if some women in the target audience have had previous negative experiences (e.g., the clinic was unattractive, staff were rude) at the clinic, then they might not readily go back for yearly mammograms. Another example relates to using the Internet as the place to distribute the product, as social marketers using this channel must ensure that their target audience has access to the Internet and will somehow be exposed to the website delivering the product.

One example of how place was not considered adequately in the marketing mix was the 5-A-Day social marketing campaign designed to foster increased public consumption of fruits and vegetables. Unfortunately, after much money spent and many social marketing campaigns implemented across communities in the United States, research suggested that the social marketing campaign did not result in significant increases in the percentages of people consuming fruits and vegetables five or more times per day (Serdula et al., 2004). One explanation was that for many people, especially those who live in low-income neighborhoods, access to affordable fruits and vegetables was not feasible and thus, the distribution channel was not addressed. As we stated previously, an upstream approach should have been implemented in this instance; campaign implementers should have worked to alter the environments in which the campaign was operating. For example, targeting local government officials to influence them to create subsidies for grocery store operators to open a store in low-income areas, or trying to influence the local

Each element of the marketing mix is interconnected.

police departments to address high crime rates so that supermarket chains would consider opening a larger retail store in these areas, may have solved the problem. These are but a few ideas that may have worked to place the product more effectively, so that eating "5-a-day" for the targeted communities would have been a more realistic and obtainable goal.

Promotion

Promotion is defined as "communication strategies that inform, persuade, and influence beliefs and behaviors *relevant* to the product" (Winett, 1995, p. 347). These strategies consist of an integrated use of different channels, such as the media or interpersonal communication or delivery systems, to promote the product and get the word out. As in classical marketing, the focus of promotion is to create demand for the product (Weinreich, 2006). Promotion is vital to the success of a social marketing initiative and communication is a key component of the promotion element; however, social marketers have tended to focus the most attention on promotion, while neglecting the other key elements.

These communication strategies can take the form of public service announcements, media events, DVDs, swag (promotional merchandise), advertising, public relations, direct mail campaigns, editorials, and the use of point-of-purchase programs. Almost anything goes in promotion if it gets the message to the intended target audience, but it is important that research and theory inform the promotion strategy. First, messages pertaining to the product need to be developed. Table 8-4 indicates that several of the value–expectancy theories, social cognitive theory, and protection motivation theory can inform this crucial step. These theories suggests that the social marketer create a sense of vulnerability or perceived threat surrounding the health issue through the messages. It is also important to portray the use of the product as resulting in more benefits than costs and that those benefits are of value. A reason for attending to the message should also be provided, such as "your loved ones would want you to" or "doctors recommend" or "people like you do it."

Formative research with the target population is necessary to determine the specific messages and to pilot test them before launching. Once the message strategy has been developed, the next step is to determine the most effective and efficient vehicles to convey the messages so that they reach the target audience and increase demand (Weinreich, 2006). This step is equally critical and will entail more research with the target audience. If the messages are not received, then the product cannot be adopted. Unfortunately, this was the case with a social marketing campaign targeting teens in Boston called "See It and Stop It" (Rothman, Decker, & Silverman, 2006). The social marketing campaign's goal was to encourage teens to visit the project website, where they would receive information about dating violence, helping abused or abusive friends, and organizing prevention projects. A pre–post quasi-experimental design was used to evaluate the campaign. Although campaign promotional ads (TV, radio, print) were professionally produced and exposure to promotional ads reached 59% among surveyed teens, only 3% reported going to a website about teen dating violence and none could name the website.

In essence, effective social marketing cannot be one-dimensional; it should consider how all elements are connected and which factors might "make or break" the initiative. Because social marketing is consumer-oriented, implementing a successful social marketing initiative to enhance the health of a community also requires a bottom-up approach, engaging members of the community in the process so that the intended behavior is possible and will be maintained after the initiative has ended and funding is gone. Of course, social marketing should expand its focus to target those individuals who constitute the environmental structures and organizations that also influence behavior. Social marketing alone may not be able to change systemic problems related to health, such as poverty or lack of access to health care, but social marketing done correctly should include a systematic exploration of all the relevant ecological factors that contribute to engaging in healthy behaviors and the strategies that could be used to influence these factors. Well-designed social

Social marketing done correctly should include a systematic exploration of all the relevant ecological factors that contribute to engaging in healthy behaviors.

marketing, therefore, should help individuals better understand their own and their communities' needs so that appropriate action on multiple levels is taken to maximize the efforts of the initiative and better public health is achieved.

New Developments in Health Communication: Tailored Communications

Most media-based approaches in health communication, including social marketing, make use of **audience segmentation** and **message targeting** practices. Indeed, in the field of health promotion, selecting a defined target population is standard practice. In health communication, the target population may be segmented further if it is believed that different portions of the audience require different types of messages (audience segmentation). For example, a health communication campaign that attempts to affect safer sexual behavior may segment on gender and develop different messages for males and females. The development of messages for a particular group such as males (vs. females) is a practice referred to as message targeting (Kreuter, Strecher, & Glassman, 1999).

Although most programs and campaigns in the health-promotion field use message targeting (which operates at the group level), a newer practice in health communication is referred to as **message tailoring** (which operates at the individual level). Message tailoring has been defined as "any combination of strategies and information intended to reach one specific person, based on characteristics that are unique to that person, related to the outcome of interest, and derived from an individual assessment" (Kreuter, Strecher, & Glassman, 1999, p. 277). Thus, tailored communications are uniquely individualized to each person, whereas targeted messages are developed to be

effective with an entire segment of the population. Targeting and tailoring can be thought of on a continuum from mass audience communications (the most generic) to targeted communications and finally to the individualized communications (the most customized). Because tailored communications are the most customized, they require an assessment of the individual (see **FIGURE 8-4**).

Message tailoring operates on the premise that, although targeting (at the group level) may enhance the perceived relevance of a health message for members of a group, there will still be a substantial mismatch between a message designed for an entire group and some members of that group. Interestingly, while most advertising utilizes group-targeting practices, some advertisers have recognized this mismatch problem and have begun using individualized communications. For example, websites such as Amazon.com assess your book browsing and buying tendencies and make tailored recommendations for books you may be interested in buying. Netflix and TiVo use similar tailoring practices, making personalized suggestions for movies you should rent or television programs you should record and watch. Even supermarket scanning technology is now capable of assessing the kinds of items you typically buy and providing customized coupons at the checkout that reflect your buying tendencies. Thus, the concept of individualized tailoring is becoming increasingly common both within and beyond the health communication domain.

In the health-promotion area, a perfect storm of major insights occurred that ultimately led to the development of tailored communication interventions. These included the observance of poor outcomes of many health-promotion programs utilizing print materials (e.g., self-help manuals) and an understanding that people are often at differing stages in the change process (see Chapter 6); as such, they require individualized messages per the stage-based theories such as the transtheoretical model and the development of new technologies that made tailoring on a largescale basis possible. The first studies in the message tailoring area compared the ability of print materials tailored on determinants from health behavior theories (e.g., transtheoretical model, health belief

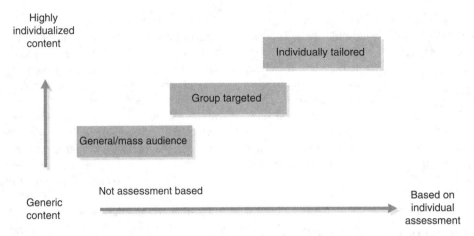

FIGURE 8-4 Level of customization of health content for mass audience, group targeted, and individually tailored interventions

Modified from Kreuter, M. W., Strecher, V. J., & Glassman, B. (1999). One size does not fit all: The case for tailoring print materials. *Annals of Behavioral Medicine, 21*(4), 276–283; Hawkins, R. P., Kreuter, M., Resnicow, K., Fishbein, M., & Dijkstra, A. (2008). Understanding tailoring in communicating about health. *Health Education Research, 23*(3), 454–466

model, social cognitive theory) to materials that were more generic or targeted in nature. The success of these early studies in demonstrating behavior change in areas such as smoking cessation and dietary practices ultimately led to a burgeoning literature on tailored health communication. Tailoring has since been applied across many other communication channels, to over 20 health behaviors, and to a number of populations (Noar, Harrington, & Aldrich, 2009). The most recent and rapidly growing area in tailoring is the development and evaluation of web-based and mHealth (i.e., mobile health) health-promotion programs (Lustria, Cortese, Noar, & Glueckauf, 2009).

For example, in one mHealth study researchers provided 27 sedentary type 2 diabetes patients with a smartphone app pedometer and personalized physical activity plans (Yom-Tov et al., 2017). The smartphone app ran in the background of their phones and tracked their physical activity, then stored their data in a central server. Then, a computer algorithm created a personalized SMS message based on the patient's physical activity that encouraged them to adhere to their physical activity regimens. Patients in the treatment group received personalized SMS message every day and each week. Compared to patients in the

control group who did not receive the personalized messages, those receiving them increased their physical activity and their walking pace and lowered their blood glucose levels over time (Yom-Tov et al., 2017). Given that the Internet and mobile devices have become such popular tools, and because each are capable of assessing individuals and providing instant tailored feedback, the application of tailoring over the web or through smartphones is ideal.

A key question often asked by those considering the use of tailoring (over targeting) is whether the extra burden of assessing individuals is worth the payoff in terms of program impact (i.e., attitude/behavior change), because, if not, targeting practices are likely to be both easier to implement and more cost effective. An investigation attempted to answer this question through a synthesis of 57 studies of tailored print communications (Noar, Benac, & Harris, 2007). The results revealed that tailored interventions have been useful in changing health behaviors, and have indeed been more effective than the targeted/generic health interventions to which they have been compared. Although synthesis of the growing research in this area is needed, particularly with newer applications of tailoring to web-based interventions, the evidence suggests that tailoring is an effective health communication strategy.

By way of example, this is how tailored interventions work:

Step 1: Assessment. Any tailored intervention begins by assessing an individual on a variety of characteristics (e.g., demographic, behavioral, psychosocial) that are relevant to the behavior under study. Assessments can be made in a variety of ways, such as through telephone, face-to-face interviews, mail, and computer or web-based surveys; for example, a smoking cessation study might utilize a telephone survey to assess an individual's stage of change for quitting smoking, attitudes about quitting, and self-efficacy to quit.

Step 2: Feedback. Computer algorithms are then used to drive decision rules that have been developed and programmed to select particular messages that are most appropriate for an individual, based on the assessment. These messages are derived from a message library, which consists of hundreds or even thousands of messages that have been created by the tailored program developers. A feedback report is then compiled (again by the computer program), printed out, and presented to the participant through the appropriate channel. In the current example, the computer software would compile the feedback report, which would subsequently be mailed or emailed to the individual. The report would contain messages specific to the stage of change the person is in, as well as specific messages regarding that individual's attitudes and self-efficacy for smoking cessation.

▶ Applied Examples

Applied Example of a Marketing Mix Strategy

As an example, the marketing mix strategy for a bystander education sexual assault and alcohol use risk reduction campaign targeting college students might include the following elements:

- The **product** could be behaviors such as getting the target audience to intervene in risky situations in which sexual assault might be at risk or decreasing their alcohol use so they can be more alert and aware of their surroundings, and therefore more likely to notice risky situations in which sexual assault might be at risk.

- The **price** of engaging in these behaviors includes comparing the costs (e.g., potential risk of putting oneself in danger by intervening if someone in the situation gets violent, the potential discomfort of intervening with strangers, potential cost of getting someone home safely such as paying for a rideshare service or gas) to the benefits (e.g., helping someone get home safely, preventing sexual assault, decreasing risk of danger).

- The **place**, which would be designed to change behaviors, might be social media websites such as Facebook, Instagram, and Twitter, printed posters and flyers in off-campus locations such as bars, restaurants, and retailers surrounding the campus and on-campus locations such as dorms, sorority/fraternity houses, academic buildings, and student recreation centers. The needs of the target audience drive the places designated to change behaviors.

- **Promotion** could be done through social media posts, stickers, campus bus advertisements, ads in bars and restaurants, and community outreach.

See **FIGURE 8-5** for an actual social marketing social media post for this target population.

Each element of the marketing mix should be taken into consideration as the program is developed and attention should be paid to how each is interconnected. Research and theory would be used to elucidate and shape the final product, price, place, promotion, and related decisions.

Applied Example of Tailoring

A promising avenue for tailored HIV behavioral intervention research is computer technology–based

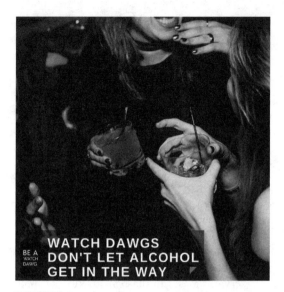

FIGURE 8-5 Social marketing campaign Instagram post targeting college students

Schipani-McLaughlin, A. M. (2017). *Developing and testing the preliminary efficacy of Be a Watch Dawg: A college-wide sexual assault and alcohol use risk reduction social media marketing campaign.* Unpublished doctoral dissertation.

interventions. Computer technology–based interventions are those programs that use computers as the primary or sole medium to deliver an intervention. Perhaps the greatest advantage of such interventions is that the cost of implementing these interventions once they are developed is likely to be minimal compared with human-delivered interventions, thus potentially facilitating their dissemination. Recall from Figure 8-1 how the net effect of certain interventions that can be easily disseminated far exceeds those that may be larger in effect size, but difficult to disseminate. Other advantages include the following: intervention fidelity is maintained through the standardization of content; computerized interventions can individually tailor intervention content; computer technologies include engaging user features such as interactivity and multimedia; computerized interventions are flexible in terms of dissemination channels; and opportunities to apply new technologies to HIV prevention will only grow in the future, including among African Americans.

Given the many advantages of such interventions and the great need for novel intervention strategies for African Americans, a computer-delivered,

individually tailored intervention for heterosexually active African Americans was developed by Noar, Harrington, Van Stee, and Aldrich (2011). The intervention is called the Tailored Information Program for Safer Sex (TIPSS).

The primary theoretical basis for TIPSS is the attitude–social influence–efficacy (ASE) model (Fishbein & Ajzen, 1975). This theory is an integration of the theory of reasoned action, social cognitive theory, and the transtheoretical model, and it suggests that three sets of proximal factors—attitudes, social influences, and self-efficacy—are critical determinants of health behavior change. In addition, the theory takes a broad view of these concepts. Attitudes include positive and negative aspects of a behavior and consideration of cognitive and emotional beliefs; social influences include perceived behavior of others (descriptive norms), as well as direct pressure or support to perform a behavior (injunctive norms); and self-efficacy includes confidence in one's ability to perform the behavior and/or the difficulty of performing the behavior. These proximal factors are thought to influence progression through the transtheoretical model of change's five stages of change, and ultimately are theorized to impact behavior and behavioral change. The TIPSS program encourages individuals (particularly those in later stages of change) to use these newly acquired negotiation skills.

The TIPSS program works as follows: Individuals are asked questions about sexual partners that determine which module(s) they receive. Assessment of all ASE variables is conducted separately by partner type, allowing for partner-specific beliefs to be assessed and appropriate feedback to be provided. Different approaches to condom negotiation were integrated into both the feedback messages as well as the negotiation interactive activity.

The TIPSS program comprises two content mechanisms. The first is tailored feedback, which is the core mechanism in any computer-tailored intervention. The second is a set of interactive exercises, which, as indicated earlier, was used for skills training purposes. Stage of change was used as the key organizing construct for the tailored feedback. Thus, once individuals move down a particular path (e.g., main partner), they are staged for consistent condom use with that partner and they receive feedback on their stage of change and level of condom use. Then, all of the feedback that they subsequently receive (on condom attitudes, norms, self-efficacy, and negotiation strategies) is sensitive to which stage of change they are in. After someone is placed in a particular stage, he or she remains on that path throughout the entire module.

Once an individual completes the assessment for a particular theoretical construct, the program computes the score and compares it to the predetermined cut point for that construct. This determines whether the individual receives above-cutoff or below-cutoff feedback on that particular construct. In all cases except for cons (where the situation is reversed), above-cutoff indicates that individuals have scored adequately on the construct, while below-cutoff indicates that they have a deficit on that construct.

> *An elegant feature of tailored interventions is the fact that they are sensitive to where individuals are located relative to these theoretical constructs.*

TABLE 8-5 Examples of Feedback Messages Developed for an Individual in the Precontemplation Stage for Consistent Condom Use with a Main Partner

Theoretical Concept	Messages
Stage of change	You told us that you never use condoms when you have sex with your main partner. Your answers also indicate that you are not ready to use condoms every time you have sex with your main partner. This is common, as using condoms with a main partner can be difficult. This program will give you ideas to think about when it comes to condom use and your main partner.
Attitudes (pros): Above-cutoff	You told us that you recognize some of the benefits of using condoms with your main partner. That's great! For a minute, think about these benefits of using condoms. Using condoms with your main partner can show respect for your partner and can build trust in the relationship by showing that you want to protect one another and do the right thing. Using condoms can also allow you and your partner to enjoy sex more, because you won't have to worry so much about pregnancy, STDs, or HIV/AIDS. Put simply, condoms mean protection for both you and your partner.
Attitudes (pros): Below-cutoff	You told us that you do not currently recognize all of the benefits of using condoms. For a minute, just think about these benefits of using condoms with your main partner. Click on one of these to learn more: 1. Using condoms can show respect for your partner and can build trust in the relationship. 2. Using condoms can allow you and your partner to enjoy sex more.
Attitudes (pros): Below-cutoff—click to learn more 1	Using condoms can show respect and build trust by showing that you want to protect one another and do the right thing. This is something that can strengthen a relationship. The key is to communicate to your partner that condoms are a symbol of caring for them and for your relationship.
Attitudes (pros): Below-cutoff—click to learn more 2	Using condoms can allow you to enjoy sex more because you won't have to worry so much about pregnancy, STDs, or HIV/AIDS. In fact, did you know that condoms reduce the risk of pregnancy by 98.5% and reduce risk of contracting HIV/AIDS by 95%? Put simply, condoms mean protection for both you and your partner.

Above-cutoff feedback thus provides positive evaluation and briefly reinforces aspects of the theoretical construct, and below-cutoff feedback communicates that they are not where they need to be, and this feedback is more in-depth and detailed. **TABLE 8-5** provides examples of both above- and below-cutoff feedback that is delivered to participants. An elegant feature of tailored interventions is the fact that they are sensitive to where individuals are located relative to these theoretical constructs, and this responsiveness in feedback is thought to play to the efficacy of these interventions. As you can imagine, then, TIPSS provides the dual advantage of tailoring combined with easy dissemination, thereby magnifying effect sizes, as described in Figure 8-1.

Ultimately, the goal of this chapter was to provide you with an overview of health communication, its mission, strategies, theories, and approaches. As a discipline, health communication uses principles of persuasion to convey important messages that will influence health behavior and influence decision-makers and policymakers, who in turn can influence the public's health behavior.

▶ Take Home Messages

- Health communication is a growing field of research replete with applications capable of producing large overall net effects in public health.
- Attitude change is the core target of health communication theories and persuasion is the technique often used to affect attitudes.
- Core constructs include attention, reception, cognitions, routes of processing, message quality, credibility of the source, and characteristics of the receiver.
- Social marketing can be used to affect large-scale behavior change health products if it is implemented correctly and based on extensive formative research.
- Targeted messages are designed for segmented subgroups of a population, whereas tailored messages are designed for individuals.

▶ References

Anderson, A. R. (2006). *Social marketing in the 21st century.* Thousand Oaks, CA: Sage.

Bull, F. C., Holt, C. L., Kreuter, M. W., Clark, E. M., & Scharff, D. (2001). Understanding the effects of printed health education materials: Which features lead to which outcomes? *Journal of Health Communication, 6,* 265–279.

Fishbein M., & Ajzen, I. (1975). *Belief, attitude, intention, and behavior: An introduction to theory and research.* Reading, MA: Addison-Wesley.

Hastings, F., & Donovan, R. J. (2002). International initiatives: Introduction and overview. *Social Marketing Quarterly, 8*(1), 3–5.

Hoda, J. (2015). Identification of information types and sources by the public for promoting awareness of Middle East respiratory syndrome coronavirus in Saudi Arabia. *Health education research, 31*(1), 12–23.

Hovland, C. I., Janis, I. L., & Kelley, H. H. (1953). *Communications and persuasion: Psychological studies in opinion change.* New Haven, CT: Yale University Press.

Kreuter, M. W., Strecher, V. J., & Glassman, B. (1999). One size does not fit all: The case for tailoring print materials. *Annals of Behavioral Medicine, 21*(4), 276–283.

Lefebvre, R. C. (1992). *Social marketing and health promotion.* In R. Bunton & G. MacDonald (Eds.), *Health promotion: Disciplines and diversity* (pp. 154–181). London, England: Routledge.

Lefebvre, R. C. (2001). Theories and models in social marketing. In P. N. Bloom & G. T. Gundlach (Eds.), *Handbook of marketing and society* (pp. 506–518). Newbury Park, CA: Sage.

Lustria, M. L. A., Cortese, J., Noar, S. M., & Glueckauf, R. (2009). Computer-tailored health interventions delivered over the web: Review and analysis of key components. *Patient Education & Counseling, 74*(2), 156–173.

McGuire, W. (1968). *Personality and attitude change: An information-processing model.* In A. G. Greenwald, T. C. Brock, & T. M. Ostrom (Eds.), *Psychological foundations of attitudes* (pp. 171–196). New York, NY: Academic Press.

McGuire, W. J. (2013). McGuire's classic input-output framework for constructing persuasive messages. In R. E. Rice & C. K. Atkin (Eds.), *Public communication campaigns* (4th ed., pp. 133–146). Thousand Oaks, CA: Sage Publications, Inc.

Noar, S. M., Benac, C. N., & Harris, M. S. (2007). Does tailoring matter? Meta-analytic review of tailored print health behavior change interventions. *Psychological Bulletin, 133*(4), 673–693.

Noar, S. M., Harrington, N. G., & Aldrich, R. S. (2009). The role of message tailoring in the development of persuasive health communication messages. In C. S. Beck (Ed.), *Communication Yearbook 33.* New York: Lawrence Erlbaum.

Noar, S. M., Harrington, N. G., Van Stee, S. K., & Aldrich, R. S. (2011). Tailored health communication to change lifestyle behaviors. *American Journal of Lifestyle Medicine, 52*(2), 112–122.

Petty, R. E., Barden, J., & Wheeler, C. (2002). The elaboration likelihood model of persuasion: Health promotions that yield sustained behavior change. In R. J. DiClemente, R. A. Crosby, & M. C. Kegler (Eds.), *Emerging theories in health promotion practice and research* (pp. 71–99). San Francisco, CA: Jossey-Bass Wiley.

Petty, R. E., Jarvis, W. B. G., Evans, L., & Bakker, A. (1995). *Using persuasion related strategies to modify AIDS-related attitudes and behaviors.* Paper presented at the annual meeting of the American Psychological Association, New York, NY.

Rothman, E. F., Decker, M. R., & Silverman, J. G. (2006). Evaluation of a teen dating violence social marketing campaign: Lessons learned when the null hypothesis was accepted. *New Directions for Evaluation, 110,* 33–44.

Serdula, M. K., Gillespie, C., Kettel-Khan, L., Farris, R., Seymour, J., & Denny, C. (2004). Trends in fruit and vegetable consumption among adults in the United States: Behavioral risk factor surveillance system, 1994–2000. *American Journal of Public Health, 94*(6), 1014–1018.

Taylor, L. E., Swerdfeger, A. L., & Eslick, G. D. (2014). Vaccines are not associated with autism: An evidence-based meta-analysis of case-control and cohort studies. *Vaccine, 32*(29), 3623–3629. http://doi.org/10.1016/j.vaccine.2014.04.085

U.S. Department of Health and Human Services. (2000). *Healthy people 2010: Understanding and improving health* (2nd ed.). Washington, DC: U.S. Government Printing Office.

Weinreich, N. K. (2006). *What is social marketing?* Weinreich Communications. Retrieved from http://www.social-marketing.com/Whatis.html

Winett, R. A. (1995). A framework for health promotion and disease prevention programs. *American Psychologist, 50*(5), 341–350.

Yom-Tov, E., Feraru, G., Kozdoba, M., Mannor, S., Tennenholtz, M., & Hochberg, I. (2017). Encouraging physical activity in patients with diabetes: Intervention using a reinforcement learning system. *Journal of Medical Internet Research, 19*(10), e338. http://doi.org/10.2196/jmir.7994

Chapter Opener: © Hero Images/Getty Images; © lzf/Shutterstock; © Henrik Sorensen/Getty Images; © MeskPhotography/Shutterstock

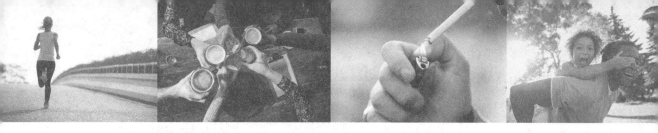

CHAPTER 9

Ecological and Structural Approaches to Improving Public Health

Richard A. Crosby, Laura F. Salazar, and Ralph J. DiClemente

It's bizarre that the produce manager is more important to my children's health than the pediatrician.

—**Meryl Streep**, actress

PREVIEW

In stark contrast to individual-level approaches to health promotion, ecological approaches target multiple influences of health behavior, because changing individuals and their behaviors may be temporary without corresponding changes to the environment in which they are embedded. Using an ecological approach, supportive environmental factors are considered when designing effective and sustainable health-promotion programs.

OBJECTIVES

1. Describe the basic considerations of ecological models of health and behavior.
2. Articulate differences and similarities between various ecological models.
3. Describe the application of ecological thinking to a health problem or behavior.
4. Understand the differences between ecological approaches, multilevel approaches, and structural-level approaches to health promotion.

▶ Introduction

Just as the world has changed rapidly, the approaches used in public health have also taken a dramatic turn in recent years. As the prevention of disease continues to be a primary challenge of public health, health-promotion professionals have increasingly turned their attention to solutions that can make positive, sustainable changes. Ecological approaches to health-promotion target multiple environmental influences of health (e.g., the availability of fresh foods, access to outdoor recreation facilities, and the walkability of sidewalks) and often involve long-standing changes to physical, legal, economic, and social environments; thus, they are quite strong and enduring.

This chapter is perhaps one of the most important chapters in this text. As such, we want to begin with the poignant example of America's obesity epidemic. The following text is taken directly from a Centers for Disease Control and Prevention (CDC) report:

> Approximately two-thirds of U.S. adults and one-fifth of U.S. children are obese or overweight. Being either obese or overweight increases the risk for many chronic diseases (e.g., heart disease, type 2 diabetes, certain cancers, and stroke). Reversing the U.S. obesity epidemic requires a comprehensive and coordinated approach that uses policy and environmental change to transform communities into places that support and promote healthy lifestyle choices for all U.S. residents. Environmental factors (including lack of access to full-service grocery stores, increasing costs of healthy foods and the lower cost of unhealthy foods, and lack of access to safe places to play and exercise) all contribute to the increase in obesity rates by inhibiting or preventing healthy eating and active living behaviors.
>
> (Centers for Disease Control and Prevention [CDC], 2009)

As you can quickly see from this CDC report, obesity may be an epidemic that is only amenable with an ecological solution. Although the value–expectancy theories you learned about in Chapter 4 may provide some direction in changing both diet and exercise behavior, programs of this type generally fail to produce long-term behavior change because of the countervailing environmental influences. Considering the new public health perspective, which takes into account the impact of the environment on individual health, it is clear that the obesity epidemic will require organizational and policy changes that reach deep into society. **FIGURE 9-1** illustrates specific ecological determinants that should be targeted.

The basic premise of ecological thinking is that health, behavior, and their determinants are interrelated. Ecological thinking has always been an important influence on health promotion. Bronfenbrenner's (1979) contribution to an ecological approach in health promotion is one of the most important, and perhaps the best known ecological model would be the PRECEDE–PROCEED planning model (developed by Green & Kreuter (2005), see Chapter 3). According to these and other models, ecological approaches foster behavior change through targeting the environmental factors that are most likely to influence people's decisions and actions. The purpose of this chapter is to describe the characteristics of ecological models, introduce several models or frameworks that describe ecological relationships, and discuss how ecological thinking and models can be used to guide health promotion.

The primary function of an ecological approach is the use of every available means that has a reasonably strong potential to ultimately contribute to lasting behavior change. Although intervening with individuals, families, and even entire communities may not be a novel idea in public health, the concept of changing key aspects of the environment is an emerging paradigm. In many cases, changes to the

One increasingly important role taken on by the public health practitioner is to become an advocate for changes in policy, regulation, and legislation that enhance people's long-term adoption of health-protective behaviors.

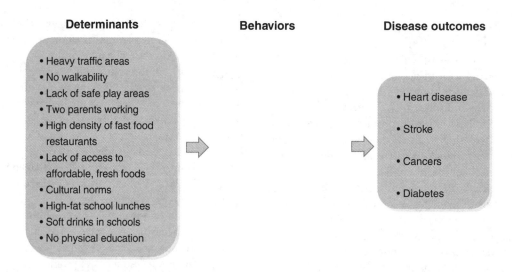

Determinants	Behaviors	Disease outcomes
• Heavy traffic areas • No walkability • Lack of safe play areas • Two parents working • High density of fast food restaurants • Lack of access to affordable, fresh foods • Cultural norms • High-fat school lunches • Soft drinks in schools • No physical education		• Heart disease • Stroke • Cancers • Diabetes

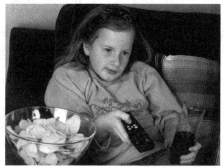
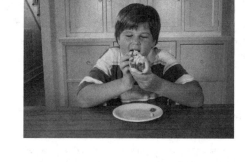

FIGURE 9-1 Ecological determinants of diet and exercise

Photos left: © Ivonne Wierink/Shutterstock, right: © D. Anschutz/Digital Vision/Thinkstock.

environment can become powerful influences on health behavior; thus, one increasingly important role taken on by the public health practitioner is to become an advocate for changes in policy, regulation, and legislation that enhance people's long-term adoption of health-protective behaviors.

One way to understand and develop an appreciation for ecological thinking is to consider the limitations of an alternative model, the medical model. In the medical model way of thinking, obesity is viewed as a medical condition amenable to medical intervention (e.g., gastric bypass, gastric stapling, or fat-blocking drugs). Note that these types of medical interventions are delivered by physicians at the individual level, that is, each patient is treated in the office, one at a time. These medical treatments may be effective for each of those individuals; however, the population as a whole will not benefit and the underlying root causes remain unaddressed. Thus, the obesity epidemic continues and is not ameliorated. As we stated earlier, there are many other factors involved in the obesity epidemic other than "people eating too much." Environmental factors such as the ubiquity of fast food restaurants; the shift from outdoor play/recreation to more sedentary, indoor activities such as video games and computer screen time; and neighborhoods lacking in walkability and safety are all significant contributors. The ecological

The ecological and contemporary perspective is that behavior is influenced by many factors at multiple social levels, and therefore changes directed at multiple levels are needed.

approach, unlike the medical approach, avoids blaming the person and emphasizes the complexity of certain health behaviors. The ecological and contemporary perspective is that behavior is influenced by many factors at multiple social levels, and therefore changes directed at multiple levels are needed. **FIGURE 9-2** provides an example of an ecological model highlighting various factors pertaining to sexual violence perpetration on college campuses across multiple levels. As shown, the model illustrates that at the highest level, factors such as gender inequality, rape culture, and gender norms are contributors to sexual violence perpetration by the individual in addition to the individual's level of knowledge, attitudes, and normative beliefs.

Ecological models have evolved over the past several decades as a consequence of lessons learned in earlier health-promotion programs. Some of these lessons have been learned the hard way—through failure. For example, in the 1980s and 1990s, the U.S. federal government spent a large sum of money testing community-level intervention programs designed to prevent heart disease. Some of the larger studies were titled the Multiple Risk Factor

Intervention Trial (Stallones, 1983) and the Community Intervention Trial for Smoking Cessation (Anonymous, 1995). The unfortunate reality was that none of these large-scale trials actually worked because they failed to target relevant environmental factors. However, on the positive side, failure can be constructive when the reasons for failure are brought to the surface. In fact, failure is often a vital part of the scientific process and can be a catalyst for change. Thus, for these large, community-level intervention studies, essential lessons should and can be learned. For example, intervention efforts, albeit large-scale initiatives, that do not attempt to alter relevant environmental factors will not succeed in changing behavior. In the absence of creating supportive environments, behaviors such as overeating may become normative, thereby perpetuating a risk environment. The concept of a "risk environment" was captured eloquently by Link and Phelan (1995) when they described how environments contribute significantly to behavior because they essentially set the stage for people to engage in the unhealthy or risky behavior. The concept is actually quite simple: some environments foster more risk behaviors than others.

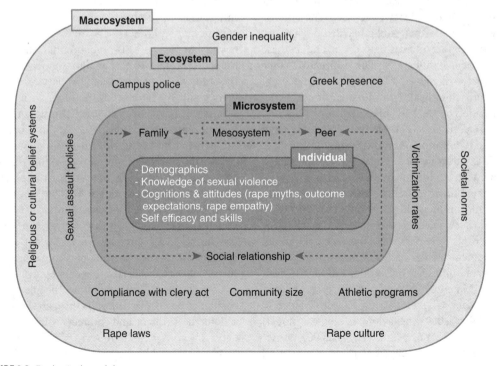

FIGURE 9-2 Ecological model

In the absence of creating supportive environments, behaviors such as overeating may become normative, thereby perpetuating a risk environment.

A good example is the lack of environmental tobacco smoke laws. In the absence of workplace policies that prohibited smoking, it was easy for people to light up, even if they had attempted to quit. Thus, not targeting the social environment is a likely reason for the failure of some of these large-scale heart disease prevention programs. Environmental factors exert tremendous (and unmitigated) influence on people to engage in risk behaviors, despite the best efforts of the intervention program (McKinlay & Marceau, 2000).

In thinking about the concept of people being at risk for unhealthy behavior, it is immediately obvious that many diseases may in fact have a **social etiology**, meaning that the underlying cause of the disease lies in the sociocultural environment. Heart disease, for example, has social etiologic roots in the structure and lack of regulation of the food industry, the tobacco industry, and the cultural tradition of sedentary lifestyles. The important point here is that public health scholars and practitioners are increasingly cognizant of these environmental influences. The desire to change these factors is indeed a key aspect of an ecological approach to health promotion. For additional information on the basis of ecological approaches, please refer to: Glass and McAtee (2006), Link and Phelan (1995), and Susser and Susser (1996).

In contrast to most of the theories presented in this text, ecological models tend to be more conceptual than theoretical, although theory certainly informs them. In this text we have chosen to focus on a few selected models. First, we will introduce Bronfenbrenner's (1979) model of human development, which has provided sustained and widespread influence on thinking about the multiple and interacting social influences on human development. The models by Hovell, Wahlgren, and Adams (2009) (behavioral ecological model) and Cohen, Scribner, and Farley (2000) (structural model of behavior) emphasize the structural aspects of the environment and originate mainly

from operant conditioning and social cognitive theory. Next, minority stress theory will be described as an ecological approach to understanding health disparities. Subsequently, we introduce intersectionality theory as an emerging framework for understanding multiple oppressions that greatly detract from the health of marginalized populations. The chapter concludes by describing the use of purely structural-level interventions in public health practice and by introducing the concepts of microenvironments and macroenvironments.

▶ Key Concepts

Bronfenbrenner's Model of Human Development

Bronfenbrenner (1979) was primarily interested in how human development is influenced by the social system. In this context, development refers mainly to psychological and social dimensions of development, which of course are important aspects of health. He noted the substantial influences of parents and family on child development, in addition to the broader societal influences of community and other social and structural influences. Furthermore, Bronfenbrenner stated that the social ecology of human development involves the study of mutual transactions between human beings and the properties of the environmental systems in which they interact throughout their life. Bronfenbrenner suggested that the fit between the person and the environment influences successful development and identified four important system levels: microsystem, mesosystem, exosystem, and macrosystem. **TABLE 9-1** provides a description of these four environmental systems. You may recall that we first introduced you to this model in Chapter 2 (you may want to look at Figure 2-2, the diagram of Bronfenbrenner's socioecological model, in that chapter again).

According to Bronfenbrenner, people develop positive and negative behaviors through their interactions, both direct and indirect, with these systems. These systems may serve to constrict and/or promote healthful development. Consider, for example, intimate partner violence (IPV). Much

TABLE 9-1 Outline of Bronfenbrenner's Ecological Levels		
Ecological Level	**Description**	**Example**
Microsystem	This level refers to the immediate environment in which a person is operating; it is a dynamic system in which the person is affected and in turn affects the environment.	Family, classroom, peer group, neighborhood.
Mesosystem	This level refers to the interaction of two microsystem environments.	Family affecting an adolescent's peer group.
Exosystem	This level refers to aspects of the environment in which an individual is not directly involved, which is external to his or her experience, but nonetheless affects him or her.	Parents' workplace, economic state of community, parents' marriage.
Macrosystem	This level refers to the larger cultural context, including issues of cultural values and expectations, in which the other systems function.	Values, laws, resources, customs of a particular culture.

research in the past 30 years has been conducted to understand why men perpetrate violence against their loved ones. Findings suggest that although some men who commit IPV may exhibit some type of psychopathology, most researchers agree that cultural factors such as patriarchy and lack of social and legal sanctions for batterers contribute to the behavior. Also, in some cultures, IPV is normative and acceptable.

Using Bronfenbrenner's model, addressing IPV would entail enacting new laws and policies that punish the behavior (macrosystem); promoting the emergence of new social norms that are unsupportive of IPV, perhaps through a national media campaign (macrosystem); implementing workplace policies that support court-ordered temporary restraining or protective orders so that an abusive husband would be arrested if he came to his wife's place of work (exosystem); and implementing school-based educational programs that promote egalitarian relationships and zero tolerance for IPV (microsystem). In many ways, Bronfenbrenner's thinking about these multisystem influences on development has become a fundamental framework guiding many areas of social science and practice, including health education and health promotion, social work, child development, and sociology.

Structural Model of Health Behavior

The structural model of behavior (Cohen et al., 2000) emphasizes environmental influences of behavior. Four categories of environmental factors are viewed as critical in shaping health behaviors: (1) availability/accessibility, (2) physical structures, (3) social structures and policy, and (4) media and cultural influences.

Availability/Accessibility

Behavior is influenced by access: the greater the access, the more likely the behavior is to occur. This principle is well illustrated by a series of studies focused on the number of stores that sell alcoholic beverages in a given community. Neighborhoods with greater density (number per square mile) of alcohol sales outlets had higher rates of alcohol-related problems, such as motor vehicle accidents (Scribner, MacKinnon, & Dweyer, 1994), interpersonal violence (Scribner, MacKinnon, & Dweyer, 1995), and gonorrhea (Scribner, Cohen, & Farley, 1998). The structural model of behavior suggests that implementing policies that reduce the density of alcohol outlets or even fast-food outlets would improve related health behaviors and health outcomes. Similarly, it has been demonstrated that the distribution of free condoms can lead to an increase in condom use (Cohen et al., 1999).

Physically limiting the product is one way to affect its availability; however, availability can also be achieved through modifying the price of the product. The concept of price elasticity suggests that people will buy less of a product as the price goes up and more as the price goes down. Studies have demonstrated that price hikes for cigarettes due to tax increases translate into reduced consumption as a result of restricted access (Flewelling et al., 1992; Ross & Chaloupka, 2003). Evidence suggests that this same effect also applies to alcohol consumption (Leung & Phelps, 1993). These two examples provide evidence that government policy changes, such as increasing taxes on tobacco and alcohol, can have a tremendous health-protective effect at the population level.

Physical Structures

The physical environment can influence a range of health behaviors and health-related outcomes such as substance use, diet, physical activity, and unintentional injury. A classic example is the Children Can't Fly program, developed in New York City (the Bronx) in response to the high rate of childhood injuries due to falls from low-income high-rise structures. Many local apartment buildings had windows with wide openings rather low to the floor, and all too often children fell through these openings. Ultimately, the community provided inexpensive window guards to 42,000 families, leading to a dramatic reduction in childhood falls and injuries (Spiegel & Lindaman, 1977).

Similarly, the fluoridation of water, fortification of salt with iodine, and convenient and safe pedestrian and bicycle routes are examples of effective environmental solutions to important health problems. Another example is creating defensible space to reduce neighborhood crime and drug dealing. A program known as Crime Prevention Through Environmental Design is credited with reducing crime by helping communities eliminate unsupervised and poorly lit spaces in urbanized areas by creating community gardens and the like (Newman, 1996).

In this example, changes were made only to the built environment and were successful in achieving significant behavior changes.

Social Structures

"Rules and organizations behind them are the social structures that mold the world we live in. In more ways than we realize, rules and organizations create an invisible structure that profoundly shapes how we live our lives and how healthy we are" (Farley & Cohen, 2005, p. 96). A striking example of the importance of social structures is the relationship between state seat belt laws and the actual use of seat belts. The national average for seat belt use was less than 40% until the federal government made highway funding contingent upon states' adopting mandatory safety belt laws in the 1980s; this quickly resulted in an increase in use rates approaching 60%. States with primary enforcement laws that enabled police to ticket nonusers had higher rates of use than states with secondary enforcement laws. States in which enforcement of these laws was vigorous had still higher rates of use. Tobacco policies have shown similar success. States and communities that adopt policies that forbid smoking in public places report lower overall rates of smoking.

Effects of Media

Media (Internet, movies, music, television, print, video games, etc.) have a profound influence on health behavior. Advertising is often used to shape social norms about the acceptability and attractiveness of engaging in certain health-related behaviors such as smoking, drinking alcohol, risky sexual behavior, high-sugar soft drinks, and high-fat diets. These negative influences are due primarily to the ubiquitous nature of media messages and partly to the ingenious use of communication theories in crafting those messages.

Behavioral Ecological Model

The behavioral ecological model (BEM) (Hovell et al., 2009) focuses on the effect of **metacontingencies**, extending the concept of operant conditioning to the societal level.

Operant conditioning, which is a cornerstone of behaviorism, was postulated by B. F. Skinner to explain how people learn new behaviors. **Operant conditioning** involves a process of reinforcement through consequences or contingencies. New behaviors are acquired as a result of being either positively or negatively reinforced via contingencies in the environment. Borrowing heavily from operant conditioning, Hovell and colleagues defined metacontingencies as social reinforcements that transcend the individual to affect large segments of a population or subpopulation.

The strength of a metacontingency can be defined by the probability of encountering social consequences for a given behavior. Hovell and colleagues also argued that societal patterns and norms are operant, in that they provide general reinforcement for certain types of behavior, and thereby they shape the context within which behavior operates. The aggregate outcomes of cultural influences on behavior are described as metacontingencies because they have generalized effects on behavior. Metacontingencies may include general cultural patterns and standards, public policy, taxes, and regulations. For example, in California, there are strong and dense (i.e., pervasive) metacontingencies against smoking in public places due to the strict antismoking laws and policies, as well as a strong social norm that frowns upon smoking (see **FIGURE 9-3**). Given this reality, the probability of coming into contact with these metacontingencies would be high (e.g., there is no smoking allowed in restaurants or bars).

Traffic regulation techniques provide a familiar example of the effect of metacontingencies on behavior. Traffic lights can be programmed so that those who drive according to the posted speed limit will not have to stop often. The effect of this metacontingency is to reinforce safe speed limits and also reduce pollution. Similarly, many communities have installed cameras

> *The strength of a metacontingency can be defined by the probability of encountering social consequences for a given behavior.*

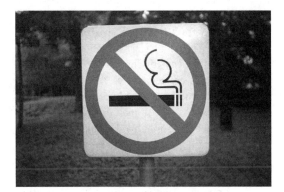

FIGURE 9-3 Example of no smoking sign
© L. Watcharapol/Shutterstock

with lasers that detect and retain photographs of speeding vehicles, resulting in tickets mailed to the registered vehicle owner. These metacontingencies have been demonstrated to reduce speeding and may serve to shift social norms toward lower speeds, even in areas without cameras and timed traffic lights. Of course, these public safety measures can only be adopted in communities where the public and policymakers share social norms favoring these safety devices over the minor infringement on civil liberties involved.

Minority Stress Theory. Minority stress theory has become increasingly important in public health research and practice. This is particularly true given the utility of this theory to address social equity issues. The basis of minority stress theory is predicated on three central tenets: (1) minority status is linked to distal sources of daily stress, (2) minority status is linked to proximal sources of daily stress through distal sources, and (3) minority group members experience disproprotionate health risks caused by exposure to proximal and distal stressors. Minority stress theory suggests that social situations do not directly influence the health of minority group members. Rather, challenging social environments lead to long-term, daily stress. In turn, this chronic daily stress creates physical and mental conditions that accumulate to the point of deteriorating health.

Of foremost importance, minority stress theory differentiates distal from proximal sources of stress. You may recall learning about distal and proximal influences in Chapter 2. Briefly, proximal influences are located closer to the person (internal). Examples of proximal sources relative to minority stress theory include constructs such as internalized homophobia, internalized racism, and feeling of hopelessness. Distal influences are located in the larger structures of society and economics (external to the person). Examples of distal sources relative to minority stress theory include constructs such as discrimination based on sexual orientation, experienced racism, and gender-based employment discrimination. Minority stress theory (see **FIGURE 9-4**) uses both proximal and distal influences as central tenets to understand how minority status may result in poor health outcomes. As such, this ecological-based theory provides a roadmap outlining the empirical pathway that explains the link between minority status and health disparities.

Minority stress theory is important to achieving social equity because chronic-daily stress is often the putative risk factor for the looming health disparities of minority members in the United States and elsewhere. For example, it has been well established that chronic psychological stress and accompanying depression impair antiviral immune responses and contribute to inflammation (Glaser & Kiecolt-Glaser, 2005). Inflammation is a significant contributor to degenerative diseases including cancer, heart disease, diabetes, Alzheimer's, and many others.

In a prospective study, minority stress was assessed among 74 bereaved men who have sex with men (MSM) (Hatzenbuehler, Nolen-Hoeksema, & Erickson, 2008). Men were assessed both before and after the loss of a partner or close friend who died of AIDS. The researchers found significant effects of minority stress on substance use and depression whereas bereavement-related stressors (e.g., length of partner illness) were largely unrelated to these health outcomes. Thus, their findings suggest the utility of minority stress theory, given its predictive ability was superior to that of a major life stressor (i.e., bereavement). Similarly, Hatzenbuehler and Pachankis (2016) found evidence supporting minority stress theory as applied to a population of lesbian, gay, bisexual, and transgender youth. They reported evidence

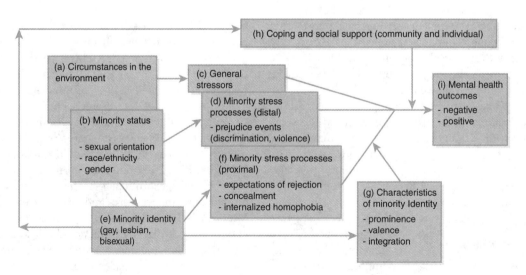

FIGURE 9-4 A conceptualization of minority stress theory applied to mental health

Reproduced from Meyer IL. Prejudice, social stress, and mental health in lesbian, gay, and bisexual populations: Conceptual issues and research evidence. Psychological Bulletin 2003; 129:674–697.

suggesting important associations between stigma-inducing mechanisms and health-risk behaviors of LGBT youth. Their findings suggest that stress reduction should be a key objective of multilevel interventions for LGBT youth. For example, stress-reduction interventions using mind-body therapies including tai chi, qi gong, meditation, and yoga have received increasing awareness in the past two decades and have shown significant effects in reducing minority-related stress and accompanying negative health behaviors and outcomes (Burnett-Zeigler, Schuette, Victorson, & Wisner, 2016).

Intersectionality. As a paradigm for facilitating a better understanding of social inequities, intersectionality theory is used to explain both oppression and privilege as they occur in members of minority populations. Social "super-structures" such as the meaning a society places on race, ethnicity, sex, gender, and economic class form the main drivers of oppression and privilege. As the name implies, it is the intersection of these drivers that form group memberships that result in either extreme oppression (e.g., homeless, African American transwomen) or privilege (wealthy, white men).

We urge you, throughout your career in public health, to constantly consider resolving social inequities as a public health imperative. As a lens of understanding these inequities, intersectionality provides insight into how an individual's membership into one or more sociodemographic categories may lead to co-occurring forms of oppression. For example, consider the health risks of a person who: (1) is black, (2) resides in an impoverished area, and (3) identifies as a sexual minority. Depending on the sociopolitical context of the environment/community, people in each of these three categories are likely to be the target of stigma, prejudice and discrimination by those in society who have social privilege and power. When, however, any one person is in all three categories, they are likely to be at extreme risk for experiencing co-occurring oppressions. **BOX 9-1** provides an example of the health risks

experienced by a sample of black men who have sex with men, residing in an impoverished area of the southern United States More importantly, Box 9-1 demonstrates how a third "layer" of intersectionality (identification as transgender woman) exacerbates the risk levels.

A highly recognized champion of this theory (Dr. Kimberle Crenshaw) recently founded the Columbia University Law School's Center for Intersectionality and Social Policy Studies. This Center is highly focused on using intersectionality theory to guide social policy, in the United States and elsewhere. Indeed, a key aspect of intersectionality theory is that laws and social policies typically apply to a specific category of people who may experience discrimination/oppression. Employment opportunities that even subtly limit hiring of minority members, for example, are in violation of equal employment opportunity law in the United States When a second form of group membership is "layered" over race/ethnicity—such as being identified as gay, bisexual, or lesbian—the level of oppression may be magnified. The intersection between minority race and sexual minority status is unlikely to carry legal/policy protection. Thus, in this example, the intersection of race and sexual minority status creates multiple oppressions that are more extreme than the oppression of being a racial minority alone or a sexual minority alone. As you can imagine then, other memberships in socially stigmatized groups may lead to a further magnification of oppression.

Of importance, we wish to emphasize that where a person resides also significantly affects the degree of oppression. For example, being a black gay man in Washington DC is probably far less likely to result in multiple oppressions than being a black gay man in Little Rock, Arkansas. Consider the likely differences in health-risk behaviors between a Latina woman who is also a sexual minority (lesbian) and a second woman who is also Latina and a lesbian but who is earning an income far below the federal poverty level and also injects drugs. In the former case, only two forms of oppression are co-occurring; whereas in the latter case four forms of oppression are co-occurring.

BOX 9-1   A Comparison of Risk Profiles Based on the Intersection of Transgender Identification

Young black men who have sex with men (YBMSM) is a common term in public health used to denote what has become the U.S. subpopulation experiencing the greatest burden of HIV. A recent study of 600 YBMSM included a question asking participants whether they identified as transgender. Thirty-two of the 600 YBMSM (all biological males) identified as transgender women. This study then compared these 32 *young black transgender women having sex with men* (YBTWSM) with those not identifying as transgender, relative to selected sexual risk behaviors. Key findings from this analysis are as follows:

Risk Behaviors	Prevalence	Prevalence	RR[1]	P
	YBTWSM	YBMSM		
Had anal sex for money/drugs	9/30 (30.0%)	36/566 (6.4%)	4.69	<0.001
Had anal sex for money	9/32 (28.1%)	36/577 (6.2%)	4.53	<0.001
Depend on sex partner for money, food, etc.	11/30 (36.7%)	69/562 (12.3%)	2.98	<0.001
Sex partner recently released from prison	8/32 (26.7%)	10/566 (1.8%)	14.8	<0.001
Had sex with a guy without knowing his name	16/30 (53.3%)	142/566 (25.1%)	2.12	<0.001
Had sex once with a guy and never saw him again	17/30 (56.7%)	177/566 (31.3%)	1.82	0.004

As shown, for each of the six selected risk behaviors, the added layer of identification as a transgender woman greatly exacerbated the contrast in levels of risk. Thus, this brief analysis provides an empirical demonstration of intersectionality augmenting risky health behaviors.

Reproduced with permission from Laura Beauchamps

FIGURE 9-5 provides a visual illustration of the differences in co-occurring oppression between these two hypothetical women. As depicted by this figure, the value of intersectionality theory lies in its ability to help prioritize populations experiencing co-occurring oppression. By prioritizing a given population, opportunities may arise for structural-level interventions (see next section).

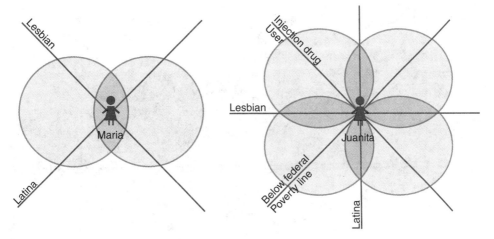

FIGURE 9-5 Intersectionality of co-occurring oppression

Finally, we urge you to consider the importance of viewing the "solution" at social/policy level and avoiding the mistake of trying to "fix the person" who is experiencing co-occurring forms of oppression. An example is a study reported by Velez, Moradi, and DeBlaere (2014). This study investigated the additive and interactive effect of these dual oppressions relative to self-esteem, among 173 sexual minority Latinas/os. The study found that high internalized racism was associated with poor self-esteem among those reporting high levels of racial discrimination. Also, the study found that low internalized heterosexism was associated with greater self-esteem among those with higher levels of racial discrimination. Finally, low internalized racism was associated with greater self-esteem among those experiencing high levels of heterosexist discrimination. We offer this example here to illustrate the interactive effect of multiple intersectionalities, as well as the usefulness of also understanding minority stress theory when using the lens of intersectionality.

Structural Interventions: A Derivative of Ecological Approaches

Structural-level interventions transcend many of the limitations of interventions based solely on the social and behavioral sciences. Defined as a planned change to the physical, social, policy, or legal environment, structural-level interventions are a derivative of ecological thinking. One aspect of ecological thinking is that the environment provides important influences on health and behavior. As stated previously, some environments set the stage for individuals to engage in risky behavior, and in addition to individuals, entire communities can also be thought of as being at risk. Of course, the converse is equally true! Environments can be "structured" to foster the adoption and maintenance of healthy behaviors. **BOX 9-2** provides an excellent example of this concept, using a highly successful transportation

Structural-level interventions transcend many of the limitations of interventions based solely on the social and behavioral sciences.

The logic behind structural interventions is that the physical, legal, economic, and regulatory structures within an individual's environment can be altered to support the adoption and maintenance of health-protective behaviors.

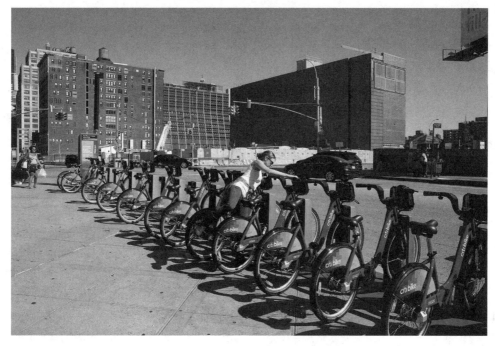

© Tim Clayton/Corbis/Getty Images

BOX 9-2 Structured Changes in Cities Can Have a Profound Impact on Health Behaviors

Faced with ever-present and overwhelming issues with traffic management, the city of New York recently created a massive system that allows people to use public bicycles to move around the city. Cast as "Unlock a bike—Unlock New York (faster than walking, cheaper than a taxi, and more fun than a subway)" this program is revolutionizing commuting in NYC while also getting people to be physically active. This structural-level intervention included the redesign of road surfaces to very clearly delineate lanes set aside specifically for cyclists, thus greatly raising the safety factor.

With hundreds of bike "pick-up/drop-off" stations throughout the city and its boroughs (including Jersey City), residents can purchase a yearly pass that allows them to take a bike for an unlimited number of 45-minute rides. Bikes are "checked out" with a key and returned into an automatic locking system. The city investment in this transportation alternative may not have been intended to raise the fitness levels of New Yorkers, but the rapid popularity of the program is very much a structural-level approach to improving cardio-vascular health. The city has effectively promoted the program as well. From the website for Citi Bike, *"Citi Bike is a fun and affordable way to get around the city, and a great alternative to the subway, taxis, buses, and walking. It's designed for quick trips with convenience in mind. Use it to commute to work or school, run errands, get to appointments, and more."* At the cost of $163 per year, the program operates in way that is sustainable for the city and economical for the residents—potentially saving money for those who use the system of thousands of bikes to replace their commute by car, taxi, bus, or subway.

---

intervention in New York City. Please note as you read this box that all four previously mentioned elements that define structural-level interventions (i.e., planned change to the physical, social, policy, and legal environment) are represented by this example.

When any given part of the environment becomes a target for change, it is known as structural intervention. Structural interventions have become increasingly popular and can be subsumed under an ecological approach. In essence, the logic behind structural interventions is that the physical, legal, economic, and regulatory structures within an individual's environment can be altered to support the adoption and maintenance of health-protective behaviors. One example of a structural intervention is providing supportive housing for homeless and unstably housed persons living with HIV/AIDS. The rationale is that by providing a stable home environment, people living with HIV/AIDS will engage in fewer risk behaviors, reducing the transmission of HIV (Kidder, Wolitski, Campsmith, & Nakamura, 2007).

Microenvironmental and Macroenvironments

Another way of conceptualizing ecological approaches is captured by the concepts of microenvironments and macroenvironments, articulated by Swinburn and Egger (2002). Similar to Bronfenbrenner's microsystem, microenvironments include social and physical factors that are proximal and persistent. These include social influence by peers, parents, and family, as well as immediate resources such as money, equipment, and facilities. Macroenvironments (also similar to Bronfenbrenner's macrosystem) include factors somewhat more distal than microenvironmental factors, affecting health and behavior in an indirect way by creating what Hovell would call metacontingencies. Macroenvironmental influences include policies, regulations, taxes, and resource allocation.

The availability of fresh foods in the home would be a microenvironmental factor, whereas the number of fast-food outlets in a community would be a macroenvironmental factor. The concept of micro- and macroenvironmental influences on behavior has

Microenvironments include social and physical factors that are proximal and persistent.

been used to explain health behaviors of various sorts, including those that lead to obesity. Accordingly, modern U.S. society provides an obesogenic environment, which is thought to contribute to the epidemic of childhood and adult obesity (Swinburn & Egger, 2002).

To illustrate these micro and macroenvironmental influences on behavior, consider this fictitious example of Tommy. To assist with this example, we provide a side-by-side comparison of these influences in **TABLE 9-2**.

Tommy is a typical 10-year-old boy attending elementary school in a suburban neighborhood of the Midwestern United States. Tommy's parents each work full-time jobs. Each morning for breakfast Tommy quickly consumes sugary breakfast cereals that he has asked his parents to buy for him. Not surprisingly, Tommy favors cereals advertised on television, designed to appeal to children like Tommy, while his parents give in to his desires because these types of cereals are often cheaper. Although Tommy lives fairly close to school, most days he gets a ride from one of his parents, who are uncomfortable letting him walk or ride his bike to school due to the lack of sidewalks. Tommy is not athletic and during physical education classes he generally stays on the sidelines with other overweight children to avoid being made fun of by other students or the teacher. At lunchtime, Tommy often consumes a cheeseburger, fries, and chocolate milk. Sometimes he takes an apple, but after eating his favorite things he usually has no appetite for the apple. After school, Tommy has a sugary toaster treat, a dessert left over from the previous evening, or some other high-fat snack. Rather than play outside, Tommy watches TV or plays video games until dinner. He would like to play outside with friends in his neighborhood, but there are no parks or other open spaces and his parents do not want him to play in the street. After dinner and dessert, Tommy does his homework, has another snack while he watches TV, and then goes to bed.

Tommy's food intake is influenced by the food industry and the school lunch program, which both promote and provide high-fat and high-calorie foods. Tommy's parents are also influenced by the food industry and are not able or are not willing to provide Tommy with

TABLE 9-2 Micro- and Macroinfluences of Diet and Exercise

Microenvironmental Influences	Macroenvironmental Influences
Parents allow or encourage a high-fat diet, provide few alternatives to high-fat food, and do not encourage physical activity	Sidewalks not provided so walking to school not safe
Affiliation with other overweight peers may affect self-perception and norms	Local community priorities favor roads over recreational areas and programs
School lunch provides high-fat diet, contributing to weight and norms	National agricultural policies funnel high-fat, commodity foods to school food services
School physical education fails to engage Tommy and other overweight children, wasting the opportunity for exercise and calorie expenditure and encouraging the sedentary norms	Federal policies fail to regulate advertising on children's programs
Lack of local green spaces, parks, and recreation facilities reduce opportunities for physical activity	Regulation of food industry fails to emphasize healthful diet Lack of organized community sports and recreation activities minimizes opportunities for physical activity School district policies do not favor healthful school environment, providing high-fat meals and physical education that does not adequately support fitness goal

a well-balanced diet. The lack of sidewalks and convenient outdoor recreation areas reduces opportunities for physical activity. The availability of electronic games, television, and Internet compete with more physical activities. Given his diet and lack of regular physical activity, Tommy will continue to gain weight; by the time he reaches high school he may be obese, and this condition is unlikely to be reversed in his adulthood. Tommy's parents are well intentioned, but are also susceptible to the same environmental influences as Tommy. They tend to buy and serve foods that are advertised and have a rather sedentary lifestyle, thereby encouraging Tommy's obesity unwittingly. Consider the environmental influences on Tommy's diet and physical activity behavior.

Is Tommy's behavior the product of individual choice or environmental influence? The answer, of course, is that individual choice and environmental influence are highly interrelated. Tommy's behavior can be understood as the product of micro- and macroenvironmental factors that generally encourage his high-fat, high-calorie diet and infrequent physical activity. However, not all children exposed to the same environmental influences become obese, so clearly there is an interaction between the individual and the environment. There is also little question that the environment influences behavior. Therefore, it makes sense to create healthful environments as often as possible. While thoughtful school curricula designed to teach Tommy the importance of skills for eating healthy foods may influence Tommy's motivation to eat fewer calories, without concomitant environmental support, Tommy's behavior is unlikely to change. After all, dietary behavior is influenced by the access to foods, advertising, the density of fast-food outlets, and other environmental factors. Changing these in ways that support healthful eating are important and necessary influences on motivation and behavior.

One of the important implications of ecological thinking is that change strategies should create environments that facilitate healthy behavior. One way of thinking about this is to create, when possible, environments where the healthful "choice" is the default option. Loewenstein, Brennan, and Volpp (2007) described this concept as asymmetric paternalism, where micro and macroenvironments are engineered to promote the adoption of health-protective behaviors, especially for those less prone to adopt them, while also not harming those who already engage in them. Simply stated, the paternalism aspect means granting access to the healthy choice while inhibiting access to the unhealthy choice. The goal is to make it easy to do the "right" thing and more difficult to do the "wrong" thing. What if, for example, general practitioners routinely scheduled a colonoscopy for their patients turning 50 years of age (the age of first recommended colonoscopy)? What if fast-food restaurants replaced the soda in their value meals with bottled water? The same concept can be applied to myriad behaviors, including dietary choices and exercise. For example, school food services and even restaurants could highlight low-fat, low-sodium foods and deemphasize highly processed, high-fat foods. Stairs could be located centrally and elevators off to the side of new buildings. Roads could be planned so that pedestrian and bicycle routes were safely integrated rather than added on later. The density of fast-food restaurants and alcohol outlets could be greatly limited through zoning regulation. Of course, these kinds of changes are not going to happen overnight or by chance, but there are ways of making incremental changes.

> *The goal is to make it easy to do the "right" thing and more difficult to do the "wrong" thing.*

▶ Applied Examples

Here we provide several examples of structural and multilevel approaches applied to a variety of health behaviors. These examples serve to illustrate the fundamental principle that small structural changes can influence large numbers of people.

Example 1: New Zealand French Fries

Morley-John, Swinburn, Metcalf, Raza, and Wright (2002) provided a fascinating study that serves as an excellent illustration of this principle. In a study in New Zealand, they found that the fat content of restaurant-prepared french fries varied from as little as 5% of the weight to as much as 20%. This variation is attributable to frying practices and the thickness of the french fry. Thinking from an ecological intervention perspective, it would be quite easy to imagine that requiring all fast-food restaurants to use thicker fries (Swinburn & Egger, 2002) would result in fat content being reduced to the lower end of the range. This small change in one practice, when magnified through large chains such as McDonald's and Burger King, could indeed have profound and lasting impacts on the mean level of daily fat intake across extremely vast populations worldwide. In turn, the net effects of this lowered mean daily intake could become part of a larger mosaic effort to engineer clinically meaningful reductions in obesity. Clearly, similar small effects magnified to meaningful levels could be achieved by mandating and enforcing frying practices that limit the absorption of fat into the potato slices.

Example 2: Smoking Control Policies and Practices

An excellent example of the power of policy is found in the adoption and enforcement of laws that prohibit the sale of tobacco to minors. More strict and comprehensive smoking policies are associated with lower rates of smoking among adolescents (Botello-Harbaum et al., 2008). An analysis found a strong relationship between merchant compliance with laws prohibiting sales to minors and the use of tobacco among minors. For every 1% increase in merchant compliance, there was a 2% decline in tobacco use among young people (DiFranza, Savageau, & Fletcher, 2009).

A widely publicized example of a program guided by the goal of modifying behavior through changes in policy and related metacontingencies is the California Tobacco Control Program. The overall objective of the program was to transform the public image of tobacco use, making it a socially unacceptable behavior. One program emphasis focused on passing laws to discourage smoking, including banning smoking in public places (environmental tobacco smoke laws). Such laws not only limit opportunities for smoking and make smoking inconvenient, but also contribute to a social climate supportive of nonsmoking behavior. Ultimately, many policies were adopted to restrict sales to minors, limit tobacco product advertising, and increase the cost of cigarettes via tax levies. Some of the funds generated by these taxes were used to support smoking cessation programs for pregnant women and to provide tobacco use prevention programs to school children. In addition, the overall program provided support for smoking prevention media and school-based programs. The expansive program emphasis on the metacontingencies of smoking policies and social norms was credited with altering societal reinforcement for smoking, thereby reducing overall smoking rates (Hovell et al., 2002).

Example 3: Encouraging Stair Use

Another example of the effects of a small structural change on behavior is the simple posting of signs on stairs and elevators to encourage greater use of the stairs (Brownell, Stunkard, & Albaum, 1980; Russell, Dzewaltowski, & Ryan, 1999). Of course, stairs that are attractive and accessible are more likely to be used, but beyond this, education and media may also foster social norms favoring stair walking and other physical activity. This is one successful example of simple structural changes that encourage healthful behavior and can be implemented in conjunction with health-promotion campaigns designed to motivate these behaviors.

Example 4: HIV Prevention in Brazil

An example of an ecological intervention is the remarkable success of the government of Brazil in the prevention of HIV and in the long-term control of AIDS. In the early 1990s, the AIDS epidemic in Brazil was not much different than the AIDS epidemic in most African countries. By the year 2000, AIDS incidence in Brazil had leveled off to about 25,000 cases per year (Okie, 2006), less than one-half the rate reported by the United States for 2006. In the short time between 1996 and 2002, Brazil achieved a 50% reduction in AIDS-related mortality and an 80% decline in AIDS-related hospitalization (Anonymous, 2005). The vast majority of this public health success story is a direct consequence of changes to the macroenvironment leading to changes in social norms.

Potentially the most significant macroenvironment change occurred in conjunction with Brazil's adoption of a constitutional right to universal access to health care in 1988. Brazil pioneered the world's first government-sponsored program that provided free access to antiretroviral therapy for all its citizens with HIV/AIDS. Clearly, this bold move also involved a huge financial investment by the government; however, it appears that the investment was wise, Brazil is estimated to have saved approximately $2.2 billion between 1996 and 2004 (Okie, 2006). Brazil effectively reduced costs in this venture by working with manufacturers to make available low-cost generic versions of antiretroviral medications. Arguably as important as the economics of this plan has been the commitment to comprehensive public education programs to prevent HIV infections. Brazil's national AIDS program has aggressively pursued the agenda of preventing HIV infection through a web of government programs, including widespread condom promotion campaigns utilizing state-of-the-art social marketing techniques.

The model efforts of Brazil exist in stark contrast to the lack of government support for condom promotion and sex education in the United States. Brazil has been credited with great success in promoting condom use among commercial sex workers, a population that is blatantly ignored and marginalized in the United States. The same is true for injection drug users, as the Brazilian government has supported effective needle and syringe exchange programs, while similar efforts in the United States have largely languished. With just these few examples in mind, it is quite clear that a truly effective ecological approach is highly dependent on active government support and sponsorship because public health is ultimately a function of social norms, which both influence and are influenced by government programs and policies. Notably, one of the greatest achievements of the National AIDS Program in Brazil is the nationwide destigmatization of AIDS. By the free provision of antiretrovirals, people were far less reluctant to be tested for HIV and to "come out" with their HIV-positive status, given the lifesaving advantages of treatment. In essence, this single change to the macroenvironment created a social norm that fostered a national attitude of compassion and caring rather than marginalization and discrimination. AIDS is not disappearing in Brazil, but it is safe to assert that their epidemic is under a level of control that is simply not possible in the absence of the broad-sweeping ecological changes made in that country.

▶ Summary

Ultimately, the goal of this chapter has been to provide you with new ways of thinking about health behavior. Collectively, ecological approaches emphasize environmental influences on health behavior and suggest the importance of multilevel programming. Even though attempting to change environmental factors may be a daunting challenge, the returns to public health may be substantial. Although it is not always possible to alter macroenvironmental influences such as public policies, it is usually possible and useful to target interventions to microenvironmental factors, such as local social and physical environmental factors.

▶ Take Home Messages

- Ecological approaches may be most applicable and effective with health behaviors that permeate daily living, such as eating and exercise behaviors, but environment and individual factors interact with respect to all health behaviors.

- We do not suggest in this chapter that health promotion should focus exclusively on structural-level changes. We do, however, suggest that the structural environment influences behavior and that health-promotion planning should always consider including structural-level intervention when feasible.

- Ecological and structural approaches provide additional perspectives that may be useful in constructing a "theory of the problem" (see Chapter 1) and suggest a variety of micro and macroenvironmental goals worth including as part of multilevel programming.

- Racial/ethnic, gender and sexual minorities experience significant and unique stressors stemming from racism, transphobia and homophobia that contribute to numerous negative health outcomes. Societal level changes are warranted; however, until significant social change occurs, mind-body interventions may provide some attenuation of negative effects.

- Intersectionality theory posits that the intersection of two or more social structures such as race/ethnicity, gender, social class, gender identity, and sexual orientation results in significant oppression of certain groups who are on the minority side of these structures.

- Multiple examples exist to support the idea that simple structural changes in the environment can have lasting and profound effects on the behaviors that greatly influence the onset of chronic diseases, including diabetes, heart disease, and cancers, as well as infectious diseases such as AIDS.

- The processes of behavior change are the same whether the behavior is personal (e.g., one's diet, physical activity, or substance use), supportive (e.g., parents provide opportunities for healthful diet and physical activity), structural (e.g., schools and communities provide healthful environments with open spaces for exercise and play and safe areas for walking and biking), or public policy (e.g., taxes on cigarettes and smoke-free public places). The key is to identify who controls or influences these goals or outcomes and then create interventions to alter their behavior.

▶ References

Anonymous. (1995). Community intervention trial for smoking cessation (COMMIT): Cohort results from a four-year intervention. *American Journal of Public Health, 85*, 183–192.

Botello-Harbaum, M., Haynie, D. L., Iannotti, R. J., Wang, J., Gase, L., & Simons-Morton, B. G. (2008). Tobacco control policy and adolescent cigarette smoking status in the United States. *Nicotine & Tobacco Research, 34*, 675–681.

Bronfenbrenner, U. (1979). *The ecology of human development.* Cambridge, MA: Harvard University Press.

Brownell, K. D., Stunkard, A. J., & Albaum, J. M. (1980). Evaluation and modification of exercise patterns in the natural environment. *American Journal of Psychiatry, 137*, 1540–1545.

Burnett-Zeigler, I., Schuette, S., Victorson, D., & Wisner, K. L. (2016). Mind-Body approaches to treating mental health symptoms among disadvantaged populations: A comprehensive review. *Journal of Alternative Complementary Medicine, 22*(2), 115–124. doi:10.1089/acm.2015.0038

Centers for Disease Control and Prevention. (2009). Recommended community strategies and measurements to prevent obesity in the United States. *MMWR, 58*(RR07), 1–26. Retrieved from http://www.cdc.gov/mmwr/preview/mmwrhtml/rr5807a1.htm?s_cid=rr5807a1e

Cohen, D. A., Farley, T. A., Bedimo-Etame, J. R., Scribner, R., Ward, W., Kendall, C., Rice, J. (1999). Implementation of condom social marketing Louisiana, 1993–1996. *American Journal of Public Health, 89*, 204–208.

Cohen, D. A., Scribner, R. A., & Farley, T. A. (2000). A structural model of health behavior: A pragmatic approach to explain and influence health behaviors at the population level. *Preventive Medicine, 30*, 146–154.

DiFranza, J. R., Savageau, J. A., & Fletcher, R. E. (2009). Enforcement of underage sales laws as a predictor of daily smoking among adolescents—a national study. *BMC Public Health, 9*, 107.

Farley, T., & Cohen, D. A. (2005). *Prescription for a health nation: A new approach to improving our lives by fixing our everyday world.* Boston, MA: Beacon Press.

Flewelling, R. L., Kenney, E., Elder, J. P., Pierce, J., Johnson, M., & Bal, D. G. (1992). First-year impact of the 1989 California cigarette tax increase on cigarette consumption. *American Journal of Public Health, 82*, 867–869.

Glaser, R., & Kiecolt-Glaser, J. K. (2005). Stress-induced immune dysfunction: Implications for health. *Nature Reviews Immunology, 5*, 243–251.

Glass, T. A., & McAtee, M. J. (2006). Behavioral science at the crossroads in public health: Extending horizons, envisioning the future. *Social Sciences & Medicine, 62*, 1650–1671.

Green, L. W., & Kreuter, M. W. (2005). *Health program planning: An educational and ecological approach* (4th ed.). New York, NY: McGraw-Hill.

Hatzenbuehler, M. L., & Pachankis, J. E. (2016). Stigma and minority stress as social determinants of health among lesbian, gay, bisexual, and transgender youth. *Pediatrics Clinics, 63*, 985–997.

Hatzenbuehler, M. L., Nolen-Hoeksema, S., & Erickson, S. J. (2008). Minority stress predictors of HIV risk behavior, substance use, and depressive symptoms: Results from a prospective study of bereaved gay men. *Health Psychology, 27*(4), 455–462. http://dx.doi.org/10.1037/0278-6133.27.4.455

Hovell, M., Wahlgren, D., & Adams, M. (2009). The logical and empirical basis for the behavioral ecological model. In R. J. DiClemente, R. A. Crosby, & M. C. Kegler (Eds.), *Emerging theories in health promotion research and practice* (2nd ed., pp. 451–510). San Francisco, CA: Jossey-Bass.

Hovell, M. F., Wahlgren, D. R., & Gehrman, C. (2002). The behavioral ecological model: Integrating public health and behavioral science. In R. J. DiClemente, R. Crosby, M. Kegler (Eds.), *New and emerging theories in health promotion practice & research.* San Francisco, CA: Jossey-Bass, Inc.

Kidder, D. P., Wolitski, R. J., Campsmith, M. L., & Nakamura, G. V. (2007). Health status, health care use, medication use, and medication adherence in homeless and housed people living with HIV/AIDS. *American Journal of Public Health, 97*(12), 2238–2245.

Leung, S. F., & Phelps, C. E. (1993). My kingdom for a drink . . . ? A review of estimates of the price sensitivity demand for alcoholic beverages. In M. E. Hilton & G. Bloss (Eds.), *Economics and the prevention of alcohol-related health problems.* NIAAA Research Monograph No. 25, NIH Publication # 93-3513.

Link, B. G., & Phelan, J. C. (1995). Social conditions as fundamental causes of disease. *Journal of Health and Social Behavior, Spec. Nos.*, 80–94.

Loewenstein, G., Brennan, T., & Volpp, K. G. (2007). Asymmetric paternalism to improve health behaviors. *Journal of the American Medical Association, 298*, 2415–2417.

McKinlay, J. B., & Marceau, L. D. (1995). Upstream healthy public policy: Lessons from the battle of tobacco. *International Journal of Health Services, 30*, 49–69.

Morley-John, J., Swinburn, B., Metcalf, P., Raza, F., & Wright, H. (2002). Fat content of chips, quality of frying fat and deep-frying practices in New Zealand fast food outlets. *Australian New Zealand Journal of Public Health, 26*, 101–107.

Newman, O. (1996). *Creating defensible space.* Washington, DC: Department of Housing and Urban Development. Retrieved from http://www.huduser.org/publications/pubasst/ defensib.html

Okie, S. (2006). Fighting HIV—Lessons from Brazil. *New England Journal of Medicine, 354*, 1977–1981.

Ross, H., & Chaloupka, F. J. (2003). The effect of cigarette prices on youth smoking. *Health Economics, 12*, 217–230.

Russell, W. D., Dzewaltowski, D. A., & Ryan, G. J. (1999). The effectiveness of point-of-decision prompt in deterring sedentary behavior. *American Journal of Health Promotion, 13*, 257–259.

Scribner, R. A., Cohen, D. A., & Farley, T. A. (1998). A geographic relation between alcohol availability and gonorrhea rates. *Sex Transmission Diseases, 25*(10), 544–548.

Scribner, R. A., MacKinnon, D. P., & Dweyer, J. H. (1994). Alcohol outlet density and motor vehicle crashes in Los Angeles county cities. *Journal of Student Alcoholism, 55*, 447–453.

Scribner, R. A., MacKinnon, D. P., & Dweyer, J. H. (1995). The risk of assaultive violence and alcohol availability in Los Angeles County. *American Journal of Public Health, 85*(3), 335–340.

Spiegel, C. N., & Lindaman, F. C. (1977). Children can't fly: A program to prevent childhood morbidity and mortality from window falls. *American Journal of Public Health, 67*, 1143–1147.

Stallones, R. A. (1983). Mortality and the multiple risk factor intervention trial. *American Journal of Epidemiology, 117*, 647–650.

Susser, M., & Susser, E. (1996). Choosing a future for epidemiology: From black box to Chinese boxes and eco-epidemiology. *American Journal of Public Health, 86*, 674–677.

Swinburn, B., & Egger, G. (2002). Preventive strategies against weight gain and obesity. *Obesity Reviews, 3*, 289–301.

Velez, B. L., Moradi, B., & DeBlaere, C. (2014). Multiple oppressions and the mental health of sexual minority Latina/o individuals. *The Counseling Psychologist, 43*(1), 7–38.

Chapter Opener: © lzf/Shutterstock; © Henrik Sorensen/Getty Images; © MeskPhotography/Shutterstock; © Hero Images/Getty Images

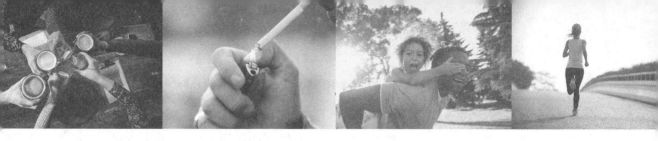

CHAPTER 10
Social Network Theory

Laura F. Salazar, Richard A. Crosby, Jamal Jones, Krishna Kota, and Ralph J. DiClemente

Social networks are these intricate things of beauty, and they're so elaborate and so complex and so ubiquitous that one has to ask what purpose they serve.

—**Nicholas A. Christakis**

PREVIEW

This chapter describes social network theory, which posits that information, knowledge, ideas, and attitudes spread through interconnected networks of nodes/actors. Information and even health behaviors spread through networks because the ties between nodes/actors represent friendships, relationships, etc. One individual within a social network may have a high degree of influence on other individuals within his/her social network, so much so that this one person is able to affect the health behaviors and health outcomes of the people to which he/she is connected. The degree of influence one has within a social network or the impact of an entire social network on individual health behaviors can depend on various aspects and characteristics of the social network understudy. An understanding of social network theory and its basic concepts provides an exciting opportunity to intervene within different populations and promote health.

OBJECTIVES

1. Obtain an overview of the history and foundations of social network theory.
2. Understand the components of social networks and how these components shape social networks.
3. Define the properties of social networks in the context of social network analysis.
4. Describe how health is affected by social networks and how social networks can promote positive outcomes.
5. Describe applications of social network research in the health-promotion literature.
6. Comprehend an emerging model in the context of social network theory.

▶ Introduction

Because of the Internet and other forms of communication, we live in a global society where people from different countries, backgrounds, cultures, religions, and mindsets share ideas, opinions, and friendships and form **networks**. A network in informal terms is "a set of relationships." But, more formally, "a network contains a set of objects (in mathematical terms "nodes") and a mapping or description of relations between the objects or nodes" (Kadushin, 2012, p. 14). However, despite this global society, it often takes us by surprise when we meet someone for the first time and then discover we have a common friend or acquaintance. In fact, we often remark "what a small world it is." Indeed, even before the advent of a global society, it was famously promulgated that each of us is connected to everyone else by only "six degrees of separation." This idea was based on the research of Stanley Milgram and Jeffrey Travers in the 1960s where they conducted an experiment to answer the question, "Two people, A and Z, who may not know each other directly, however, may both have acquaintances. How many such acquaintances are needed to link them?" Researchers asked 296 volunteers in Nebraska to send envelopes addressed to a stockholder in Boston, only by sending the envelopes to someone they know by the first name. This process is continued until the envelope reaches the stockholder in Boston area. They found that an average of six such acquaintances were needed for the envelope to reach from the volunteer in Nebraska to the stockholder in Boston area—hence the six degrees of separation (Milgram, 1967; Travers & Milgram, 1969). Thus, although it may be difficult to conceive, almost every individual is essentially connected to another, either directly or indirectly and these interconnections form social networks.

Social networks have been at the core of human society since hunter and gatherer times although in modern times the context has changed dramatically. Social network theory, which is the subject of this chapter, is one of the few theories in social science that can be applied to a variety of levels of analysis from small groups to entire global systems. Essentially, the same concepts can be applied to small groups, organizations, nations, and even international systems. Social network theory more recently has been extended to public health to explain health behaviors, morbidity, and mortality. For example, one can readily understand how an infectious agent such as the bacterium *Mycobacterium tuberculosis* that causes the disease tuberculosis can easily spread through a social network; however, Christakis and Fowler (2007) examined how obesity spreads among those with close ties to other individuals within their social network. They observed that an individual was more likely to become obese if he or she had a friend who also became obese. **BOX 10-1** describes the classic study conducted by Christakis and Fowler (2007) that demonstrated, for the first time, that obesity is a social phenomenon but one that spreads in similar ways to tuberculosis.

In this chapter, we provide an overview of social network theory, discuss a brief history and development of social network theory, describe key components and concepts of social networks, provide examples of how social network theory and analyses are applied to public health and health behavior research, and introduce the network-individual-resource model.

▶ Intellectual Foundations and a Brief History

The concept of social structures and connections between these structures were discussed as early as the late 1800s. The initial contributions to this concept were made by Auguste Comte, Sir Henry Maine, Ferdinand Tönnies, Emile Durkheim, Sir Herbert Spencer, Charles Horton Cooley, Gustave LeBon, and Georg Simmel, who had written "Society exists where a number of individuals enter into interaction." The paradigm shift in this concept came from the works of Jacob Levy Moreno and Helen Hall Jennings in 1934, who developed an innovative approach, sociometry, which involved the application of experimental techniques and empirical methods, to analyze the dynamic

BOX 10-1 The Social Spread of Obesity

Christakis and Fowler utilized a social network analysis to ascertain the spread of obesity among a cohort of offspring from the Framingham Heart Study. The researchers queried over 5000 **egos**, persons whose behavior was being analyzed and their connections to **alters**, individuals connected to an ego who may influence the behavior of the ego. Longitudinal statistical models were used to examine whether weight gain in an individual was associated with weight gain in his/her friends, siblings, spouse, and neighbors. Christakis and Fowler also examined three different kinds of friendships: an "ego-perceived friendship," in which an ego identifies an alter as a friend; an "alter-perceived friendship," in which an alter identifies an ego as a friend; and a "mutual friendship," in which the identification is reciprocal. It was hypothesized that the degree of influence on health behavior is associated with the type of friendship one perceived he/she was in. For example, ego-perceived friendships may have the greatest influence on individual health behaviors of the ego because this person may esteem the alter and try to emulate his/her friends. Whereas in alter-perceived friendships, the ego may not esteem his/her friends as high and thus will not wish to emulate their behavior.

The authors report that among 5000 offspring from the Framingham Heart Study, a person's chance of becoming obese was 57% higher if he/she had a friend who became obese during the follow-up period. Similar results were observed for individuals who had obese siblings and obese spouses. However, these effects were not observed for individuals with obese neighbors in immediate geographic locations. The authors also found that people of the same sex had greater influence on each other as opposed to people of the opposite sex. The authors concluded that social networks influence biological and behavioral aspects of obesity. Obesity spreads through social ties.

interactions between groups and individuals within (Borgatti, Mehra, Brass, & Labianca, 2009; Freeman, 2004; Wellman, 1997).

Later, Mark Granovetter in 1973 published his work *"The strength of weak ties,"* which explained the relation between the networks at micro and macro levels. The inter-personal relations at the micro level form networks, which then, in turn become large-scale patterns at the macro level. In this study, participants who started new jobs through contacts were asked how often they "saw" their contacts. The findings suggested that 27.8% of participants rarely (once a year or less) saw their contacts, and 55.6% occasionally saw their contacts (more than once a year but less than twice a week), compared to 16.7% participants who saw their contacts often (at least twice a week). These results indicated that weak ties among social networks played an important role in diffusion of information and growth of networks (Granovetter, 1973).

In the later decades, Stephen P. Borgatti, Martin G. Everett, and Linton C. Freeman were among few who have made extensive contributions to apply social network theory into various

fields. Today social network approaches have been extended to a myriad of public health outcomes, including violence perpetration, obesity, condom use, and smoking, among others (Barrington, Latkin, Sweat, Moreno, Ellen, & Kerrigan, 2009; Bond & Bushman, 2017; Christakis & Fowler, 2007, 2008).

As an example of the power that social networks have over health behavior, consider a study suggesting that the perpetration of violence may be promoted through the influence of social networks. Using data from the National Longitudinal Study of Adolescent Health, Bond and Bushman (2017) investigated the spread of violence through social networks. Simply stated, adolescents who had friends perpetrate violence were more likely to also engage in violent behavior. This friend-to-friend association with violence extended beyond immediate friends to four degrees of separation (i.e., friends of friends of friends, of friends) for serious fights. For violence that caused serious injury, the authors found a similar effect, but with two degrees of separation. For violence defined as "pulling a weapon on somebody" the effect extended to three degrees of separation.

▶ Key Concepts

Components of Social Networks

Actors/Nodes. The major components of social network theory are **nodes** or **actors** and ties that connect the nodes where together they form a *network*. Nodes could be individual persons, schools, industries, states, or any other structure that could form a tie or relationship with other structures (Stephen & Borgatti, 2010). Similarly, ties could be of several types, such as friendships, trade agreements, communications, and contacts between two structures. Another important aspect of social networks is the position of nodes in their network. Nodes that are placed in a critical position, which receive more flow, have a higher control or influence in the network, and are distinct from those that are positioned to receive less (Borgatti et al., 2009). Actors/nodes form dyads or *pairs* (two individual nodes connected together) that may have weak or strong ties. Information is passed through interconnected pairs in the form of knowledge, attitudes, beliefs, and social support to engage in health behaviors. Dyadic relationships within a social network are particularly important in sexual-network and injection-drug-use research. In these instances, disease can spread through dyads due to unprotected sex or needle sharing if one individual is infected with a disease within the dyad (Gyarmathy et al., 2010; Peterson, Rothenberg, Kraft, Becker, & Trotter, 2009).

Similarly, nodes may also form **triads** (three interconnected nodes). Triads form the foundation of social network theory and analysis. The researcher or public health practitioner may be concerned with two concepts related to triadic relationships: balance and transitivity. In terms of **balance**, if a dyad shares agreement with a third actor or if one person within the dyad likes the third actor, then both actors within the dyad

> *Nodes could be individual persons, schools, industries, states or any other structure that could form a tie or relationship with other structures.*

are more likely to form a tie with the third actor (Kadushin, 2012). In other words, two individuals who have a close relationship will likely form ties with a third individual to form a triadic relationship than two individuals who do not have a close relationship to each other. However, imbalance may occur in a triadic relationship if two nodes have unfavorable views or attitudes toward a third actor. If actor A is an enemy of actor C and actor B is an enemy of actor C, then balance theory posits that actors A and B form a tie within the triadic relationship of A, B, and C to isolate actor C.

Transitivity is the second critical concept related to triadic relationships. The concept of transitivity posits that within a triad if there is a tie between actor A and actor B, and a tie between actor B and actor C, then actor A will likely form a tie with actor C (Kadushin, 2012).

Researchers typically examine the types of relationships between network actors to describe various characteristics of the network such as network **density** (to be discussed in more detail) and centrality of a node. In social network research, **centrality** refers to "popularity" or number of connections a particular node (or actor) has within a social network (Kadushin, 2012). An actor/node with a high degree of centrality has far more connections than an individual located within the periphery of a social network, and thus he/she can disseminate information within the social network much more efficiently and have a greater influence on health behavior outcomes. For example, Amirkhanian, Kelly, Kabakchieva, McAuliffe, and Vassileva (2003) used social networking approaches for an HIV prevention intervention program for young men who have sex with men (YMSM) and relied upon network leaders to disseminate HIV/AIDS prevention information to other YMSM within their social networks. Upon evaluation of the intervention, the researchers were able to show that network leaders significantly helped to improved HIV prevention communication within a social network, significantly increased network members' HIV/AIDS knowledge and risk reduction steps, improved perception that peer group norms supported safer sex, improved attitudes toward condom use and safer sex, improved self-efficacy for making risk reduction behavioral changes, and improved favorable intentions to enact risk reduction behavioral changes. These improvements in HIV behavioral outcomes were due in part to the influence of network leaders among YMSM.

Homophily. You have perhaps heard the expression, "birds of a feather flock together?" This expression nicely describes the concept of **homophily**. Homophily is from the Greek, meaning, "love of the same," and is the tendency of individuals of similar characteristics to form ties. Homophily plays an important role in the formation of ties and in turn social networks. Homophily can occur among those with similar backgrounds, occupational statuses, gender, racial/ethnic groups, and persons with shared belief systems. This phenomenon explains the social relationships where people are more likely to form ties with people who are similar to them (McPherson, Lovin, & Cook, 2001). Again, an applied example may be useful. In a study examining the health behaviors of older adults within a social network, homophily was observed for nodes with close contacts within their social network (Flatt, Agimi, & Albert, 2012). Older adults who smoked were more likely to have close contacts with other individuals who smoked within their social network. Further, older adults who were inactive were more likely to have close ties to other individuals who were also inactive within their social network even when accounting for demographic variables such as race and age. The degree of homophily can vary across relationship types and subpopulations for behaviors of interest that are related to health outcomes (Daw, Margolis, & Verdary, 2015). As Daw and colleagues stated: "…some relationships could be more homophilous for certain behaviors than others, meaning that homophily may be greater within networks where that behavior occurs. Behaviors that are

> *Homophily is from the Greek, meaning, "love of the same," and is the tendency of individuals of similar characteristics to form ties.*

more social (drinking and smoking), may be more similar among friends, while behaviors that occur at home (TV watching) may be more similar for siblings, and exercise may be more similar among club-mates, since exercise often occurs in club settings" (Daw et al., 2015, p. 34).

The degree of influence that homophily has on one engaging in a health behavior may be moderated by the salience of emotional support and the frequency of interaction between nodes. Furthermore, descriptive norms may motivate individuals within a social network to engage in certain health behaviors because others within the network convey the idea that the behavior is normal, which inspires others to do the same (Cialdini, Reno, & Kallgren, 1990). Injunctive norms, for instance, would preclude individuals from engaging certain health behaviors to avoid group sanctions.

Homophily exists within structural interactions. There are three primary types of structural interactions: (a) dyad level—the focus in on the characteristics of nodes or actor, (b) node level—analysis is focused on number of connections for a node, position of node in network, and (c) group level—focus is at network level on factors such as density of nodes, centralization. **BOX 10-2** describes a study in which multiple levels of structural interactions were assessed to explain injection drug use (IDU).

Mutuality. **Mutuality** in dyadic relationships is another important concept to understand. Mutuality implies that relationships are reciprocal and involve a give and take between two entities (Kadushin, 2012). The flow of information, resources, and emotional support flow both ways between actors A and B. Relationships that are one-sided are asymmetric, such as the relationship between a provider and a patient. Mutuality in a dyadic relationship (or a lack thereof) may have effects on various outcomes, such as perceived stress and depression. For example, Powell, Denton, and Mattsson (1995) found that high mutuality and internal locus of control were significantly related to low levels of depression for adolescents when examining mother–adolescent dyads. Mutuality is likely to occur among pairs with similar attributes. The principle of mutuality

BOX 10-2 Measurement and Assessment of Structural Interactions Among Injection Drug Users in St. Petersburg, Russia

In a social network research study, Gyarmathy and colleagues investigated how individual attributes, dyad characteristics, and social network characteristics influenced receptive syringe sharing, distributive syringe sharing, and sharing cookers in injecting partnerships of injection drug users in Russia (Gyarmathy et al., 2010). Individual level characteristics measured included demographic variables such as age and marital status, as well as other variables such as homelessness and HIV status. The researchers also collected nominated egocentric network data by asking participants to name people with whom they had contact within the previous 6 months who provided physical assistance, material aid, health advice, drugs, and with whom they used drugs or had sexual intercourse. The researchers also asked participants which of their nominated network members injected drugs. Note: Please keep in mind that social network studies, because participants are expected to convey information about others who are not necessarily enrolled in the study, warrant special oversight by institutional review boards and a high degree of safeguarding of confidential information. Typically, participants are asked to use initials of their network members rather than names. Gyarmathy and colleagues defined an "injecting dyad level" as a dyad where the IDU participant reported that another network member was also an IDU and they used drugs together in the past 6 months. At this level, the researchers ascertained receptive needle sharing, distributive needle sharing, and the sharing of cookers. Social-network–level variables assessed included binary variables to ascertain the density of the injecting network and the density of the non-injecting network. The researchers found that all three levels were associated with injection equipment sharing. Characteristics at the dyad level were modified by social network characteristics.

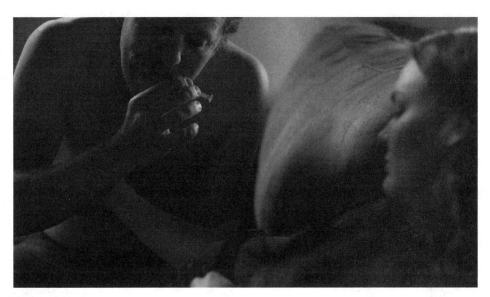

© Mark Andersen/Getty Images

can be extended to coalition building. In the realm of public health, mutuality may allow for coalition building by creating mutual flows between pairs that may not have similar attributes (Kadushin, 2012) to enact behavior change among individuals in various populations. This is especially true for drug and alcohol use prevention programs that build coalitions between various entities in an attempt to decrease drug and alcohol consumption (Kadushin, 2012).

▶ Three Assets of Social Network Models

Three important assets of social network models are **communication, information**, and **relations**. Communication within a social network allows actors/nodes to maintain relationships to people with whom they are connected over time. Frequent communication between two actors of a dyad can prevent decay and maintain the relationship within the larger social network (Oswald & Clark, 2003). Communication is an important aspect of social networks because it is the key driver of how information, ideas, and knowledge are spread through the network. For example, Barrington and colleagues examined the relationship between social network norms and condom use among male partners of female sex workers in La Romana, Dominican Republic, and assessed network level factors such as composition of the social networks of male clients as well as network density in addition to social support, communication about condom use, condom use norms, and condom use behaviors (Barrington et al., 2009). The researchers asked various questions on how frequent a participant communicated with other individuals within his social network about using condoms and whether any male contacts within his social network ever said that they disliked using condoms (Barrington et al., 2009). Results from this study indicated that male clients who talked about condoms to all of their social network contacts used condoms more consistently with female sex workers compared to men who did not communicate with their contacts about condom use. This example illustrates the importance of communication within a social network and its influence on health behavior outcomes. It is important to note that communication patterns within a social network can

Frequent communication between two actors of a dyad can prevent decay and maintain the relationship within the larger social network.

be affected by the size of the social network, the emotional closeness of actors within a social network, and the type of relationship that forms the ties of the social network. For instance, Roberts and Dunbar (2011) examined the communication patterns (operationalized as the time to last contact) in the social networks of 251 women. The researchers found that large network sizes, emotional closeness and the type of relationship (kinship vs. friendship) affected the time to last contact between actors within the social networks of women. Specifically, large kinship networks had longer times to last contact, participants with high levels of emotional closeness with other members within their social network had shorter times to last contact, and the effect of emotional closeness was greater for kinship ties than for friends.

Relationships form a key aspect of social networks. According to Haythornthwaite (1996), relationships indicate the connection between two or more people or things and are a specific kind of interaction between network actors. Haythornthwaite (1996) further stated that investigators might be concerned with the type of relationship (friendships, kinships, intimate partners, injection drug use partners, etc.) as well as how often the interaction takes place, or how much information and/or resources is exchanged. As we previously discussed, these relationships represent ties between two actors. Social network theory is concerned with the content as well as the pattern of relationships to determine how and what resources flow between actors. Specifically, when examining relationships in a social network the public health practitioner may be concerned with the content that is shared in a relationship, the direction of information flow between network actors, and the strength of the relationship. The type of relationship can

Relationships that are asymmetrical typically have information flow in one direction while the flow of information may not be relevant or measured in undirected relationships.

affect the health outcomes of an individual within a social network (as in the case of homophily). Also important, is the direction of information and resource flow between two network actors as well as the perceived relationship between network actors. Relationships that are asymmetrical typically have information flow in one direction while the flow of information may not be relevant or measured in undirected relationships. Finally another important aspect of relationships is the strength. Strength represents the intensity of the relationship and may represent the value of the link between two actors. Examining tie strength is important to assessing the overall connectedness of actors. Information and behaviors are likely to flow between network actors who have strong ties. However, weak ties allow for the transfer of new innovative information within social networks (thus, "the strength of weak ties").

Another asset of social networks is their ability to spread information to individuals within the network. Social network structures can influence the spread of information and who utilizes the information within a social network. Haythornthwaite (1996) described five principles of how information can be studied using social network approaches. The principles are:

- Information needs
- Information exposure
- Information legitimation
- Information routes
- Information opportunities

As we previously noted, relationships are an important asset to social networks and have an impact on what information is exchanged, between which actors the information is exchanged, and the extent to which the information is exchanged within a social network. Understanding the type of relationship (or tie) between two actors allows the researcher to have a better understanding of the information needs of the two actors and the social network more broadly. Assessment of an actor's prominence or position within a group can help the researcher understand information exposure. For instance, the strength of the relationship between actors or if actors are centrally located

within a social network can influence whether they receive information. Actors who are located at the periphery of a social network may not be exposed to information circulating *within the network*; however, actors in a central position within a network may not be exposed to new and innovative information from actors *at the periphery*.

The strength of a relationship between actors can indicate the degree to which actors can lend credibility to the information they deliver to other actors. Further, this strength can affect whether recipients use the information they receive. Network ties serve as a mechanism to legitimate the sender as a source of information. Patterns of forwarding and receipt allow the researcher to better understand information routes to determine where information travels within a network environment.

Finally, information opportunities depend largely on the principle of **brokerage**. Brokerage refers to lack of connection within a network. These can also represent connections between disorganized others. Usually measured as **betweeness** (the extent to which an actor sits between others in a network), brokerage may allow for some actors to serve as intermediaries between other network actors or two different networks. This concept is more commonly referred to as **bridging.** Bridging refers to connection across networks within a social system. As Haythornthwaite (1996) described an actor can maintain a central role without being connected to other individuals within a social network. An actor who sits between peripheral groups within a network or between two networks occupies a central position and therefore serves as a gatekeeper and who filters and imports important information between network members or between two networks.

Also important is the point that networks reside within

> *An actor who sits between peripheral groups within a network or between two networks occupies a central position and therefore serves as a gatekeeper.*

a larger social system. Social systems and the networks within them can be **traditional** (e.g., physical contact and connections occur in person) or **virtual** (e.g., via social media). Information and health behaviors flow within larger social systems. Social systems are the patterns of network relationships constituting a whole between individuals, groups, and institutions. Within social systems, social structure refers to the social arrangements of a society that emerge from, and determine the actions of, individuals. Essentially, individual actors are characterized by the roles they play in social systems (Merton, 1938, 1957). Roles are the set of expectations and patterns of behavior associated to positions in a social structure. Social systems increase their complexity by becoming increasingly insensitive to the complexity of the environment; however, another principle of social systems is that their increased complexity is associated with their dependency on environmental complexity (Valentinov, 2014).

Because of the increasing complexity of the environment, networks tend to self-organize and exert influence on the health outcomes of various populations at various levels. Two levels of network organization are the **meso** and the **macro** levels. Meso-level networks can constitute organizations or involve randomly distributed networks and scale-free networks. A discussion on the randomly distributed networks and scale free networks is beyond the scope of this text, but you are encouraged to read for more understanding of these types of networks (Cranmer & Desmarais, 2011; Moreira, Paula, Costa Filho, & Andrade, 2006). Macro-level networks can include large-scale networks and complex networks (Bailón, Wang, & Borge-Holthoefer, 2014). The use of the modular structure of networks to define brokerage at the local and global levels can help to capture role differences than alternative approaches that only consider local or global network features. An opportunity and challenge to public health is addressing the basic question, "how can we catalyze the characteristics of networks to so they evolve more quickly to achieve a specific outcome?"

▶ Health Effects of Social Networks

Evidence increasingly suggests that social networks may have profound effects on a range of health-related attitudes, behaviors, and disease outcomes. Examples include smoking, food choices, the perpetration of violence, and even divorce. The idea that "birds of a feather flock together" (i.e., homophily) is certainly part of this overarching influence (**FIGURE 10-1**); however, a companion to homophily is known as induction.

Induction occurs when one member of a network has a direct or indirect influence on the attitudes, beliefs, or behaviors of another person in the network. This is in contrast to joining a network based on preexisting similarities. Regardless of the existence of homophily and/or induction, the potential for social networks to magnify both positive and negative health behaviors is one that warrants the full attention of public health professionals. Consider, for instance, the all-so-critical behavior of tobacco use. Christakis and Fowler (2008) used data from the Framingham Study to investigate, over 32 years, several possibilities relative to the decline of smoking in the past several decades. Specifically, they investigated possible influences of:

- Clusters of those who smoked and did not smoke
- The influence of social contacts on individual-level smoking behaviors
- Whether social contact influence varied based on "type" (siblings, spouses, friends, co-workers, or neighbors)
- The influence of education and smoking intensity
- The role of large sub-networks in smoking cessation
- Whether people who continue to smoke "move" to the periphery of their network

They found that the decline in the number of people that smoked was associated with several of the preceding bullet points. For example, people who continued to smoke were more likely to be

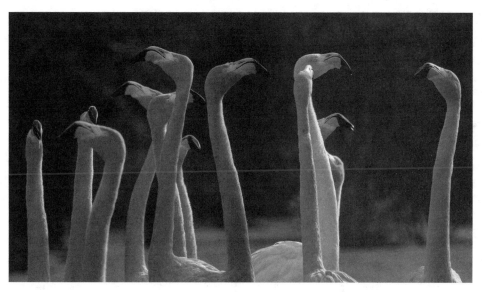

FIGURE 10-1 Homophily can be commonly understood as "birds of a feather flock together"
© Tino Schning/EyeEm/Getty Images

located in the periphery of a network as opposed to its core. Also, smokers were more likely to have ties to other smokers rather than non-smoking network members; this created a tendency toward segregation of clusters based on smoking.

Another example relates to food selection, specifically the selection of antibiotic-free animal products. Smith and Carpenter (2017) investigated the likelihood of people in a network to persuade others to adopt the practice of selecting and consuming antibiotic-free animal products. In this study, the concepts of homophily and behavioral determinants (i.e., norms, attitudes, awareness, and previous behavior) as well as **superdiffuser** traits were explored as predictors of intention to persuade others relative to this food choice. Superdiffuser is a term used to describe key members of a homophilic network who are largely responsible for norm setting in the network. Superdiffuser can be defined as a highly influential person who possesses three distinct traits: connectivity (ability to reach people and form "bridges" across groups), persuasiveness (skills and motivation to convince others), and **mavenism** (a person viewed as an expert relative to a specific content area of knowledge/skill). They found that behavioral determinants, intention to purchase

antibiotic-free animal products, and mavenism each predicted intentions to persuade others. Homophily, mavenism, and connectivity predicted patterns of inter-personal persuasion. These three traits may therefore be considered as vital to the spread of behaviors within and across social networks. Although in this case, the example was relative to antibiotic-free animal products, it is entirely conceivable that these same three traits would be equally important with respect to other health behaviors. Thus, an intervention implication is that a public health effort to foster given health behaviors could be "seeded" through the use of people who possess large amounts of these three key personality traits.

At this juncture it is important to note that superdiffusers may also exist in the virtual world. In **BOX 10-3**, we provide an example suggesting that superdiffusers (known as

> *One term used to describe key members of a homophilic network is "superdiffuser"— these are people who are largely responsible for norm setting in the network.*

BOX 10-3 Superusers—An Online Counterpart to Superdiffusers in Social Network Theory

A study of four digital health social networks tested the idea that only about 1% of a network population shapes the landscape of an online social network (van Mierlo, 2014). This idea comes from the 90-9-1 principle in cyber culture. This principle explains participatory patterns and network effects within Internet communities and posits that 90% of network actors observe, but do not participate in Internet communities. Further, the principle posits that 9% of actors contribute sparingly to these communities. Finally, the principle posits that 1% of actors create the majority of Internet content within cyber communities (i.e., the superusers). Van Mierlo and colleagues examined whether the 1% rule applied to moderated Digital Health Social Networks that were designed to promote behavior change. Using data from more than 63,000 actors in these four networks, the study found that those highly frequent users (superusers) were posting about 75% of the online content. The study found that although lurkers benefited from the interactions between superusers and contributors, they did not generate network effects or contribute to network growth and thus generated little to no network value. The authors concluded that superusers generate the majority of traffic and create value within Internet communities. They also emphasized that recruitment and retention of superusers within digital health networks is vital for long-term success of health-promotion programs. These results have implications for online social media marketing campaigns that rely on superusers and popular opinion leaders to generate and disseminate health-promotion content on social networking sites.

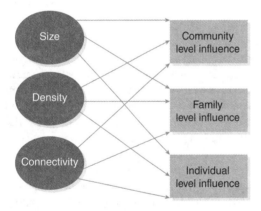

FIGURE 10-2 The influence of network properties on different levels of social networks

"superusers" in this case) generate the majority of content viewed across various digital social network sites.

A useful way to visualize how broadly a social network can influence communities, families, and individuals is shown in **FIGURE 10-2**. As shown, each of three components are linked to each of these three levels of influence (Carrington, Scott, & Wasserman, 2005). The first is **size** of the network. The size of the network represents the number of actors that constitute the network. The second is **density** of the network.

Density represents the number of direct (actual) connections divided by the number of possible connections in a network. The density of a social network can facilitate the transmission of ideas, knowledge, information, and other resources. The greater the density of a social network, the more likely the network is to be considered cohesive, a source of social support and an effective transmitter of ideas and resources. The third is **connectivity** within the network. The connectivity of the social network calculates the number of nodes that would have to be removed in order for one actor to no longer be able to reach another. Connectivity is high when there are different pathways that connect two actors. That is, there are multiple pathways for information or other resources to reach from actor to another.

▸ Social Network Analysis

The use of social network theory requires the use of a specialized set of analytic techniques, broadly referred to as social network analysis. The two major empirical methodologies in social network analysis are, **whole network analysis**, and **egocentric network analysis** (Wellman, 1997). In whole network analysis, researcher starts with selecting a set of nodes that is then considered as the study population. The researcher then measures ties between these nodes. In this method, a predefined structure such as an organization is selected as the population. This approach provides information about a few types of ties between many pairs of nodes.

In egocentric network analysis, individuals (known as focal nodes) are randomly selected from a population and data are collected about the number, nature, and characteristics of individuals who are connected to the sample of focal nodes. In this approach, the information obtained is in-depth regarding the many ties between the focal nodes. The network analysis is in reference to the sample individual (ego) and focuses mainly on the composition of ties with nodes.

Special software tools were developed to conduct social network analysis, such as UCINET (Borgatti, Everett, & Freeman, 2002). For example, in a study examining how risk networks contribute to racial/ethnic variation in HIV prevalence, Kottiri, Friedman, Neaigus, Curtis, and Des Jarlais (2002) utilized UCINET network analysis software to assess the risk networks of IDUs in the Bushwick neighborhood of New York City, NY. Using this software, they identified 92 component networks that varied in size from 2 IDUs to 230 IDUs. Although HIV prevalence was higher among black and Puerto Rican respondents (compared to respondents who self-reported being white/non-Hispanic), the researchers found no racial/ethnic differences in the size and structure of risk networks of IDUs. Further, egocentric sexual and drug risk networks were racially/ethnically homogenous.

Although social network analysis is far beyond the scope of this chapter and text, we do feel that you should become familiar with the basic terminology thereby enabling you to be a consumer of the peer-review literature regarding social network theory and health behavior. Typically, researchers are interested in reporting a variety of metrics related to the properties of the social network. **TABLE 10-1** summarizes these key network properties.

▶ Application Potential of Social Network Theory

A critical concept in network theory is to understand that networks are constantly evolving. This evolution can be natural, as occurring when actors/nodes within the network are the sole influence on any change in network composition. The evolution, however, can also be facilitated by formal intervention. Consider, for instance, an entering class of freshman on a large college campus that draws students from all over the world. On the first day of the opening semester it is safe bet that the density of the freshman class social network is close to zero. Because college/university administrators, however, recognize the value of social networks to the spread of information across students, planned social events are typically provided as a method of catalyzing the evolution of the network thus increasing the density factors progressively toward 1. Thus, planned intervention can be designed to foster the evolution of a network in a positive way. This, of course, can be applied to public health practice. One form of a positive intervention method is based on what is known as a key player analysis. Key players are network members who are closely connected to others (few degrees of separation) and high in persuasiveness, connectivity (i.e., a high level of degree centrality), and mavenism. Once key players are identified, intervention efforts with the people may be especially productive in that they may become superdiffusers to others in the network. This also has implications for any researcher using Respondent Driven Sampling to recruit members of otherwise hidden populations. Through formative research, it may be possible to identify who these key players are; thus, recruit them as seeds. The researcher first identifies seeds or "initial respondents" to participate in the study.

> *A critical concept in network theory is to understand that networks are constantly evolving.*

TABLE 10-1 Key Network Properties

Strong versus weak ties refers to a degree of association between two actors/nodes. A strong tie is when two actors know each other well and information flows freely between them. A weak tie is when two actors have infrequent contact and may not share similar views, attitudes, or behaviors. Although counterintuitive, weak ties are the conduits for novel information to flow into a network. This is because strong ties are confounded by homophily, thus leaving little opportunity for novelty. In contrast, weak ties may occur across people with very different attitudes, behaviors, etc. thereby creating opportunity for the exchange of novel information and ideas. Moreover, weak ties may bring different networks of strongly tied people together thus forming new connections and increasing betweeness centrality of the network.

Degree centrality is the number of nearest neighbors (direct connections to another node—connections that do not "pass through" another node). The average number of ties classified as nearest neighbors is used to calculate degree centrality.

Distance is the number of connections and paths between two nodes. The mean distance between nodes is best thought of in terms of degrees of separation (it is an average degree of separation for the entire network). Degrees of separation apply here in that most social networks (unlike a family, for example) comprise people whom may not all know each other (even through weak ties). Thus, for example if person A and person D are only connected through persons B and C, then the distance between A and D is defined by three degrees of separation (i.e., A $\rightarrow$ B = 1, B $\rightarrow$ C = 2, C $\rightarrow$ D = 3).

Closeness centrality is the average distance from a given starting node to all of the other nodes in the network is known as closeness centrality.

Betweeness centrality refers to ties between network members that are only possible between a third actor/node. The more an actor/node appears between other actors/nodes, the greater the betweeness centrality.

Density is the number of actors/nodes divided by the possible number of ties. The values of density can range from 0 (nobody knows anyone) to 1 (everybody knows everybody else).

Induction assumes a certain degree of susceptibility of alters to behavior change efforts by egos—this may be particularly common with adolescents who have not yet fully formed their own set of values, attitudes, and corresponding practices.

Structural holes occur when a possible tie between two people (each of importance to the network) is not realized.

After participating in the study, seeds are then asked to identify other individuals (who may be interested and eligible) to participate in the study. Seeds are given a finite number of coupons and asked to distribute their coupons to those individuals whom they know or are acquainted with and is also a member of the target population under study. Respondents who come into the study with a coupon are screened for eligibility and asked to participate. If these respondents agree and participate in the study, they are given a set of coupons and asked to recruit other potential respondents to participate. This peer recruitment cycle continues until the sample sized is reached.

A clear form of intervention would involve creating shorter distances between network members as this is optimal in terms of being protected by network norms, enhancing communications, etc. (and in a corresponding fashion, with short distances being of greatest risk regarding the spread of unhealthy behaviors through a network, e.g., opioid use). Another form of intervention would involve disseminating health communication messages through social networks. This could be realized through two concepts based on social cognitive theory: modeling and verbal persuasion. Modeling refers to the imitation of behavior one views and then perceives as normative. For instance, the use of popular opinion leaders (POLs) to model health behaviors among their network members. As part of this approach, verbal persuasion could be used by the POLs to affect behavior change as well. Ko et al., (2013) used this approach to affect HIV risk behaviors, but they used online networks and Internet POLs (iPOLs). iPOLs were recruited to deliver HIV prevention information via an intervention webpage (Ko et al., 2013). Because of their influence within online social networks, they were able to reach over 950,000 individuals online and affect HIV risk behaviors of other individuals within their online social networks. Individuals who viewed the intervention webpage reported HIV-risk reduction behaviors including being more likely to test for HIV within 6 months and consistently use condoms during anal sex with online sex partners compared to individuals who viewed a nonequivalent control webpage.

One important use of network theory also involves the advantage of reaching hidden or "closed" populations. As is common in public health, those populations that are in greatest need may often be the same populations that are marginalized by society to the point of becoming difficult to reach through traditional public health efforts. An excellent example of using social network theory to reach a marginalized population occurred in Russia (Amirkhanian et al., 2003). This study recruited 14 intact social networks of young men who have sex with men (YMSM) and subsequently employed social network theory to identify key players in each network. These men were then provided with a six-session education program designed to give them skills needed to serve as an HIV prevention intervention agent

with other men in the network. This approach to reaching YMSM in these otherwise hidden networks turned out to be highly effective. For example, the study found favorable changes in men's frequency of discussing AIDS prevention, HIV-risk reduction attitudes/norms, and self-efficacy to engage in safer sex practices, and increased frequency of condom use. The concept of reaching entire networks through key players is grounded in social cognitive theory (see Chapter 7), especially through two concepts: modeling and verbal persuasion.

▶ The Network-Individual-Resource Model

One specific social network model recently developed to explain the influence of social and sexual networks on individual HIV risk taking behavior is the Network-Individual-Resource (NIR) model. The model accounts for network ties and how the dynamics of various social and sexual networks influence the transmission of HIV (Johnson et al., 2010). The model focuses on two levels of HIV transmission: the individual level and network level, which is "composed of two or more individuals who share a characteristic in common, interacting either momentarily or permanently over time." The network level can include a dyad of intimate partners, family members and peers, a community, or society. The NIR model posits that the individual as well as social/sexual networks rely on mental resources and tangible resources to guide risk taking or preventive behaviors. Mental resources at the individual level include attitudes, perceived norms, perceived and actual control over the behavior, and intentions to engage in the behavior. Whereas mental resources at the network level include social support, trust, relationship equity, social capital, shared norms and expectations, possession, and power wielding. Tangible resources for an individual include: income, physical health, access to medical care, and life expectancy. Tangible resources within a social network include:

partner income and joint possessions, dyadic and/or family physical health, mutual trust within a family or levels of trust within a community, pooled tangible resources to benefit network members and allies, and power wielded by stakeholders. Tangible resources within a network may also include the physical health of the dyad and family.

The NIR model utilizes four postulates to explain how individuals and their networks use resources to engage in health behaviors. The postulates are as follows:

1. Resources enable surviving and thriving
2. Resources that satisfy pressing needs are most valued
3. Networks are actual or potential resources for individuals
4. HIV spreads through networks

Thus, to understand and intervene within certain populations, public health practitioners must first understand the resources available to an individual and those within his/her social or sexual network; understand the needs of the individual or network to identify which resources are most valued and thus more likely to be utilized; make sure intervention efforts are trusted and valued by the individual and his/her network; and target high prevalence networks to minimize the spread of HIV.

One study examined predictors of condom use among men who have sex with men (MSM) in Ghana using the network-individual-resource model as their theoretical framework (Nelson et al., 2015). In this study, the researchers conducted a cross-sectional survey with 22 peer social networks of MSM in Ghana. Autonomy, competence, and relatedness were operationalized as mental resources for using condoms within peer networks of Ghanaian MSM. The authors also examined STD knowledge, HIV knowledge, sense of community within the peer network, HIV stigma, gender nonconformity, and attitudes toward gender equitable and gender inequitable norms as additional resources for the men. Although there were no differences in reports of condom use in the past 3 months between social networks, the researchers found that networks with higher levels of consistent condom use had higher STD and HIV knowledge, norms more supportive of gender equity, and experienced more autonomy support in their healthcare encounters compared to networks with lower levels of consistent condom use.

▶ Take Home Messages

- Almost every individual is essentially connected to another, either directly or indirectly, and these interconnections form social networks.
- Major components of social network theory are nodes or actors and the ties that connect them.
- Nodes or actors can be individuals, schools, industries, states, etc., where together they form a *network*.
- Information, knowledge, ideas, and attitudes as well as infectious and chronic disease can spread through interconnected networks of nodes/actors.
- The characteristics of social networks such as the position of an actor/node within a network, the similarity between network actors, and cohesiveness of the network can facilitate the spread of ideas, attitudes, behaviors, and information and affect a variety of health behaviors and outcomes.
- Social networks reside within a larger social system, and these social systems as well as the networks within them can be traditional in the form of physical contact or virtual such as connections on social networking sites.
- Networks are constantly evolving, and this evolution can be facilitated in a positive way through public health interventions by relying upon key players or superdiffusers who are closely connected to others, have a high degree of centrality, and have high persuasiveness.
- The Network-Individual-Resource (NIR) model explains the influence of social and sexual networks and posits that to intervene in a particular network, it is important to understand what resources are available within the network, which resources are most valued and

thus more likely to be utilized, and to ensure that intervention efforts will be trusted and valued by the individuals within the network.

▸ References

Amirkhanian, Y. A., Kelly, J. A., Kabakchieva, E., McAuliffe, T. L., & Vassileva, S. (2003). Evaluation of a social network HIV prevention intervention program for young men who have sex with men in Russia and Bulgaria. *AIDS Education and Prevention, 15*(3), 205–220.

Barrington, C., Latkin, C., Sweat, M. D., Moreno, L., Ellen, J., & Kerrigan D. (2009). Talking the talk, walking the walk: social network norms, communication patterns, and condom use among the male partners of female sex workers in La Romana, Dominican Republic. *Social Science & Medicine, 68*(11), 2037–2044.

Bond, R. M., & Bushman, B. J. (2017). The contagious spread of violence among US adolescents through social networks. *American Journal of Public Health, 107*(2), 288–294. doi: 10.2105/AJPH.2016.303550. Epub 2016 Dec 20

Borgatti, S. P., Everett, M. G., & Freeman, L. C. (2002). UCINET 6 for Windows: Software for Social Network Analysis. Harvard, MA: Analytic technologies.

Borgatti, S. P., Mehra, A., Brass, D. J., & Labianca, G. (2009). Network analysis in the social sciences. *Science, 323*(5916), 892–895. doi:10.1126/science.1165821.

Carrington, P. J., & Scott, J., Wasserman S. (2005). *Models and methods in social network analysis.* Cambridge, England: Cambridge University Press.

Christakis, N. A., & Fowler, J. H. (2007). The spread of obesity in a large social network over 32 years. *New England Journal of Medicine, 357*(4), 370–379. Epub 2007 Jul 25

Christakis, N. A., & Fowler, J. H. (2008). The collective dynamics of smoking in a large social network. *New England Journal of Medicine, 358*(21), 2249–2258. doi: 10.1056/NEJMsa0706154

Cialdini, R., Reno, R., & Kallgren, C. (1990). A focus theory of normative conduct: Recycling the concept of norms to reduce littering in public places. *Journal of Personality and Social Psychology, 58*(6), 1015–1026.

Cranmer, S. J., & Desmarais, B. A. (2011). Inferential network analysis with exponential random graph models. *Political Analysis, 19*(1), 66–86. doi:10.1093/pan/mpq037

Daw, J., Margolis, R., & Verdery, A. M. (2015). Siblings, friends, course-mates, club-mates: How adolescent heath behavior homophily varies by race, class, gender, and health status. *Social Science & Medicine, 125*, 32–39.

Freeman, L. (2004). *The development of social network analysis.* Vancouver, BC, Canada: Empirical Press.

Flatt, J. D., Agimi, Y., & Albert, S. M. (2012). Homophily and health behavior in social networks of older adults. *Family and Community Health, 35*(4), 312–321. doi: 10.1097/FCH.0b013e3182666650

González-Bailón, S., Wang, N., & Borge-Holthoefer, J. (2014). The emergence of roles in large-scale networks of communication. *EPJ Data Science, 3,* 32. https://doi.org/10.1140/epjds/s13688-014-0032-y

Granovetter, M. S. (1973). The strength of weak ties. *American Journal of Sociology, 78*(6), 1360–1380. doi:10.1086/225469

Gyarmathy, V. A., Li, N., Tobin, K. E., Hoffman, I. F., Sokolov, N., Levchenko, J., … Latkin, C. A. (2010). Injecting equipment sharing in Russian drug injecting dyads. *AIDS & Behavior, 14*(1), 141–151. doi:10.1007/s10461-008-9518-6. Epub 2009 Feb 13

Haythornthwaite, C. (1996). Social network analysis: An approach and technique for the study of information exchange. *Library & Information Research, 18*(4), 323–342.

Johnson, B. T., Redding, C. A., DiClemente, R. J., Mustanski, B. S., Dodge, B., Sheeran, P., … Fishbein, M. (2010). A network-individual-resource model for HIV prevention. *AIDS & Behavior, 14* (Suppl 2), 204–221. doi:10.1007/s10461-010-9803-z

Kadushin, C. (2012). *Understanding social networks: Theories, concepts, and findings.* New York, NY: Oxford University Press.

Ko, N. Y., Hsieh, C. H., Wang, M. C., Lee, C., Chen, C. L., Chung, A. C., & Hsu, S. T. (2013). Effects of Internet popular opinion leaders (iPOL) among Internet-using men who have sex with men. *Journal of Medical Internet Research, 15*(2), e40. doi:10.2196/jmir.2264

Kottiri, B. J., Friedman, S. R., Neaigus, A., Curtis, R., & Des Jarlais, D. C. (2002). Risk networks and racial/ethnic differences in the prevalence of HIV infection among injection drug users. *Journal of Acquired Immune Deficiency Syndromes, 30*, 95–104.

McPherson, M., Lovin, L., & Cook, J. (2001). Birds of a feather: Homophily in social networks. *Annual Review of Sociology, 27*(1), 415–444. doi:citeulike-article-id:3022278, 10.1146/annurev.soc.27.1.415

Merton, R. K. (1938). Social structure and Anomie. *American Sociological Review, 3*(5), 672–682.

Merton, R. K. (1957). *Social theory and social structure.* New York, NY: Free Press.

Milgram, S. (1967). The small world problem. *Psychology Today, 2,* 60–67. doi:citeulike-article-id:1288399

Moreira, A. A., Paula, D. R., Costa Filho, R. N., & Andrade, J. S., Jr. (2006). Competitive cluster growth in complex networks. *Physical Review. E, Statistical, Nonlinear, and Soft Matter Physics, 73*(6 Pt 2), 065101. Epub 2006 Jun 1

Nelson, L. E., Wilton, L., Agyarko-Poku, T., Zhang, N., Zou, Y., Aluoch, M., … Adu-Sarkodie, Y. (2015). Predictors of condom use among peer social networks of men who have sex with men in Ghana, West Africa. *PLoS One, 10*(1), e0115504. doi: 10.1371/journal.pone.0115504.

Oswald, D. L., & Clark, E. M. (2003). Best friends forever? High school best friendships and the transition to college. *Personal Relationships, 10,* 187–196.

Peterson, J. L., Rothenberg, R., Kraft, J. M., Beeker, C., & Trotter, R. (2009). Perceived condom norms and HIV risks among social and sexual networks of young African American men who have sex with men. *Health Education Research, 24*(1), 119–127. doi:10.1093/her/cyn003. Epub 2008 Feb 16

Powell, J. W., Denton, R., & Mattsson, Å. (1995). Adolescent depression: Effects of mutuality in the mother-adolescent dyad and locus of control. *American Journal of Orthopsychiatry, 65*(2), 263–273. http://dx.doi.org/10.1037/h0079617

Roberts, S. G. B., & Dunbar, R. I. M. (2011). Communication in social networks: Effects of kinship, network size, and emotional closeness. *Personal Relationships, 18*, 439–452.

Smith, R. A., & Carpenter, C. J. (2017). Who persuades Who? An analysis of persuasion choices related to antibiotic-free food. *Health Communication*, 1–11.

Stephen, P., & Borgatti, B. O. (2010). Overview: Social network theory and analysis. In A. J. Daly (Ed.), *Social network theory and educational change* (pp. 17–30). Cambridge, MA: Harvard Education Press.

Travers, J., & Milgram, S. (1969). An experimental study of the small world problem. *Sociometry, 32*(4), 425–443. doi:10.2307/2786545

Valentinov, V. (2014). The complexity–sustainability trade-off in Niklas Luhmann's social systems theory. *Systems Research and Behavioral Science, 31*, 14–22. doi:10.1002/sres.2146

van Mierlo, T. (2014). The 1% rule in four digital health social networks: An observational study. *Journal of Medical Internet Research, 4*, 16(2), e33. doi:10.2196/jmir.2966

Wellman, B. (1997). Structural analysis: From method and metaphor to theory and substance. *Contemporary Studies in Sociology, 15*, 19–61.

Chapter Opener: © Henrik Sorensen/Getty Images; © MeskPhotography/Shutterstock; © Hero Images/Getty Images; © lzf/Shutterstock

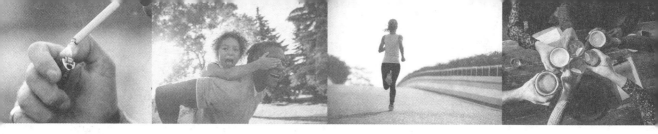

CHAPTER 11

Diffusion of Innovations Theory

Richard A. Crosby, Ralph J. DiClemente, and Laura F. Salazar

Make everything as simple as possible, but not simpler.

—**Albert Einstein**

PREVIEW

This chapter describes diffusion of innovations theory (DOI), which posits large-scale health behavior change is possible by developing an approach or physical device that is viewed as novel. This theory also posits that diffusion occurs in a predictable pattern through established social systems. Because the new public health implies changing health behaviors of entire populations—not just individuals identified as being "at risk" (see Chapters 1 and 2), understanding this theory in its entirety is one of the most important skill sets you will acquire.

OBJECTIVES

1. Understand the concept of diffusion and be able to describe the four main elements of diffusion theory.
2. Identify and describe the key characteristics of a successful innovation.
3. Explain the implications of the S-shaped diffusion curve and adopter categories.
4. Distinguish between opinion leaders and change agents and describe the role of each in the diffusion of innovations.
5. Apply the principles of diffusion to health promotion.

▶ Introduction

In the previous chapter, you learned the basic principles of health communication and how they can be utilized to favorably influence health behaviors. By this point, it is likely that you have begun to appreciate the value of cognitive theories and the importance of information and social influences in health promotion. As you have acquired this information and the corresponding skills, you also learned about the importance of building social equity into your work as a health-promotion professional. Your task now is combine all of what you have learned so far ad apply this to a greatly expanded theory—one that is frequently used to change the health behaviors of entire populations. This chapter presents a unique approach to understanding how information and social ties can profoundly influence behavior change.

The best way to think about DOI is to begin with a basic observation of human behavior: people tend to follow the lead of others. This simple observation is one of many primary tenets underlying DOI. Basically, people are more likely to adopt an innovation if they observe others having also adopted the innovation, and this is especially likely if they also observe others experiencing a positive outcome. Diffusion theory suggests that the highly visible influence of peer modeling can indeed ignite a chain reaction of behavioral adoption that results, over time, in increased adoption of the innovation. Stated informally, DOI suggests that behavior can be contagious. Indeed, some innovations spread very rapidly, while other innovations languish. Diffusion theory provides a framework for understanding how innovations diffuse, and—therefore—these principles can be used to promote the adoption of healthful innovations.

DOI suggests that behavior can be contagious.

▶ Key Concepts

Diffusion theory was originated by Everett Rogers (1983, 1995). Historically, this theory has deep roots that extend back in time and it has been applied to a broad range of behaviors, including health behaviors. The foundations of diffusion theory can be traced back to research on innovations in agriculture. Rogers (1995) described an early study (Ryan & Gross, 1943) as one of the single best illustrations of diffusion. In this classic study, the adoption rates of growing hybrid varieties of corn (a risk proposition when your livelihood is at stake) by Iowa farmers were plotted over several years (see **FIGURE 11-1**).

Results showed that over a 15-year period virtually all Iowa farmers gradually adopted this innovation. Surprisingly, some farmers adopted the hybrid seed right away and some much later; ultimately, cumulative rates of adoption created an **S-shaped curve**, with about 10% of farmers planting the hybrid corn in the first 5 years, followed by an increase to 40% in the following 3 years, and then a much slower rate of adoption over the next 10 years or so. Moreover, the researchers found that timing of adoption varied by the attitudes of the farmers: farmers who reported being more eager to take chances were more likely to adopt the planting of hybrid seed, while those who were more cautious about risk, more committed to conventional ways. Further, those who were less connected with other farmers adopted the innovation much later. (This logic, for which attitudes in general and attitudes specifically about the relative advantages of a particular innovation are associated with behavior, should be familiar to readers of Chapter 4.) This phenomenon, where some people adopt new practices early while others do so much later or not at all, can be observed with respect to numerous innovations, including health behaviors such as the use of contraceptives, breast cancer screening, bicycle helmets, regular exercise, low-fat diets, and many other health-related innovations.

Given this background, it is quite easy to see how DOI later came to be applied to health promotion. In effect, the decision to adopt a newly recommended health behavior, practice, or program is not much different than a farmer's decision to plant a new variety of seed corn. In both cases, there is an inherent fear of the unknown and a probable concern about social norms (what will other people think about my decision and

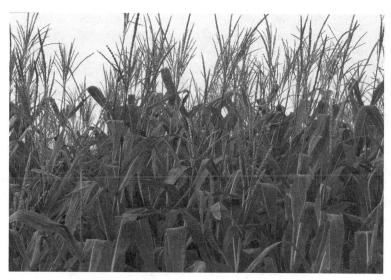

FIGURE 11-1 Hybrid corn field
© Scott Bauer/USDA Agricultural Research Service.

consequent action?). Increasingly, the principles of diffusion theory are being applied to different types of health-promotion programs (Cooke, Mattick, & Campbell, 1999; Luepker et al., 1996; Oldenburg & Parcel, 2002; Simpson et al., 2000).

Four Elements of Diffusion Theory

Rogers (1995, p. 10) defined diffusion as "the process by which an innovation is communicated through certain channels over time among members of a social system." Using this definition, we can extract four key elements:

1. Innovation
2. Communication channels
3. Time
4. The social system

Element 1: Innovation

Rogers (1983) defined innovation as "an idea, practice, or object that is perceived as new by an individual or other unit of adoption." The word "perceived" in this definition is vital. For example, the concept of using long-acting hormonal contraceptives (implants or injectables) may be quite novel to some populations of women, particularly those residing in resource-poor, developing countries. Try to imagine how novel the idea of such a practice might be to women when they first learn of it, and the uncertainty that women might experience when they first consider adopting a long-acting contraceptive. Depending on the perceptions of the women about the innovation, they may quickly reject or embrace it. How people develop perceptions about an innovation and then make decisions about adoption are the primary concerns of DOI.

Please bear in mind that innovations can include concepts, policies, practices, and objects (products). Something does not need to be totally new to be an innovation—it just needs to be

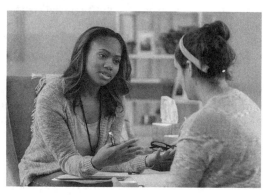

© Steve Debenport/E+/Getty Images

Simply expecting these deeply ingrained and unquestioned cultural values to change because of a new public health recommendation would be unrealistic when viewed through the lens of diffusion theory.

relatively novel in a particular subgroup. For example, hand washing to prevent the spread of disease, eating a vegetarian diet to reduce the risk of cancer and heart disease, or eliminating table salt from the diet to reduce the risk of high blood pressure are common practices in many parts of the world, but in some population groups these practices could be viewed as novel. In each case, the public health suggestion of a new practice has the potential to be in direct conflict with current practices and cultural beliefs of any given population. Simply expecting these deeply ingrained and unquestioned cultural values to change because of a new public health recommendation would be unrealistic when viewed through the lens of diffusion theory.

A contemporary example of a practice that is perceived as novel and is being promoted as an innovation to reduce the death rate from colorectal cancer (CRC) is annual self-screening for the preliminary symptom of this neoplasia—known as a polyp (a growth inside the colon). A newly approved innovation in the field of early CRC detection is the Fecal Immunochemical Test (FIT). This is a greatly improved method of detecting polyps, as it does not require the person to avoid eating red meat before the specimen is collected and it does not require any special collection procedures (other than to simply pass a small paintbrush-like tool over a fresh stool specimen before it is flushed down the toilet). This test offers the advantage of 98% specificity as it does not detect the presence of nonhuman blood (i.e., from the ingestion of meat products). More importantly, FIT uses an antibody-based method of detecting human occult (meaning "not normal") blood that thus provides a greatly enhanced ability to detect smaller cancers and more pre-cancerous polyps, with far greater specificity than past methods of at-home screening for CRC.

Element 2: Communication Channels

A key tenet of DOI is that any innovation can be diffused through a social system via two distinct communication channels. The first channel is the **media**. Media is a formal channel, and television, radio, Internet, and print media all serve as effective agents to convey information to people regarding a given innovation. One type of knowledge conveyed through media is **awareness knowledge**. Simply stated, awareness knowledge lets people know that the innovation exists (see **FIGURE 11-2** for an example).

The second channel is an **interpersonal channel**, which is generally a more informal channel. People's interactions can serve as a viable mechanism for transmitting information about innovations that may lead to their ultimate adoption. The key here is that a person who has adopted the innovation may convey a **subjective evaluation** (i.e., a personal favorable opinion) of that innovation to other people who have not adopted the innovation. Such conveyance may not necessarily be intentional. By simply adopting an innovation, a person models the innovation. The attitudes or behavior of a close peer tends to shape subjective evaluations and can be a significant factor influencing another person's adoption of the innovation. One example of the influence of knowing someone who has adopted a certain practice is provided by the FIT kit screening program, previously described. In a study occurring in rural Appalachia one of the chapter authors (Crosby) found that the return rate of completed FIT kits was greater for people receiving the kit based on a referral from a family member, compared to people receiving kits without a family-member referral. In rural Appalachia, "family members" commonly extend far beyond the traditional nuclear family to broadly defined familial relations such as second and third cousins. Because some families may have upwards of 100 members in this area of

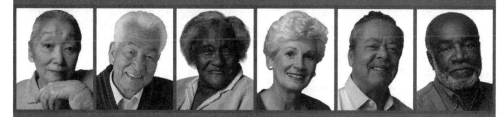

When we heard that **1** out of **3** people 60 years old and older get shingles...

we got the **shingles vaccine!**

What is shingles?

- Shingles is a disease that causes a painful, blistering rash. One in five people with shingles will have **severe, long-term pain** after the rash heals.

- **Almost all older adults can get shingles.** About one in three people will develop the disease during their lifetime.

- Shingles is **more common and more serious in older adults.** Nearly 1 million Americans get shingles every year and about half of them are 60 years old and older.

How can the risk of shingles and long-term pain from shingles be reduced?

- A new vaccine against shingles has been developed and is recommended for people 60 years old and older.

- You can reduce your risk of shingles and long-term pain by **getting the vaccine**.

- In a clinical trial involving people 60 years old and older, the shingles vaccine **prevented long-term pain** in two out of three people who got vaccinated and **prevented the disease** in about half of them.

Reduce **YOUR** risk of shingles. **GET VACCINATED.**

For more information, ask your healthcare provider, call 800-CDC-INFO (800-232-4636), or visit www.cdc.gov/vaccines/vpd-vac/shingles/default.htm.

FIGURE 11-2 Example of print media to increase awareness of shingles vaccine
Courtesy of the CDC

the country, the informal communication channel for this particular innovation was deemed to be of great value.

A key principle associated with interpersonal channels of communication involves the concept of **homophily**. Homophily means that any two

Homophily means that any two people are very similar in their views, perceptions and beliefs within their larger social system.

people are very similar in their views, perceptions and beliefs within their larger social system. When two people share a predominance of values or norms, they are said to be homophilous. As you might imagine, if two people are largely homophilous, and one has adopted the innovation while the other has not, then the conditions for adoption of the innovation are ideal. Think for a moment about what the concept of homophily means to a health educator who is seeking to change behavior in a given population. The degree of homophily between **change agents** (i.e., those who actively attempt to promote adoption of an innovation) and members

of the target population is an important consideration in designing health-promotion programs. In other words, the higher the degree of homophily between change agents and members of the target population, the more receptive the target population will likely be to the innovation. Opinion leaders are people who are admired and respected by other members of their community; thus, they can be effective change agents because of the high degree of homophily between them and the target population.

Element 3: Time

As diffusion is a process, it takes time. Innovations diffuse through populations at variable rates as a consequence of several factors. The first factor is largely tied to the innovation itself: some innovations are better suited to quick adoption than others. A new product that provides great benefit and is safe and easy to use (e.g., a bike helmet) would be adopted more quickly than something more complicated with less perceived benefit (e.g., adopting a vegan diet). The social system is the second factor that can affect the rate of diffusion. Each of these aspects will be discussed in more detail in subsequent sections of this chapter.

To understand how diffusion occurs over time it is useful to consider the **innovation–decision process**. How quickly, or slowly, people progress through this process is a critical determinant of the rate of diffusion (the time it takes for the innovation to be adopted). This process was described by (Rogers, 1995) as comprising five discrete stages:

- Knowledge
- Persuasion
- Decision
- Implementation
- Confirmation

Stage 1: Knowledge. One must know about the existence of something before adopting it. When you first find out about something of interest—a new application for your smartphone or a new program for social networking, for example—you might adopt it at your earliest convenience. But, how do you learn about the innovation? What

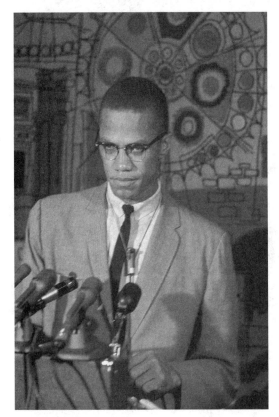

Malcolm X
© Robert Parent/The LIFE Images Collection/Getty Images

is it you would want to know before adopting it? Obtaining information is a fundamental part of the adoption process. Diffusion theory has identified the following three forms of knowledge that are particularly important: **awareness**, **acquisition**, and **principles knowledge**. It is important that you learn to distinguish these three types of knowledge.

Awareness knowledge, or knowledge of the existence of the innovation, can occur by coming into contact with others who know about the innovation, and so those with a broader social network are more likely to find out about certain innovations. Awareness knowledge can also come about through media and other promotions. Providing information to people is seen as necessary and fundamental to the adoption of an innovation. Rogers cautioned that selective exposure to a new innovation may be a strong barrier against obtaining awareness knowledge (Rogers, 1995); in essence, people may be unlikely to pay much attention to messages promoting a new innovation unless they first feel a need for the innovation. Thus, breaking through this barrier is an initial challenge in mass media campaigns promoting an innovation.

How-to-knowledge and principles knowledge each follow the acquisition of knowledge regarding how the innovation is to be used (**how-to knowledge**). Moreover, how-to knowledge is thought to precede knowledge about the principles that underlie the innovation (**principles knowledge**). Respectively, these two forms of knowledge propose two goals for planned interventions: (1) to facilitate understanding of how to use the innovation (or at least learn that it is easy to use), and (2) to promote understanding of how the innovation works. Condom use is one example that can be used to illustrate these concepts quite nicely. Potential adopters will most likely need to know how to select condoms that fit well and feel comfortable, and how to apply condoms so as to avoid problems with breakage and slippage. This would be how-to knowledge, and it is critically important, as the lack (or perceived lack) of ability to use the product or engage in the practice is a critical determinant to adoption. (See **BOX 11-1** for an example of how complex how-to-knowledge may be in this

context.) Potential adopters may also want to gain an understanding of how condoms work to prevent pregnancy and disease and learn that they serve as an impassible barrier against sperm and even the smallest microorganisms that cause disease. This would be an example of principles knowledge.

Stage 2: Persuasion. At this stage, the primary requirement for adoption is forming a strong and positive attitude toward the practice or product. Attitude development may occur in a manner much like that described in the theory of reasoned action (see Chapter 4). Expected consequences of adopting the innovation are central to this stage. People develop their attitudes toward the innovation through their exposure to various forms of information, termed **innovation–evaluation information**. As you might imagine, people are likely to form their attitudes toward an innovation based on considerations such as perceived relative advantages and costs of adopting the innovation; in other words, people examine the relevance and acceptability of the innovation. Information from various sources, including advertisements, news articles, word-of-mouth, and promotions, can all be important influences on persuasion. However, peer influence is thought to be a particularly important contribution to attitude formation. At this stage, DOI emphasizes the tendency of successful adopters to promote the persuasion process through their open display of satisfaction with the innovation (see **FIGURE 11-3**).

Stage 3: Decision. This is the stage where people decide to accept or reject the innovation. Note that deciding is not the same as trying or implementing. Instead, deciding is a lot like intending (theory of reasoned action; theory of planned action). Intention may be strongly associated with behavior, but environmental barriers often get in the way and prevent attempts or reduce enthusiasm. One key principle of this stage is that people will be more likely to arrive at an affirmative adoption decision if they can try the innovation without being committed to it. Stated differently, a no-cost trial of the innovation may encourage people to accept the practice or product on a long-term basis. Think about the use of contraceptives, for example. Some can be tried with very little

BOX 11-1 An Example of Missing "How-to-Knowledge" Among Young Black Men Who Have Sex with Men

Frequency of Condom Use Errors/Problems Stratified by Partner-Application Among Young Black Men

Error or Problem	HIV − (n = 283)	HIV + (n = 108)	P
	% (n)	% (n)	
Errors			
Not enough time available to put on condom	14.1 (37)	7.5 (8)	0.08
Started having anal sex then put condom on later	12.9 (34)	16.1 (16)	0.058
Took condom before having your nut	19.0 (50)	26.4 (28)	0.11
Condom slipped off penis during withdraw	9.5 (25)	7.5 (8)	0.55
Gave up condom use because it got too frustrating	8.7 (23)	7.5 (8)	0.71
Condom contacted sharp jewelry, fingernails or teeth	1.5 (4)	3.8 (4)	0.18
Condom was not lubricated	9.9 (26)	6.6 (7)	0.32
Condom dried out during sex	20.9 (55)	20.8 (22)	0.97
Condom used was not in a sealed package	15.2 (40)	10.4 (11)	0.22
Condom was damaged during sex	6.5 (17)	5.7 (6)	0.77
Condom distracted attention from the pleasure of sex	16.3 (43)	20.8 (22)	0.31
Problems			
Condom break during sex	15.2 (40)	29.2 (31)	0.002
Condom slipped off during sex	9.1 (24)	16.0 (17)	0.005
Lost erection when condom was put on	18.3 (48)	18.9 (20)	0.89
Condom leaked during sex	3.8 (10)	6.6 (7)	0.24
Condom length was not right	24.3 (36)	13.9 (10)	0.07
Condom width was not right	29.1 (43)	27.8 (20)	0.84

Reproduced from Crosby, R. A., Mena, L., Yarber, W. L., Graham, C. A., Sanders, S. A., & Milhausen, R. R. (2015). Condom use errors and problems: A comparative study of HIV-positive versus HIV-negative young, black MSM. *Sex Transmitted Diseases, 42,* 634–636.

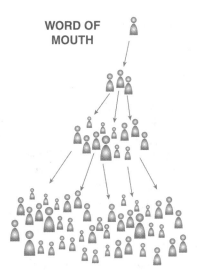

WORD OF
MOUTH

FIGURE 11-3 How word-of-mouth works toward innovation adoption
© Vlue/Shutterstock

commitment (e.g., condoms) and others require a fairly substantial commitment (e.g., intrauterine devices, pills, implants, injectables, tubal ligation, or vasectomy). Another example is a health club providing a free trial membership, designed to encourage people to use the club's facilities without having to sign a lengthy contract. The goal, of course, is to get people in the door with the underlying assumption being that once people use the club's facilities and enjoy their experience, some will join the club.

Stage 4: Implementation. This stage refers to the actual adoption or trial of an innovation. It is important to note that for many innovations, trial or implementation of an innovation does not always equate with continuation of use. Depending on the nature of the innovation, some may experience success and some may experience difficulty with implementation. Furthermore, even though the innovation may be successfully implemented, it does not mean that continued use of the innovation will occur.

Rogers (1995) also suggested that an important aspect of this stage is the extent to which people reinvent the innovation. **Reinvention** occurs when people alter the innovation to suit their own purposes. Reinvention can make an innovation more attractive because adopters can

modify it for particular purposes, but reinvention can also undermine the utility of some innovations. For instance, the innovation of a drug for men having erectile issues (erection-enhancing drugs) has been "reinvented" by thousands upon thousands of men as a "party drug" to make sex last longer. When reinvention translates into risk to health the innovation becomes problematic rather than helpful. Thus, regardless of the innovation, the potential for reinvention constitutes an important overall consideration in this fourth stage of adoption.

Stage 5: Confirmation. Confirmation represents the ultimate stage of adoption, when people decide whether to make a long-term commitment to use the innovation. For example, many people start a diet or exercise routine, but over time fail to maintain their adoption of the innovation. Maintenance of healthful behaviors, of course, is the ultimate goal of health promotion. Many studies and programs are designed to facilitate maintenance because it can be difficult to maintain certain behaviors without a lot of support, at least until the behavior can be fully integrated into one's lifestyle. The key feature of confirmation is reinforcement. People who experience positive reinforcement for their use of the new product or practice are far more likely to continue using it compared to those not experiencing reinforcement. Reinforcement can be physical,

> *The key feature of confirmation is reinforcement.*

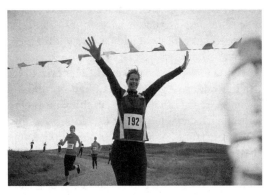

© Hero Images/Getty Images

social, or emotional. It may come from within the person (**intrinsic reinforcement**) or from other outside sources (**extrinsic reinforcement**). Innovations that are reinforcing or that can easily be reinforced are more likely to be sustained.

Element 4: Social System

The fourth and final element of diffusion theory is the social system. As you will recall from reading Chapter 10, social networks can be extremely powerful when it comes to shaping the health behaviors of a population. Considering, for example, the ability of a social network to influence obesity (Christakis & Fowler, 2007), it comes as no surprise that a wide range of health behaviors are "spread" through social systems. Every social system is characterized by norms that define the social structures within the community and established patterns of communication (**communication structures**). The social system sets the boundaries for diffusion and the communication structures spread information about the innovation. Communication structures can be formal or informal. Formal structures are well known to students in colleges and universities, as these institutions are replete with rules and policies for interacting with staff, administrators, and faculty. Informal communication structures, however, are far more amorphous. Rules for interactions between students are generally absent, thereby leaving these communication structures free to develop and change as a function of the students themselves, rather than the institution. Informal communication structures are especially important to diffusion theory. These structures typically comprise homophilous groups of people, and within these groups it is imperative that at least one member is willing to depart from the existing norm to try the innovation. Again, this is often an opinion leader. A remarkable quality of diffusion theory is that a predictable pattern of adoption within communication structures occurs, beginning first with innovators, then by opinion leaders, whose behavior tends to stimulate wide ranging adoption. The next section of this chapter greatly expands on this pattern.

Adopter Categories and the S-Shaped Diffusion Curve

The four elements of diffusion theory—innovation, communication channels, time, and the social system—help us understand how a new product or practice naturally becomes part of culturally acceptable standards in any given population. Culture is not static; it evolves over time. The question, however, is how does a cultural practice change? One answer may be that change occurs when key opinion leaders in a population establish a new norm. Thus, a key implication of diffusion theory is that opinion leaders (people who are well respected in a community) tend to be highly influential with respect to the adoption of innovations.

Key opinion leaders are located within the center of their respective social networks, tend to have elevated social status, and have frequent contact with others in the network. They are also characterized by their connection to people outside their immediate social networks. Although opinion leaders are not necessarily the first to adopt an innovation, they tend to be among the first to comprehend the advantages of an innovation and to try them out.

In the parlance of diffusion theory, five adopter categories exist:

- Innovators
- Early adopters
- Early majority
- Late majority
- Laggards

These five adopter categories can be plotted on a bell-shaped curve, as shown in **FIGURE 11-4**. This curve is vital to understanding the different rates of adoption based on category.

Innovators represent the first category of adopters. These people have a proclivity for experimentation and can be daring and bold when it comes to trying something new. They may not, however, hold a central position within communication structures, and others may not view them as opinion leaders. Innovators typically make up a relatively small proportion (approximately 2.5%) of those who ultimately adopt any particular

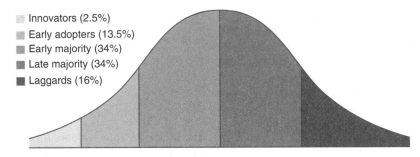

FIGURE 11-4 Diffusion of innovation adopter categorization

Data from Rogers, E. M. (1995). *Diffusion of innovations* (4th ed.). New York, NY: Free Press.

innovation. Figure 11-4 displays this percentage, along with the percentages for the other four adopter categories. Of note, the bell-shaped curve shown in Figure 11-4 can be represented as a cumulative rate of adoption, as is shown in **FIGURE 11-5**.

This cumulative rate of adoption takes the form of the classic S-shaped curve that characterizes diffusion theory. Essentially, adoption is quite slow at first because only the innovators (2.5% of a population) have made the adoption, but the rate then picks up as the early adopters (13.5%) begin adoption of the innovation. Most importantly, the rate quickly escalates when the early majority (34.0%) and the late majority (34.0%) adopt the innovation. Indeed, getting an innovation into the hands of the early majority is likely to create a momentum that ultimately assures success of the innovative product or practice.

Early adopters adopt relatively early in the process because they tend to have access to a variety of media and know people from whom they hear about innovations. They also tend to appreciate the advantages of innovations. Many early adopters hold central positions within their communication structures. They may be generally well respected and even admired by others in their social system, so many early adopters are opinion leaders whose opinions and behavior can "ignite" a diffusion effect that can rapidly spread through the social system. Change agents in the context of public health are those who seek to increase the rate and extent of adoption of an innovation. Change agents may or may not be early adopters. They often attempt to influence

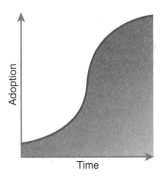

FIGURE 11-5 Cumulative rate of adoption

Data from Rogers, E. M. (1995). *Diffusion of innovations* (4th Ed.). New York, NY: Free Press.

opinion leaders to become early adopters and to be visible in their adoption decision. Change agents try to influence early adopters, thereby building toward a critical mass of adoption, which will eventually lead to rapid diffusion. Once this occurs, the process is no longer dependent on the efforts of the change agents. Stated metaphorically, change agents are the spark that ignites the flame that will eventually become a full-blown wildfire. Change agents are typically local leaders who may or may not hold formal titles or have the status of an elected official. Examples include a full-time bartender who has a large line-up of regular customers, a hairdresser who has a large clientele of local residents, and a clergy person who is highly regarded by members he/she serves.

People in the early majority may take relatively longer periods of time to pass through the innovation–decision process compared to innovators and early adopters. However, the sheer number of adoptions that occur among the early majority truly mark the successful diffusion of an innovation. A revisit to the communication structures is beneficial at this point. As the innovation first begins to spread through the early majority, it is quite likely that one adopter in the communication structure may encounter another person in the same structure who has not yet adopted the innovation. This encounter creates an interpersonal communication channel that can be effective in diffusing the innovation. Interpersonal communication channels are quite active at the point when approximately 20% of a social system has adopted an innovation. As the number of people adopting any given innovation reaches 50%, the chances of adopters encountering people who have not yet adopted the innovation begins to decline and the rate of diffusion slows down, hence the S-shaped curve (see Figure 11-5).

The late majority comprises people who may require extended lengths of time to pass through the innovation–decision process despite being surrounded by people who have recently adopted the innovation. The late majority is reluctant to adopt the innovation and tends not to have access to a variety of information sources. They have relatively homogeneous social networks and are typically skeptical about change, at least initially. Their initial uncertainty may be overcome once the innovation is well established in the population, as they may need time to gather and process information and to vicariously experience the positive benefits of the innovation before they choose to adopt it.

Finally, it must be noted that about 16% of a social system may be extremely reluctant to adopt or are impervious to the advantages of adoption. The term **"laggards"** is used to represent this category of potential adopters, as well as those who never adopt the innovation. Laggards tend to be extremely traditional and therefore quite slow to accept change. Laggards may have few ties to the key opinion leaders of a social system and the length of time needed for them to pass through the innovation–decision process may be protracted.

Key Characteristics of Innovations

BOX 11-2 provides a listing of 12 characteristics of innovations, divided into three sections. Seven characteristics best apply to the decisions that people make before they adopt the product or practice, two apply to the actual process of adoption, and three apply to the continued success of the innovation after adoption. Ideal innovations would have highly favorable characteristics. As a rule, the greater the number of key characteristics that can be satisfied, the greater the rate and depth of diffusion. The goal is to make the innovation as simple as possible for the user to adopt on a long-term basis. Referring back to the quite from Albert Einstein used at the start of this chapter, this does not necessarily, however, equate with "simpler" because improvements of an innovation may have underlying layers of complexity (e.g., Apps used to track running distances or calorie consumptions are easy-to-use on the "consumer side" but complex to construct on the technology side).

With only a small amount of effort, you can identify multiple examples of innovations that did not possess highly favorable characteristics and therefore diffused slowly and not extensively. For instance, the female condom was intended to provide women with an effective, self-controlled barrier method for both contraception and disease prevention. Unfortunately, diffusion of this public health innovation was extremely low due to its low relative advantage, high complexity, and social relations. Box 11-2 provides several possible reasons that might explain the lack of diffusion of the female condom. For example, the characteristic of relative advantage would suggest that the female condom did not provide couples with a product that was any easier to use or less detracting from the sexual experience than the male condom. Further, the cost of purchasing the female condom is substantially greater than the price of male condoms. The complexity of the female condom is also a likely cause for its lack of diffusion, as the device requires skill and practice. Another characteristic that may readily explain low diffusion is the potential impact on social relations. The female condom requires considerable application time and effort—a task that may unacceptably

---

BOX 11-2 Twelve Key Characteristics of a Successful Innovation

Characteristics That Users Think About Before Adoption

Compatibility: The innovation must be consistent with current cultural values and practices.

Communicability: Learning about the innovation should be easy—it lends itself to clarity.

Impact on social relations: The product or practice must not disrupt social customs in any way.

Relative advantage: The new product or practice must be substantially better than what it replaces.

Reversibility: Users must perceive they can discontinue use of the innovation when they desire.

Risk and uncertainty level: Users can be assured that the product or practice is low risk but effective.

Trialability: Users can try the product or practice before deciding to adopt it for the long term.

Characteristics That Apply During Adoption

Complexity: The successful innovation will be easy to use or perform.

Time: The successful innovation will require only a minimal time investment.

Characteristics That Apply After Adoption

Commitment: Use of the innovation should require minimal commitment.

Modifiability: The resource system must be able to modify the product or practice as needed.

Observability: People in the user system must be able to clearly see that the product or practice works.

---

interrupt arousal and sexual foreplay. Although other aspects of this barrier method are consistent with the characteristics shown in Box 11-2 (e.g., reversibility, commitment, risk and uncertainty levels, and trialability), it is important to note that the relative strength of only a few ill-fated characteristics can be a deal breaker for the innovation.

Although the characteristics displayed in Box 11-2 do not represent a comprehensive listing, it is important to note that Rogers (1983) determined that the majority of variance in diffusion rates could be explained by five main characteristics: relative advantage, compatibility, complexity, trialability, and observability.

Relative Advantage

The innovation must have significant appeal so that people will expend effort to change their behavior (even if the innovation is a one-time behavior, such as having a home tested for radon gas). That appeal may take the form of a perceived economic, social, personal, or physical benefit that will occur as a direct result of innovation adoption. Both actual and perceived relative advantages may be important in determining adoption; indeed, social advantages may often be key perceptions that drive people to change from the past or current practice. Consider, for example, the social advantages of smoking cessation for someone who moves from New York to California. Given the unpopularity of tobacco use in California, being a smoker may make the relocated person feel alienated in his or her new community. The social advantages alone may easily be the tipping point in a decision to adopt an innovation, such as a nicotine replacement therapy or other smoking cessation techniques, or participating in smoking cessation programs.

Unfortunately, social advantages may also work in favor of maintaining a health-compromising behavior and thus rejecting innovations designed to promote health. For example, for people who consume food high in fat, the innovation of a low-fat diet may not have relative advantage in terms of partaking in foods

A paradox of prevention is that people do not appreciate it when it works because, in essence, nothing happens.

commonly served at parties and events (cheeses, meats, fried foods, etc.). Thus, overcoming this barrier would be a challenge, and the new way of eating must appeal to advantages other than those that are social (such as weight reduction or reduced risk of adverse health conditions).

Most typical approaches to health-promotion programs focus on the physical or health advantages of an innovation or innovative practice. For example, cholesterol-lowering drugs (e.g., statins such as Lipitor) are promoted as a way to prevent heart disease, side-curtain air bags are promoted as way to avoid death or disability in the event of an auto accident, and soy products are promoted as a way to prevent cancer. The inherent problem in each example is that people have a very difficult time believing they are even susceptible to heart disease, fatal or serious auto collisions, and cancer. Moreover, the adoption of any one of these three innovations offers little if any direct evidence to the adopters that their new behavior has paid off. Indeed, a paradox of prevention is that people do not appreciate it when it works because, in essence, nothing happens.

Compatibility

This characteristic applies to sociocultural beliefs and values, previous innovations, and the needs of individuals. In short, innovations that are consistent with a person's current attitudes and behavior and do not depart too radically from past ideas or innovations of a similar nature are more likely to be adopted. Perhaps most importantly, the innovation must be perceived by the potential adopter as meeting a critical need. An example is electric toothbrushes (see **FIGURE 11-6**). Electric toothbrushes do not depart radically from manual toothbrushes in their nature; however,

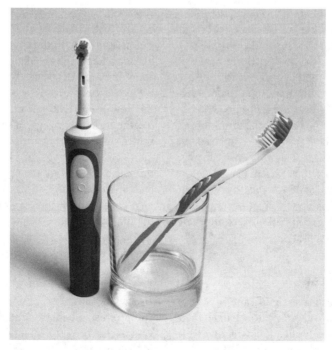

FIGURE 11-6 Old versus new toothbrush
© iStockphoto/Thinkstock

electric toothbrushes are more effective in removing plaque, removing stains, and keeping gums healthy. When various companies began to market electric toothbrushes with a range of costs, features (e.g., playing music for two minutes), and colors, the innovation suddenly became more acceptable and normative (even trendy).

In stark contrast, innovations as simple as an outhouse (latrine) in developing countries may not be readily adopted because they are not compatible or consistent with norms of the community, such as the idea that you should not defecate twice in the same place. In addition, using an outhouse may not be perceived as hygienic, and so water sanitation efforts that build latrines may not be successful. The point of these vignettes is that to enhance adoption of any innovation, the change agent should always begin his or her work by understanding the community's values, beliefs, and needs regarding the potential adoption of an innovation. This understanding, in turn, will greatly aid the adoption effort by helping communities to perceive that the innovation can be compatible for them.

An example from the Carter Center, in Atlanta, GA, serves as an excellent illustration of overcoming compatibility issues as the primary form of public health intervention. In the photo shown here children are displaying a single oral dose of medication that, taken annually, has greatly reduced the schistosomiasis epidemic in Nigeria and actually reverses up to 90% of the damage caused by the disease. The public health challenge was about convincing communities that this annual dose of medication was an important health-protective behavior. Because the innovation was not compatible with existing norms, meeting this challenge involved overcoming cultural beliefs about disease, medication, and the concept of prevention through taking a pill (**FIGURE 11-7**).

Complexity

Complex innovations—those that require extensive knowledge and skill—tend to be adopted at slower rates than innovations that are less complex. A key concept that applies to this characteristic is self-efficacy. Whether the issue is to adopt

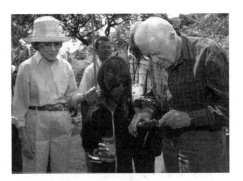

FIGURE 11-7 Child Receiving Medical Care From Outreach Conducted by the Carter Center
Courtesy of The Carter Center

the innovation or to continue its use after initial adoption, community members will need to feel confident in the use of the innovation or the performance of the innovative behavior. The issue may be especially applicable to the initial use of an innovation or the initial practice of an innovative behavior because any level of experienced frustration may quickly erode previous resolve to adopt the innovation. Aerobic exercise can be considered an innovation designed to avert the onset of heart disease for people who have never exercised, but people who have never engaged in an exercise such as running may not know the proper shoes to buy for their gait and feet, what clothing to wear, or how to pace their workout. Thus, they may lack confidence to start a running program, or they may become frustrated and reject the innovation entirely.

It is easy to think of numerous examples regarding innovations with a complexity level that may be detrimental to adoption. Infant car seats are a good example. Parents frequently complain that proper installation of the car seat requires technical knowledge and skill not conveyed in the instructions. As a result, many states set up "drive-through programs" where trained personnel (such as state

> *Any level of experienced frustration may quickly erode previous resolve to adopt the innovation.*

troopers) install the car seat for otherwise frustrated parents, which facilitates adoption.

Trialability

As previously mentioned, an innovation that can be tried without a full commitment to long-term adoption may diffuse more rapidly than one requiring an all-or-nothing decision. Innovations that can be tried at low cost and are reversible are more likely to be adopted than innovations that require expense and long-term commitment. A good example of this concept is the adoption of a daily or weekly exercise routine by working out in a gym. Gym memberships can be quite expensive and the length of contracts typically spans one year. Because people who run these businesses may know something about the concept of trialability, they frequently offer trial memberships that give people just enough time in the gym to experience some initial success, thus prompting them to consider taking the plunge and paying for a 1-year membership. Fortunately, most health-protective behaviors do have a high degree of trialability: eating a low-fat diet, eating a low-sodium diet, exercising, improved dental hygiene practices, condom use, smoking cessation programs, and other programs designed to allow individuals to try healthy behaviors before committing to anything long-term.

Some protective behaviors, however, have no level of trialability at all—they require an immediate decision. Colonoscopy, for example, is a highly effective but underutilized method of cancer prevention recommended for people 50 years of age and older. Once the colon is cleansed and the procedure begins, the adoption decision cannot be reversed. Vaccination is another example of a behavior that lacks trialability. So, the question becomes, "How can the characteristic of trialability be satisfied when the behavior is an all-or-nothing action?" The answer lies in the next characteristic: observability.

Observability

Innovations that are easily observable are more likely to be adopted than those that are not.

Returning to the vaccine example, a person may have grave concerns that a vaccine such as Gardasil (a vaccine against infection with human papillomavirus) may cause severe pain at the injection site, perhaps lasting for days. It is possible for a person to observe a friend getting vaccinated with Gardasil and being informed that no lasting pain was experienced. More importantly, observability has the potential to greatly facilitate the rate of adoption from innovators through the late majority and even into the laggards. Consider, for example, two very different innovations: the use of home water filters and the use of bicycle helmets. Adoption of the former innovation is observable only to people residing in the home or occasional friends and relatives who may visit. Adoption of the latter innovation, however, requires the purchase and use of the helmet in public. Thus, whenever the adopter is riding his or her bicycle, people can readily observe the new behavior. Modeling the behavior of helmet use is far more feasible than modeling the use of home water filtration. Consequently, the diffusion effect for helmet use, all things being equal, is likely to be much greater than the effect for home water filtration.

▶ An Applied Example

Ultimately, diffusion theory provides many good ideas that can be used to bridge the gap between innovation and adoption. One example involves the innovation of organically grown foods that are part of a "farm-to-table" program that by-passes a series of manufacturing/processing steps. Farm-to-table programs are quickly gaining popularity in the United States, and this is translating into increased numbers of programs, farmer's markets, and farm-to-table restaurants—thereby making superior quality nutrition content available to massive numbers of people. Many of these programs have also been designed to "re-capture food" for free distribution to people who cannot afford to purchase healthy meals. For instance, Food Gatherers is a Michigan-based program that reaches more than thousands of household each month with free, high quality, produce and other forms of nutritional assistance to people experiencing hunger. The innovation in this case is the act (on the part of the community agency) of acquiring large supplies of low-cost, or no-cost food that is then made available through food pantries to people most in need. Adoption of this program by people in need was greatly magnified through the use of marketing methods, including display methods that optimized the distribution of produce that was otherwise un-popular (beets, turnips, cabbage, etc.).

Engaging in speculation about how programs such as Food Gatherers can best serve the hunger needs of a community, it is important to first consider the process for selecting and recruiting popular opinion leaders to represent the agency. These committed change agents can then communicate the relative advantages of the innovation in ways that would make them socially and practically acceptable to people in need of nutritional assistance. That products such as fresh beets, turnips, and cabbage do have relative advantages over highly processed food would become a primary teaching mission for these opinion leaders. They would additionally need to demonstrate how these foods could be prepared in a way that is compatible with the cultural "food norms" of the community. As a key factor in the adoption process, the characteristic of observability will most likely work in favor of the program, especially when program recipients write testimonials about the program in various forms of social media. Ultimately, the efforts of the POLs would lead to use of the program by early adopters, with the S-shaped diffusion curve to soon follow.

▶ Summary

In sum, diffusion theory posits that people progress through five discrete stages (knowledge, persuasion, decision, implementation, and confirmation). These stages are quite different from the categories of adoption that characterize the S-shaped diffusion curve. Innovators are viewed as the leverage point for catalyzing behavioral adoption of any given innovation into the next category: early adopters. In turn, early adopters (many of whom may be quite influential socially)

catalyze adoption of the early and late majority. Of course, in any given population, a percentage of people will reject the innovation (laggards). The speed of diffusion and rate of adoption are tied to the innovation itself. You now have a good command of many key characteristics that can make or break any given innovation, and that knowledge will be important to you when you apply diffusion theory to a health-promotion program at some point in your career.

▶ Take Home Messages

- People are more likely to adopt an innovation if they observe others having adopted the innovation, especially if those adopting the innovation are experiencing positive outcomes.
- The principles of diffusion theory can be very useful in planning interventions. Understanding the elements of (1) the innovation itself, (2) communication channels, (3) time, and (4) the social system is a key first step in health-promotion planning.
- The degree to which a target population is homologous impacts its receptivity of innovations.
- Diffusion theory categorizes people based on the speed at which they adopt an innovation: innovators, early adopters, early majority, late majority, and laggards.
- In order to be successful, an innovation must be compatible with local customs, must not negatively impact social relations, and should provide an advantage over products/practices that already exist. The innovation should also lend itself to clarity and trialability, and should be low risk and easily reversible.

▶ References

Christakis, N. A., & Fowler, J. H. (2007). The spread of obesity in a large social network over 32 years. *New England Journal of Medicine, 357*, 370–379.

Cooke, M., Mattick, R. P., & Campbell, E. (1999). The dissemination of a smoking cessation program to 23 antenatal clinics: The predictors of initial program adoption by managers. *Australian and New Zealand Journal of Public Health, 23,* 99–103.

Luepker, R. V., Perry, C. L., McKinley, S. M., Nader, P. R., Parcel, G. S., Stone, E. J., ... Wu, M. (1996). Outcomes of a field trial to improve children's dietary patterns and physical activity: The child and adolescent trial for cardiovascular health (CATCH). *Journal of the American Medical Association, 275,* 768–776.

Oldenburg, B., & Parcel, G. (2002). Diffusion of health promotion and health education innovations. In K. Glanz, F. Lewis, & B. Rimer (Eds.), *Health behavior and health education: Theory, research and practice* (3rd ed., pp. 312–334). San Francisco, CA: Jossey-Bass.

Rogers, E. M. (1983). *Diffusion of innovations.* New York, NY: Free Press.

Rogers, E. M. (1995). *Diffusion of innovations* (4th ed.). New York, NY: Free Press.

Ryan, B., & Gross, N. C. (1943). The diffusion of hybrid seed corn in two Iowa communities. *Rural Sociology, 8,* 15–24.

Simpson, J., Oldenburg, B., Owen, N., Harris, D., Dobbins, T., Salmon, A., ... Saunders, J. B. (2000). The Australian national workplace health project: Design and baseline findings. *Preventive Medicine, 31,* 249–260.

Chapter Opener: © MeskPhotography/Shutterstock; © Hero Images/Getty Images; © lzf/Shutterstock; © Henrik Sorensen/Getty Images

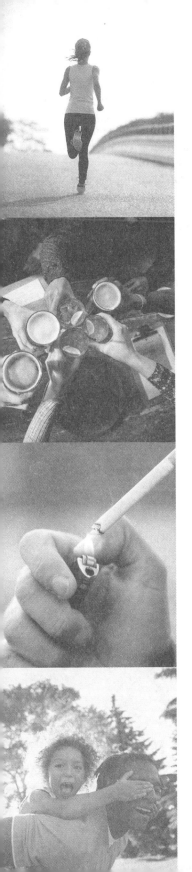

SECTION III

Application to Public Health Research and Practice

Now that you have acquired a thorough understanding of the theories most commonly used in health behavior, the next challenge is to learn core skills that are essential to health promotion practice. These are: 1) translating an empirically-tested health promotion program into widespread public health practice, 2) being "versatile" with theory such that you can combine two or more theories for a specific use, 3) becoming skilled in the measurement of theoretical constructs, and 4) accurately and thoroughly evaluating health promotion programs.

This section begins by introducing you to the field of implementation science, through the lens of translating research into practice and then "moving" the practice into broad-scale dissemination across entire populations. Because the field of health behavior is increasingly focused on translation and dissemination, you will find that this particular chapter will be one that will serve you well throughout your career in public health.

The next chapter will then introduce you to the concept on Intervention Mapping (IM). We realize that this is an "advanced skill" and thus we have placed it strategically in this textbook, as a culminating point of your education on health behavior theory in public health. The concept of IM is critical to your professional development because it places priority on resolving the public health problem at-hand and thus keeps the use of theory in perspective (i.e., theory is a tool used for the design of health promotion programs).

You will next be exposed to the basic principles of measurement. As you progress through this chapter, it will become apparent to you that measuring health behavior is indeed far from simple, yet the task is critical to understanding and changing health behavior. This core practice is vital simply because theory can only be applied with high fidelity when the constructs involved are assessed accurately. You will learn that accuracy in assessment is unquestionably vital to theory application. As you read this chapter, we urge you to master the twin concepts of reliability and validity and to take time to learn and practice identifying the four basic metrics of measurement. One caveat is in order before you begin learning about measurement: accuracy in the assessment of theoretical constructs is as important to the practitioner as it is to the researcher.

The final chapter in this section provides you with a primer on program evaluation. This chapter represents a logical endpoint to all that you have learned previously in this textbook. This seemingly broad-sweeping statement is true because evaluation is the gauge used to determine how effectively you have used your theory acumen to promote health-protective behaviors. Theory is nothing more than a means to an end—your work in public health is always

about changing behavior to prevent disease, and in the final analysis it is not about the intermediate act of skillfully applying theory. Although the traditional conceptualization of evaluation suggests it occurs last, you will learn that evaluation is better conceived as being interwoven into the entire process of program planning and measurement. We urge you to acquire and sharpen your evaluation skills, keeping in mind that this ongoing method of diagnosis is very much your lifeline to continued program improvement and, ultimately, to the economic justification for the existence of your entire health promotion program.

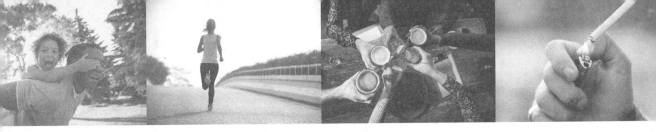

CHAPTER 12

Translating Research to Practice: Putting "What Works" to Work

Rita K. Noonan, James G. Emshoff, and Natalie Wilkins

Build a better mousetrap and the world will beat a path to your door.

A man who appears to have known little about research translation

—**Ralph Waldo Emerson** (1803–1882)

PREVIEW

There is a wide gap between public health research and everyday practice, which means that effective health innovations are not being used to reduce illness, injury, disability, and death. We can do better. Drawing from efforts in other industries and social science fields, public health practitioners can do a better job of putting "what works" to work. If we succeed in putting the best existing research into practice across our communities and clinical settings, we can create a safer, healthier population.

OBJECTIVES

1. To understand the gap that exists between public health research and public health practice.
2. To learn which factors make it more or less likely that new knowledge will be effectively disseminated and adopted into common practice.
3. To understand the importance of capacity building and partnership in order to increase integration between research and practice, and ensure that new scientific information is relevant, useful, and effectively adopted and implemented.

▶ Introduction

An untold number of scientists, doctors, researchers, and public health practitioners go to work every day hoping to make a difference in people's health. They spend a lifetime trying to find the best way to prevent heart disease, cancer, motor vehicle crashes, HIV infection, obesity, and hundreds of other public health problems. What would you say if you knew that many of the effective strategies to prevent these problems never got used? Sadly, this is what happens in public health. The best scientific discoveries often do not make it into practice settings, and those that do take more than a decade to get there! What's more, many potentially impactful innovations that emerge from public health practice (especially those that are developed at the grassroots practitioner level) are not identified for further research and evaluation, and thus remain untested in their effectiveness and largely unknown to the broader public health field. According to the Institute of Medicine, it takes 17 years for new knowledge generated from randomized controlled trials to be translated into practice (Institute of Medicine, 2001). Even after this delay of an entire generation, this new knowledge is applied unevenly and often ineffectively.

According to the Agency for Healthcare Research and Quality, roughly $95 billion dollars is spent on medical research in the United States each year. Ninety-nine cents of every research dollar is spent on new drugs and medical devices, which leaves only one penny per dollar to fund the research that ensures the safe and effective delivery of medical care to patients (Clancy, 2006). This lopsided equation is akin to investing all your money in the development of a vaccine without thinking about how you will administer the serum.

Failure to address the chasm between research and prevention practice not only means we have poorly invested in programs or strategies that are underutilized or not utilized at all; it also means we are failing to harness the best existing science to prevent illness, injuries, disabilities, and death (Brownson, Colditz, & Proctor, 2017). Let's go back to Ralph Waldo Emerson's quotation cited at the beginning of this chapter: "Build a better mousetrap and the world will beat a path to your door." Emerson does raise valid assertions on the importance of ensuring that public health strategies ("mousetraps") are sound from both a scientific and practical perspective. Indeed, if a public health program or policy is to be successful, it must be effective, as shown through research and evaluation, as well as feasible, useful, and applicable to the practice contexts in which it is to be implemented (Dearing, 2009). In this way, it is critical that the "mousetraps" we build in public health be rooted in both research- and practice-based knowledge and be informed by evidence drawn from both (Puddy, Wilkins, Thigpen, Singer, & Donovan, 2017). What Emerson does not take into account in this metaphor, however, is the true difficulty and complexity involved in identifying, testing, and ensuring the widespread adoption of public health innovations. This process is complicated and fraught with obstacles and detours. How will the world find out about these mousetraps? Will they believe they are truly better? Will they understand how to use them? Will they know where to buy them? Fortunately, public health researchers and practitioners are drawing from other industries and social science disciplines to pave the way and make the road easier to travel. What we mean is, research is being conducted and researcher–practitioner partnerships are being established that are helping to better understand *the process* involved in bridging the research–practice gap. There are studies that help us understand how to translate, support, and effectively implement **scientific innovations** (defined as any new knowledge, scientific advances, or technologies that may improve public health). We use the term "translational research" to describe this line of research, although there are many other terms, such as "discovery to delivery," "technology transfer," and "knowledge translation."

This chapter provides an overview of what is known about the process of integrating research and practice (from a variety of fields) and how we can apply lessons learned to public health. Fortunately, there is a growing body of research that public health practitioners can draw upon, including knowledge exchange, diffusion of innovations, social marketing, implementation science, and systems science. We begin by discussing the public health model's four steps to achieving widespread adoption and use (see **FIGURE 12-1**). The right-hand side of the model contains a host of unarticulated processes that we will highlight in this chapter. First, after a scientific innovation, such as a health promotion intervention has been deemed efficacious under tightly controlled research conditions, how do we **translate** it for use in real-world settings? How do we distill the information into a useable format and package the material for a large population of users? Second, what is the optimal plan to **disseminate** the

innovation to the population that needs it most? Who is our audience and how can we best reach them? What channels should we use?

Third, after the innovation is disseminated to people who are ready and willing to use it, we aim to achieve widespread **adoption**. We focus on what is known about adoption (why an individual or organization chooses to try out something new) and what happens after adoption. We also discuss ways in which we can support practitioners in integrating evidence-based interventions into the broader landscape of their work and the complex issues they are working to address. Fourth, and finally, after we have determined that a program is effective, we have translated and packaged it for easy consumption, we have disseminated it using the best messages and delivery systems, and we have organizations that have chosen to adopt this program, we now aim for high-quality **implementation** of effective interventions. How do new programs or technologies get implemented? How do we support high-quality implementation? Do users adapt/change the program or use it the way it was originally specified, implemented, and tested (i.e., with fidelity)? Thus, we also explore the tension between **fidelity** and **adaptation**. Although you learned about Diffusion of Innovations in Chapter 10, this

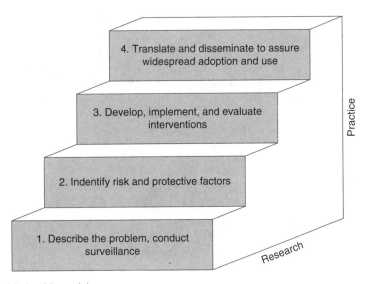

FIGURE 12-1 The public health model

Modified from Mercy, J.A., Rosenberg, M.L., Powell, K.E., Broome, C.V., & Roper, W.L. (1993). Public health policy for preventing violence. *Health Affairs, 12,* 7–29.

chapter gives you a somewhat different application of that theory, as we will apply it to adoption and use of programs by organizations.

Throughout each section, we discuss the importance of **capacity building** efforts to ensure that users of new information and strategies based on the best available evidence are adequately supported in their efforts to put those strategies in place. This includes ways in which public health strategies based on the best available evidence should be accompanied by training, coaching, and monitoring to support implementation, and ways in which partnerships between researchers and practitioners are critical for ensuring feasible, effective, and sustained implementation. We know that knowledge alone is not sufficient to change behavior, but by equipping researchers and practitioners in the field of public health with the skills, motivation, communication, and partnerships necessary to achieve effective, sustainable implementation we can make great progress in closing the gap between research and practice.

▶ Key Concepts

The Public Health Model

You have probably been exposed to the public health model, which is used to guide our prevention efforts; however, it never hurts to review. Figure 12-1 displays the four-step model. We start on the left-hand side with step 1 (etiology/surveillance), which is to understand the dimensions of a problem, such as "how big is it" and "where is it?" The next step is identifying risk factors: What populations are at greatest risk? What factors in

the environment are contributing to this risk? How can we lower the risk and/or increase protective factors? Based on these steps, we then develop and rigorously test interventions. The final step—step 4—is widespread adoption of interventions that have been shown to be effective. This last step is where some act of magic is assumed to occur. The vast majority of public health researchers go to school to understand steps 1, 2, and 3; step 4, however, is rarely studied or discussed. This is unfortunate, because widespread adoption will not happen by itself. Before we can achieve widespread adoption and use of effective interventions, we need to examine the "black box" that sits between steps 3 and 4. That box contains the processes associated with research translation (see **FIGURE 12-2**).

Why the Black Box?

The gap between steps 3 and 4, or the "black box," is a product of many different issues: (1) most public health professionals are trained in steps 1, 2, and 3, or the left-hand side of the model, and know very little about how to achieve step 4 or why it's important; (2) the system of rewards in many institutions, particularly academia, discourages work that is focused on practice settings, which is necessary for translation research and for developing and testing strategies that are feasible and relevant in practice contexts, because it is often difficult to conduct the kind of rigorous research that produces high-status publications; and (3) there is a research and development (R&D) bias in funding for health research (as evidenced by the fact that 99 cents of every medical research dollar is spent on new medicine). The driving assumption behind

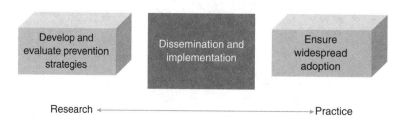

FIGURE 12-2 "Black Box" of research translation

most available funding from government institutions is that, "if you build it they will come." Apparently, most funders have read Ralph Waldo Emerson's famous mousetrap quote!

In the 1989 movie, *Field of Dreams*, Ray Kinsella (played by Kevin Costner) is a novice farmer who becomes convinced by a mysterious voice that he is supposed to construct a baseball diamond in his cornfield. The film's underlying themes are the fulfillment of dreams and that people can overcome regrets they may have about their life choices. Ray Kinsella mends his broken relationship with his deceased father by following the advice of the mysterious voice: "If you build it, he will come." Although this worked out in the end for Ray Kinsella (i.e., he gets to play catch with the ghost of his father on his baseball field), in the real world of human behavioral health interventions, "if you build it" (particularly if you build it without consideration and meaningful input from those in practice) then many potential outcomes are possible (Emshoff, 2008):

- "they might not feel invited"
- "they might not find it"
- "they might think they already have one"
- "they might want 10 more, right now"

If you think it is difficult to get people to use a better mousetrap, imagine the difficulty public health researchers and practitioners have in changing people's daily habits, which are often recalcitrant to change efforts and where many of the interventions are often complex. Public health works with "social technologies" that include all the complexity of human interaction in a variety of social settings. We are often asking people to adopt and use innovations—programs, policies, practices, or processes—that are not always easy to integrate into their current routine.

Obviously, there are many factors that determine how, when, and whether a new program gets picked up and used widely. To simplify, we can follow the model depicted in **FIGURE 12-3**. This model helps us understand the black box between what has been deemed effective and what merits further dissemination and implementation; therefore, steps 1, 2, and 3 of the public health model are outside of this figure, although it is worth

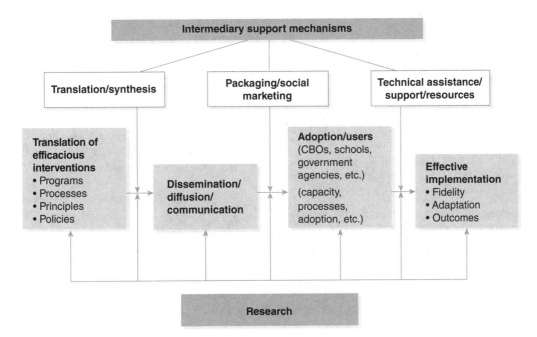

FIGURE 12-3 Science to practice flow chart

noting again that as public health interventions are being developed and tested (step 3) it is critical that practical considerations around feasibility, acceptability, and relevance be prioritized (practice to research), because this increases the likelihood of their wide-scale adoption later on (step 4; Dearing, 2009). For the four step science to practice model (depicted in Figure 12-3 and not to be confused with the 4-step public health model), we are starting with a body of interventions with known properties—those that represent the best existing evidence. Why else would we want to disseminate them? The flow chart follows these steps, with capacity building and technical assistance throughout: (1) translating an efficacious intervention into a practical prevention program, (2) disseminating innovations to key audiences, (3) adoption of effective innovations for use in appropriate settings, and (4) effective implementation. Successful execution of each step requires training, skills acquisition, capacity development, and partnership.

Throughout this chapter, we will use the terms **program**, **innovation**, and **intervention** interchangeably to refer to a wide variety of scientific advances and new knowledge that may be the subject of translation; these can include manualized programs, **processes** that are essential to public health's functions, public health **principles** (e.g., using data to make decisions), or **policies**.

Programs: These are normally behavioral change strategies that have a set of steps that should be followed. A program often has a curriculum or guide that should be implemented the same way each time. Sometimes we call these "programs in a box."

Processes: Many evidence-based processes currently exist to help public health practitioners improve community-based programming. For example, Getting To Outcomes is a 10-step process that empowers prevention practitioners to plan, implement, and evaluate their own prevention programs (Wiseman et al., 2007). Similarly, community responses to disasters often have a well-defined set of steps that should be

followed to reduce further illness and injury in the aftermath of a crisis event.

Principles: Public health principles include the emphasis on primary prevention, using data to make decisions, working across the social–ecological model, population-based efforts, and evaluating our work. (See other chapters in this book to get a fuller description of these principles.)

Policies: Policies are codified mandates to do something. These can be "big P" policies, such as federal regulations that inhibit smoking on airplanes, or "small p" policies, such as a school policy that requires a teen dating violence curriculum in all health classes. Thus, policies can have a broad effect on a whole society, or a more narrow effect on a particular organization.

Step 1: Translation

Interventions that have been shown to be efficacious using randomized controlled trials often require additional work before they can be implemented in community or clinical settings (Close, 2005). Weisz and Bearman (2014) have acknowledged the challenges facing the marriage between science and practice. Many interventions lack training materials, user manuals, and identified delivery channels to encourage adoption; others require modifications in order to reach new audiences or gain acceptance in implementation settings; innovations need to be "packaged" and prepared for a wider audience of practitioners before they are ready for a "prime time" market.

Researchers often assume that if they publish their findings in a scholarly journal, then their work is finished. However, very few end users are going to pick up the *American Journal of Public Health* to figure out which school-based violence prevention program they should implement. Practitioners need to know what programs are available, are applicable to their population, and have corresponding user-friendly manuals.

A Real Life Example: What Would Coke Do?*

Let's take an everyday example and walk through the distillation and packaging process. Let's say we are promoting a new Coca-Cola beverage instead of a public health intervention. We would not stop our efforts because we developed a wonderfully sweet, tasty beverage and then wrote about it in some trade journal (e.g., *Beverage Industry*); rather, we would figure out how to persuade people to consume as much of the product as possible. We could do this by understanding the market we are trying to reach, packaging the product in a way that is appealing to consumers, selling it in consumable amounts (not 50-gallon drums), and making it available everywhere! As you can infer from this example, R&D is the *start* of this process, not the end.

We understand that we are not selling Coke and that public health practices are different from consumer goods; however, we can learn from the business sector because they have a vested financial interest in getting this right. We can learn a lot about "technology transfer" from them. We need to get our best science translated into digestible formats and settings for end users and package the materials appropriately. Of course, this process depends greatly on the practice or intervention being translatable and scalable. Even if we are able to accomplish this part of the process, it may not be sufficient to ensure adoption and use. The next step is disseminating materials based on what known about the end users.

Step 2: Dissemination

Dissemination is defined as the intentional spreading of information for a specific purpose. This term is often distinguished from **diffusion**, which is often considered to be a more passive process that happens unintentionally or naturally. We know from decades of experience that public health prevention efforts are not always adopted or implemented, even if they are wrapped in a pretty package. We also know that knowledge, although necessary for behavior change, is not sufficient for behavior change—think about people who eat fast-food or smoke. Thus, we need to take the next step to market the innovation to key audiences and build (or identify) sufficient delivery channels. Fostering partnerships between the developers of public health strategies and those that are charged with implementing them can also help strengthen dissemination and uptake.

Because public health agencies are not exactly like McDonald's restaurants, we must engage in a different kind of marketing of our products: social marketing. Although we cover social marketing in greater detail in Chapter 9, we provide a brief overview to illustrate its specific application to dissemination.

As previously discussed, **social marketing** uses regular marketing principles to "sell" ideas, attitudes, and behaviors that benefit the target audience, and society in general, as opposed to benefiting the marketer (Weinrich, 1999). Social marketing approaches are gaining wider utilization in a variety of health improvement campaigns, including contraceptive use, drug abuse, heart disease, breast cancer screening, and teen dating violence, among others. This kind of an approach includes end users and/or those who will be charged with implementing public-health strategies in the process of dissemination. Social marketing can be thought of a process that, like traditional marketing, includes five steps (Kennedy & Crosby, 2002):

1. *Conducting formative and audience research.* Who is your end user? Who do you want to "buy" this product? What consumer habits or preferences do they have?

2. Using the research results to *divide the target audience into segments* with similar characteristics and tailoring messages to appeal to each segment.

---

* All references to commercial products in this chapter are meant to illustrate theoretical concepts and should not be understood as implied endorsements on the part of the Centers for Disease Control and Prevention.

3. *Identifying the costs and benefits* of the product or behavior from the consumer's point of view and then designing messages that minimize the costs and promote the benefits to create the perception of a beneficial exchange.

4. *Employing the four P's* analysis of campaign plans by considering the attractiveness of the program or product, the affordability and perceived reasonableness of its price or nonmonetary costs, the convenience with which it can be accessed or its placement, and the best channels and messages to use in its promotion to the target audience.

5. *Revising campaign* offerings based on ongoing consumer feedback.

Following these five steps should help public health professionals tackle a variety of questions that come up regularly during the research, development, and dissemination processes. For example, who are the most influential people for disseminating knowledge? Although many university professors may not like to hear this, most practitioners do not refer to academic journals when they are looking for a new solution to a public health or human service problem (Sorian &

Baugh, 2002). Instead, practitioners on the ground (as opposed to in academia) in real-world settings prefer to get information from peers (Wandersman et al., 2008). James Dearing, a communications expert and researcher at Kaiser Permanente, cataloged the "Top 10 dissemination mistakes," and includes one major error frequently made by public health institutions: "We use intervention creators as intervention communicators" (Dearing, 2009). Our top researchers are not necessarily the best people to communicate the innovation's benefit to the public. Formative research and reevaluation will also help public health professionals avoid other dissemination mistakes, such as assuming that scientific evidence matters in the decision making for potential adopters, or assuming that we will win over decision makers by simply providing more evidence. Public health is a field that is very committed to research and science, but successful dissemination requires that we let our audience *tell us* what they want, rather than imposing our own values or preferences on them (Dearing, 2009) This bidirectional flow of knowledge and expertise has been referred to more broadly in the translation literature as **knowledge exchange** (Conklin, Hallsworth, Hatziandreu, & Grant, 2008), and is an important principle for guiding successful dissemination (see **TABLE 12-1**).

TABLE 12-1 Top 10 Dissemination Mistakes

Dissemination Mistake	Description	Solution
We assume that evidence matters in the decision making of a potential adopter.	Interventions of unknown effectiveness and of known ineffectiveness often spread while effective interventions do not. Evidence is most important to only a subset of early adopters and is most often used by them to reject interventions.	Emphasize other variables in the communication of innovations, such as compatibility, cost, and simplicity.
We substitute our perception for those of potential adopters.	Inadequate and poorly performed formative evaluation is common when experts in the intervention topical domain engage in dissemination.	Seek out and listen to representative potential adopters to learn wants, information sources, advice-seeking behaviors, and reactions to prototype interventions.

Dissemination Mistake	Description	Solution
We use intervention creators as intervention communicators.	While the creators of interventions are sometimes effective communicators, the opposite condition is much more common.	Enable access to the experts, but rely on others whom we know will elicit attention and information seeking by potential adopters.
We introduce interventions before they are ready.	Interventions are often shown as they are created and tested. Viewers often perceive uncertainty and complexity as a result.	Publicize interventions only after clear results and the preparation of messages that elicit positive reactions from potential adopters.
We assume that information will influence decision making.	Information is necessary and can be sufficient for adoption decisions about inconsequential innovations, but for consequential interventions that imply changes in organizational routines or individual behaviors, influence is typically required.	Pair information resources with social influence in an overall dissemination strategy.
We confuse authority with influence.	Persons high in positional or formal authority may also be regarded as influential by others, but often this is not the case.	Gather data about who among potential adopters is sought out for advice and intervene with them to propel dissemination.
We allow the first to adopt (innovators) to self-select into our dissemination efforts.	The first to adopt often do so for counter normative reasons and their low social status can become associated with an intervention.	Learn the relational structure that ties together potential adopters so that influential members can be identified and recruited.
We fail to distinguish among change agents, authority figures, opinion leaders, and innovation champions.	It is unusual for the same persons to effectively play multiple roles in dissemination into and within communities and complex organizations.	Use formative evaluation to determine the functions that different persons are able to fulfill.
We select demonstration sites on criteria of motivation and capacity.	Criteria of interest and ability make sense when effective implementation is the only objective. But spread relies on the perceptions by others of initial adopters.	Consider which sites will positively influence other sites when selecting demonstration sites.
We advocate single interventions as the solution to a problem.	Potential adopters differ by clientele, setting, resources, and so on, so one intervention is unlikely to fit all.	Communicate a cluster of evidence-based practices so that potential adopters can get closer to a best fit of intervention to organization prior to adaptation.

Dearing, J. W. (2009). Applying Diffusion of Innovation Theory to Intervention Development. *Research on Social Work Practice, 19*(5), 503–518, with permission

In addition to formative research, public health efforts should glean insights from best practices in training and education to identify optimal modalities and channels for dissemination. The advancement of technology, for example, has resulted in an explosion of web-based trainings, webinars, blogs, and listservs, used as means for disseminating information to large audiences. Unfortunately, many of these passive knowledge transfer strategies—such as attending continuing medical education lectures (in person or online)—are unlikely to have a major impact on physician practice (Soumerai & Avorn, 1990). The growing field of dissemination and behavior change suggests that what's old is really what's new. People change their behavior in ways that have been predictable for many years: humans need adequate time to learn something new, they need to practice new skills in the actual setting where they will be practiced (behavioral rehearsals), and they need a supportive environment to do so. The best dissemination strategy in the world cannot create this fertile environment for change, but it can increase the likelihood that the right information gets into the right hands at the right time for the right purpose. This is a very tall order and requires that that marketing research be conducted ahead of time.

Dissemination: A Real Life Example

Revisiting the example of Coke is useful. After the tasty beverage is developed, it is then packaged nicely in consumable amounts and marketed to key audiences. But then what? How do people get it? Coke isn't dropped out of airplanes into various communities, and companies don't ask people to bring their cars to the warehouse to pick it up. Rather, there are distributors who load their product into their trucks and then drive along paved roads and highways to deliver the product to millions of stores. There is a complex infrastructure and sophisticated distribution system to get the packaged product from point A to point B. In fact, Coke's own lofty goal was that every person on earth should have a Coca-Cola product "within arm's reach of desire" (Allen, 1994). They built an infrastructure—roads, trucks, donkeys, bicycles, whatever it took—to support the realization of that goal. Public health innovations, like Coke, also require an infrastructure to move effective strategies from research into practice (see **BOX 12-1**).

BOX 12-1 Not-On-Tobacco (N-O-T): Building Widespread Dissemination into Program Design

West Virginia led the nation in teenage smoking during the mid-1990s, and, as a result, the West Virginia University's Prevention Research Center (PRC) partnered with West Virginia's Bureau for Public Health, Department of Education, and other members of the state's public health community to strengthen school-based tobacco control initiatives. West Virginia needed an effective, user-friendly, teenage smoking cessation program that could be adopted statewide and that would support a newly developed state tobacco-free school policy emphasizing prevention and cessation support rather than punitive action.

To create national distribution and outreach, the West Virginia team partnered with the American Lung Association (ALA). The partnership identified local and national needs and took on the shared goal of developing a theoretically based, scientifically tested teenage smoking cessation intervention. With funding from the Centers for Disease Control and Prevention and other organizations, the West Virginia University PRC launched a smoking cessation project characterized by: (1) teachers, students, and school health professionals providing input for program development; (2) the ALA providing program expertise, funding, and a means for disseminating programs; and (3) PRC researchers providing a scientific framework to evaluate the effectiveness of programs and a commitment to program dissemination.

Through an iterative, collaborative process, the partnership developed a smoking cessation program designed for 14 to 19-year–old daily smokers. The program was given the youth-approved name,

Not-On-Tobacco, or N-O-T. In addition to smoking cessation, other N-O-T goals include reducing smoking; increasing healthy lifestyle behaviors (e.g., physical activity, healthy eating); and improving stress management, decision making, coping ability, and social support skills. Students participate in the program on a voluntary basis, and the program includes 10 hour-long weekly sessions and 4 booster sessions in same-sex groups with same-sex facilitators (e.g., teachers, school nurses, counselors, volunteers).

Facilitators are trained by the ALA and may lead sessions in both schools and other community settings. They assist participants with (1) identifying reasons for smoking and excuses for not quitting, beliefs and behaviors that reinforce smoking and self-defeating behaviors, triggers for smoking, and other barriers to the quitting process; (2) recognizing and understanding the process of nicotine addiction, advertising ploys to encourage youth smoking, and situations that may spark relapse; and (3) developing skills in cognitive restructuring, coping with stress and peer pressure, identifying and maintaining social supports, goal setting, and assertiveness and other behavior changes.

Over a 10-year period, the N-O-T program went through several iterations, testing, refinement, and retesting. Studies have consistently shown that adolescents enrolled in N-O-T programs have significantly greater quit and reduction rates than adolescents in more conventional smoking cessation programs.

Given the N-O-T program's proven effectiveness and feasibility, the ALA has adopted it as a national best practice model and is disseminating it widely. Train-the-trainer protocols, training manuals, materials for students, and guides for initiating programs in high schools have been developed. In a mutually beneficial relationship, the ALA produces, packages, trains, disseminates, and tracks participation in N-O-T, while the PRC provides scientific oversight, technical assistance, data management, and evaluation, and takes the lead on reports and publications.

Public Health Impact

Since 2000, about 300,000 teens in the United States have participated in the N-O-T program. Recently, N-O-T was identified as the most widely used teen smoking cessation program in the nation, accounting for about one-third of all adolescent intervention efforts. Given the effectiveness demonstrated from 1999 through 2003, we can assume that about one of every six participants quit smoking as a result. Generally, studies have found that N-O-T doubles a teen's chances of quitting smoking. Translation of materials into Spanish is increasing the program's reach, as will a culturally appropriate version for American Indian youth that is under way.

After rigorous review by an independent panel of scientists, N-O-T has been recognized as an effective program by the National Registry of Evidence-Based Programs and Practices (NREPP). The program is included in the NREPP's repository of science-based programs, is listed on the Substance Abuse and Mental Health Services Administration's Model Program's website (www.nrepp.samhsa.gov), and is now a Model Program, which could increase support for its dissemination nationwide. This recognition should help make N-O-T even more widely available to help teenagers in need.

Translation Lessons Learned from the N-O-T Program

1. Involvement of multiple stakeholders, including school personnel and students, in the N-O-T program design resulted in a program that is feasible and effective and that attracts local champions to spearhead implementation in multiple locales.
2. Dissemination of the N-O-T program was a goal from its beginning, and this aim was a valuable guide to keep the program practitioner-friendly, consistent with local policies, and appealing to local funding agencies.
3. Having a partner with experience in national dissemination (the ALA) provided the capacity for widespread diffusion and adoption of the N-O-T program.

The Centers for Disease Control and Prevention. Not-On-Tobacco (NOT)—Smoking cessation program for 12–19 year olds selected as a model program. Retrieved July 25, 2011 from http://www.cdc.gov/prc/preventionstrategies/not-on-tobacco-smoking-cessation.htm

Planning for Dissemination: Diffusion of Innovation Principles (DOI)

You may be familiar with the concept of multilevel marketing; if not, it involves someone near the top of the marketing pyramid selling products to people below, who have been recruited to sell the product. Those sales people in turn sell the products to multiple sellers further down the chain, and so on, until the product gets into the hands of the consumer. Dissemination of prevention strategies often follows a similar pattern. For instance, the Federal Department of Education may put resources into a specific prevention approach, which they disseminate to state departments of education, who then "sell" the program to the school districts within their states. This process continues until the program reaches the students in the classroom. While dissemination occurs at each of these levels, it may need to be focused differently depending on the level.

The audiences at each level are different. Marketing and advertising use a concept, market segmentation, to reflect the differences between subgroups in the population of interest. Each segment of the market has its own needs, values, resources, and history, and the dissemination or marketing process should reflect these differences. Effective dissemination begins with an understanding of what the potential user wants and what he/she is capable of using. For example, there is no sense in disseminating a program to a mental health clinic if it is more expensive than the entire annual budget of the center or is inconsistent with the values or experience of that center. In fact, a study of potential users should precede not only the dissemination of the program, but also the development of the program itself.

Is the dissemination process beginning to sound like big business? The concept of social marketing refers to the use of business marketing strategies and techniques in the promotion of social good—in this case, the prevention of adverse health outcomes. As you may recall from Chapter 9, social marketing can occur at the individual level (e.g., how to persuade pregnant women to practice good prenatal health behaviors), but in this instance social marketing should be used at the organizational level (e.g., how to persuade a prenatal health clinic to adopt a new smoking cessation program).

One of our consistent themes is that public health rarely provides sufficient attention to these processes. Sometimes we take the attitude reflected above: "If we build it, they will come." Why wouldn't they? Can't they see we have a great program here? Those in the world of business know that without considerable focus on the marketing of the program, and input from end users in product development, very few products would be sold in any meaningful quantities. In fact, it is quite common to farm out the distribution of effective programs to for-profit publishing houses that engage in dissemination by mail order and may or may not offer any of the training/coaching support that led to the intervention's effectiveness in the first place. Most program developers do not have the time or resources in training others on how to use a program effectively or how to sustain it over time. One explanation is that program developers typically are recipients of grant funding obtained to develop and test the program; however, after that, the funding stream runs out and they don't have the salary support or additional resources to take it a step further.

Step 3: Adoption

We turn now to the next step in our "science to practice" model: adoption by potential users. After a program has been identified as effective, translated for real-world settings, and efforts have been made to disseminate this program to potential users, these potential users must sift through the information made available to them (assuming it has reached them) and decide whether to adopt this new program.

The literature on adoption overlaps with the literature on dissemination and diffusion because these processes are so related, as whether a program is adopted is a function of characteristics of the program, characteristics of the messages about the program, and characteristics of the adopter.

Characteristics of the Program

When you are considering what kind of car, home entertainment system, or computer to buy, what do you look for? Would you choose products that have been recently developed but are just now reaching the market? Would you wait until your friends have tested the product first? Would you look at data describing the performance of the product (e.g., how fast the computer operates)? Would you buy a new television if it meant changing all of the other components in your entertainment system (e.g., new speakers, new cable system)? How important is price?

The way you look at these products is not that different from how organizations look at new programs and decide which public health programs and practices to adopt. Those who have studied these processes (starting with Rogers, 1962) have concluded that certain kinds of programs are more likely to get adopted. In his famous body of work concerning the Diffusion of Innovations, Everett Rogers explored several factors that explain the adoption of new products in a marketplace. For starters, a program is more likely to be adopted if it is perceived to have advantages over alternatives—either current practice or other available programs. As scientists, we often believe that the program perceived to be the most advantageous is the one that has been proven to produce the best outcomes. Although this may be a factor, other elements of perceived advantage include its cost, its ease of implementation, the degree to which it requires people to change (particularly in ways they are not experienced or comfortable with), its reputation, and its face validity (does it look good to an outsider).

Second, a program is more likely to be adopted if it is compatible with the organization's culture, philosophy, or current practices. For example, a faith-based organization may not be as likely to adopt a teen pregnancy program that includes contraception as a strategy. Third, the complexity (or simplicity) of the program affects the likelihood of its adoption, as organizations naturally gravitate toward simple solutions. Fourth, if the program can be tried out before making a full commitment to its adoption, it is more likely to be adopted. Organizations, like

people, want to know what they're getting into. Fifth, programs that can be observed in action are more likely to be adopted—would you buy a house or car, sight unseen? Finally, flexible programs are more likely to be adopted. If an organization feels that a program can be adapted to fit its local needs, culture, and conditions, it is more likely to be comfortable with it and more likely to use it. We will discuss this adaptation in more detail later in the chapter.

Characteristics of the Message

What kinds of messages help sell a product? We know that effective messages highlight the aspects of a product or program that the audience (not the inventor) finds desirable and these effective messages usually don't use scientific or other jargon. When Toyota tries to sell you a car, they may mention the MPG of the car, but there is much greater focus on nontechnical aspects of its performance. In addition, effective messages are presented by credible sources. Of course, this might mean different sources for different audiences. Academics tend to place high reliance on peer-reviewed scientific journals for knowledge, while practitioners often place greater weight on messages delivered by their peers (see **FIGURE 12-4**).

Characteristics of the Adopter

In Chapter 10, you read about different kinds of adopters that were described by Rogers' Diffusion of Innovations curve. Organizations are like people. Some are eager to innovate, and others are highly resistant to change. Where an organization lies on this continuum will predict how likely it is that it will adopt new programs. In general, organizations that have more resources are more likely to adopt new programs. They may have the staff to devote to new work, the facilities for implementation, the time for training, and the ability to recruit participants. But even organizations with enough resources may not adopt new programs if they don't have leadership or a culture that encourages learning and change (Aarons & Sommerfeld, 2012; Senge, 1990). Some organizations, like some people,

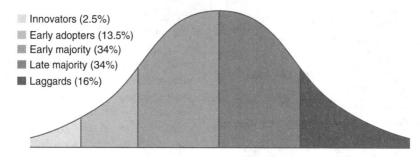

Innovators (2.5%)
Early adopters (13.5%)
Early majority (34%)
Late majority (34%)
Laggards (16%)

FIGURE 12-4 Diffusion of Innovations curve

Data from Rogers, E. M. (1995). *Diffusion of innovations* (4th ed.). New York, NY: Free Press.

just get comfortable with what they are doing and view change as threatening. Or they may not reward their staff for trying new things—or may even punish them if they try something that doesn't work. Conversely, organizations with "transformational leaders" (i.e., leaders who are inspiring and charismatic) and a high level of leadership–staff interaction and exchange are more likely to have a culture open to innovation and adoption of evidence-based programs and practices (Aarons & Sommerfeld, 2012).

Another related factor is the degree to which organizations are tuned into new information. Do they talk to their peers, do they read the literature in their field, and do they attend professional or scientific conferences? Without staying up-to-date on the state of the art in their field, it is unlikely they will change.

The environment surrounding the organization affects the likelihood of program adoption as well (Klein & Sorra, 1996; Vakola, 2013). Different disciplines are more or less resistant to change. Law tends to be fairly stable, so lawyers tend to do the same things year after year, but those working in information technology are expected to change quickly as their field changes quickly. In addition, organizations, like people, are more or less resistant to peer pressure to change. If most schools in a district are using a new substance abuse prevention program, the remaining schools may feel pressure to adopt it as well. Finally, when the environment is uncertain (e.g., it is not clear how budgets might change or if the organization might get restructured next year), innovation and adoption get stifled.

Adoption and Risk

In many ways, the act of adopting a program is the act of minimizing and managing risk. Every major purchase you make involves some risk. Will this car drive as well as I thought? Will it be reliable over time? Will it impress other people? Will it get the mileage I was promised?

Programs that have the desirable characteristics listed above (e.g., have perceived advantages and are simple, less costly, observable, and flexible) represent less risk to the adopter. But we should also consider the adopting organization. Some organizations, like some people, are early adopters. They tend to have a higher threshold of risk and are able to manage it effectively. Organizations that have a lot of administrative support and resources may find they can manage the risk of a new program more easily, and organizations with a culture encouraging change will not find new programs as risky (Aarons & Sommerfeld, 2012).

Supporting Adoption: Evidence-Based Decision-Making and Systems Thinking

As outlined in the sections above, public health practitioners have to grapple with many considerations when making decisions about the prevention strategies they want to invest their time, resources, and efforts into in order to achieve public health impact. Practitioners have to identify strategies that are not only effective based on the best available research evidence, but that also "fit" within their local context. Supporting practitioners as they engage in these adoption and decision-making efforts means supplying the necessary tools and resources to gather the information and evidence they need to make informed decisions. For example, CDC has developed **Understanding Evidence**, an interactive online tool that walks practitioners through the process of identifying public-health strategies that have been tested for effectiveness (best available research evidence), gathering information on their local context (contextual evidence), and leveraging the collective wisdom and experience of those who live and work in the communities in which strategies will be implemented (experiential evidence, Puddy et al., 2017).

Public health practitioners do not adopt and implement strategies in a vacuum; often, they must address multiple public health outcomes in shifting and often complex environments. It can be challenging to find the time, resources, and buy-in needed to adopt multiple prevention strategies to address these many different public-health issues. Systems thinking is one method that researchers and practitioners in public health are increasingly using to address some of these challenges and to identify strategies for adoption that have the potential to impact multiple public-health issues (Best, Clark, Leischow, & Trochim, 2007; Carey et al., 2015; Leischow et al., 2008; Luke & Stamatakis, 2012). Systems thinking is the practice of considering the parts, the whole, and their interconnections in order to understand an issue (or issues), as well as the possible intended (or unintended) consequences of actions taken on a part or the whole of a system (Peters, 2014; Senge, 1990). Understanding the systems in which public-health practitioners' issues and priorities are embedded, and the ways these issues are related to one another can help practitioners identify prevention approaches with the potential to solve multiple issues. This in turn can aid in adoption by helping practitioners "make the case" for adopting prevention strategies based on the best available evidence to decision makers, partners, and other key stakeholders whose buy-in may be needed. For example, the Colorado Department of Public Health and Environment was able to demonstrate how an evidence-based suicide prevention program, Sources of Strength, had the potential to impact not only suicide but also sexual violence and bullying among youth across the state. This enabled them to secure resources and buy-in from key suicide, sexual violence, and youth violence partners and scale up adoption of this evidence-based public health strategy (Wilkins, Myers, Kuehl, Bauman, & Hertz, 2017).

Step 4: Implementation

We now turn to the final step in our model—implementation. So far, we have determined that a program is effective, we have translated and packaged it for easy consumption, we have disseminated it using the best messages and delivery systems, and we have organizations that have chosen to adopt this program. Now, the "rubber meets the road": the organization is ready to use the program.

When we implement "hard" technologies, like buying a new car, we have relatively few choices about how to use it: we simply drive it the way it was intended to be driven. If we don't know how to make something work, we can consult the manual. However, with social and health technologies, the kind of programs we have discussed so far, the users have multiple choices about how to put the program into place. For example, if the program is a classroom-based curriculum, then the teacher may not teach all of the lessons or have all of the materials. Or perhaps the teacher did not receive full training on the curriculum. Or maybe the curriculum is delivered to the wrong audience (e.g., too old or too young). Or maybe the curriculum was designed to be delivered by peers, but is being implemented by teachers. The tension between adaptation and fidelity when implementing evidence-based programs is an area of great importance and attention in dissemination and implementation research and practice (Bopp, Saunders, & Lattimore, 2013; Hansen, 2013; Lize, Andrews, Whitaker, Shapiro, & Nelson, 2014). Variations in implementation may, in some cases, be critical for ensuring that the program is appropriate and "fits" with the local context, but, if the variations become too extreme, then the program's effectiveness may be compromised as it may no

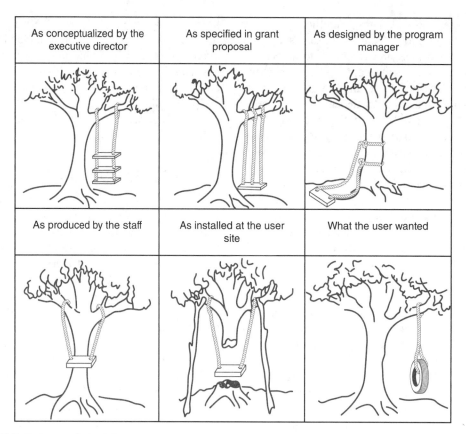

As conceptualized by the executive director	As specified in grant proposal	As designed by the program manager
As produced by the staff	As installed at the user site	What the user wanted

FIGURE 12-5 Cartoons of adaptation

longer resemble or represent the original program that was adopted (see **FIGURE 12-5**).

It may be helpful at this juncture to think of the implementation of a program as an algorithm or like following a recipe. If an ingredient is missing, in the wrong quantity, or added at the wrong time, or if the ingredients are cooked at the wrong temperature or in the wrong pan, the final product may not taste as intended. This is not a problem with the recipe, but rather with the implementation. Likewise, when programs do not achieve their intended outcomes, it may not be a problem with the program, but with its implementation (see **BOX 12-2**).

Just as with food, implementing a program effectively is as important as implementing an effective program. Unfortunately, most of the work of social scientists goes into testing

program effectiveness, not testing the feasibility of program implementation (as in the example of Arby's test kitchen given in Box 12-2). This reality is reflected in the matrix shown in **FIGURE 12-6** (Fixsen, Blase, Naoom, & Wallace, 2009; Noonan, 2010) that shows we will achieve effective health outcomes if we: (1) choose effective programs to implement, and (2) implement these programs effectively.

Let's look at the 2 × 2 table shown in Figure 12-6. On one axis you have the effectiveness of the innovation (or intervention) as high and low. On the other axis, you have effectiveness of the implementation—in other words, whether it was delivered as designed—as high and low. If you have an effective intervention that is delivered poorly (e.g., didn't include the core components), you will not get the desired result. You can

BOX 12-2 Arby's Test Kitchen

Let's continue with the recipe analogy. Arby's national test kitchen is located in a suburb of Atlanta, Georgia, in the southeastern United States. The test kitchen is charged with coming up with new recipes and products to be sold at Arby's restaurants around the country. What do you think is the biggest challenge to the kitchen scientists? Finding something that tastes good to diverse groups of consumers? Creating recipes made from ingredients that can be secured and delivered in mass quantities across the country without sacrificing freshness? Making sandwiches that are affordable to all income strata? All of these are important, but the number one challenge, dwarfing these others in importance, is to develop a product that can be produced over and over and over by thousands of (mostly teenage) employees in a consistent fashion. Essentially, the biggest challenge lies not in product development, but in product implementation.

If implementing a cheddar bacon roast beef sandwich consistently with high quality is a challenge, then imagine the issues associated with implementing complex multicomponent health promotion and prevention programs that require service organizations to restructure or delivery agents to learn new skills—all of which are designed to impact behaviors as complex as negotiating condom use, using condoms, using contraceptives, getting a colonoscopy, or adhering to complicated medical regiments (Warhop, 2006).

High Effectiveness High Implementation * Model program implemented with fidelity	High Effectiveness Low Implementation * Half of model sessions are delivered
Low Effectiveness High Implementation * Ineffective program implemented with fidelity to content and delivery format	Low Effectiveness Low Implementation * One-hour session in assembly hall delivered by a boring person

FIGURE 12-6 Effectiveness implementation 2×2 matrix

Reproduced from Noonan, R. (2010, December). *Translating "translation:" What do we know? What can we do better?* Paper presented at the expert panel meeting: Prevention of falls among older adults, Atlanta, GA.

have an ineffective intervention (e.g., the DARE program) that, no matter how well or how many times you implement it, it will not produce the desired results. There is only one box that ensures that we are getting the results we desire, and that the public deserves, which is when you have effective interventions that are implemented effectively (Fixsen, Blase, Timbers, & Wolf, 2001; Leschied & Cunningham, 2002; Washington State Institute for Public Policy, 2005).

What Are the Elements of Implementation?

Several questions apply to implementation. Examples include the following:

- Did the user use the correct content (e.g., were all of the curriculum materials used)?
- Did the user follow the right processes (e.g., was each lecture component accompanied by a role play)?

■ Did the program get delivered with the right dosage (e.g., enough sessions, with the correct amount of time per session)?

■ Were the right people involved (e.g., did the intended people deliver the program to the intended recipients)?

■ Did the intended participants fully engage with the program (e.g., did they attend all sessions)?

■ Was the program delivered in the correct setting (e.g., a classroom vs. the home)?

All of these questions (and others) are ways of asking: Did you follow the recipe? The answer to that question was examined in one study of drug prevention programs (Gottfredson & Gottfredson, 2002). The author found that only half of the curricula used and only one-fourth of the mentoring programs implemented met the dosage requirements.

If any of the questions listed previously were answered with less than "totally!," we might wonder if the intended outcomes of the program are likely to occur. In the world of program evaluation, concluding that a program is not effective, when in fact the measurement of the implementation processes suggests that it was not fully implemented—or not implemented according to the program "recipe," if you like—is called a type III error. Type III errors can be avoided by understanding what affects implementation, supporting high quality implementation, and carefully evaluating our success.

What Affects Implementation?

Durlak and DuPre (2008) identified a variety of factors, at multiple levels, that affect the quality of implementation. An example at the community level is the amount of funding given to an organization to implement a program. Without proper funding, we would expect corners to be cut. At the organizational level, we would expect organizations that are more open to change, organizations with solid communication channels, and organizations that have a strong advocate or champion for the program to implement it more effectively (Durlak & DuPre, 2008).

Characteristics of the program deliverer also matter. To achieve optimal implementation, people who are delivering the program should perceive a need for the program, believe in its benefits, have the skills necessary to deliver the program, and feel confident in their ability to do so. Finally, some innovations are more likely to be implemented well than others. Programs are more likely to be implemented correctly if they are compatible with the setting in which they are used and if the program lends itself to a certain amount of adaptation to this local setting.

Similarly, Dean Fixsen (cofounder of the National Implementation Research Network) and colleagues published a comprehensive synthesis of the implementation literature (Fixsen, Naoom, Blase, Friedman, & Wallace, 2005). In this monograph, several **core implementation components**—that is, the elements that are associated with effective implementation—are identified across a variety of human service fields such as agriculture, business, child welfare, engineering, health, juvenile justice, management, manufacturing, medicine, mental health, nursing, social services, and substance abuse, among others (Fixsen et al., 2005).

Core Implementation Components

Based on the commonalities among successful implementation programs, core implementation components have been identified (Fixsen et al., 2009). The goal of implementation is to have practitioners (e.g., care managers, foster parents, nurses, teachers, therapists, physicians) use innovations effectively. To accomplish this, high-fidelity practitioner behavior is created and supported by core implementation components (also called implementation drivers). As shown in **FIGURE 12-7**, these components are: staff selection, preservice and in-service training, ongoing coaching and consultation, staff evaluation, decision support data systems, facilitative administrative support, and systems interventions.

Due to space limitations, we will not discuss all of these components; rather, we will highlight just a few to illustrate the dominant themes in this chapter. Let's start with recruitment and staff

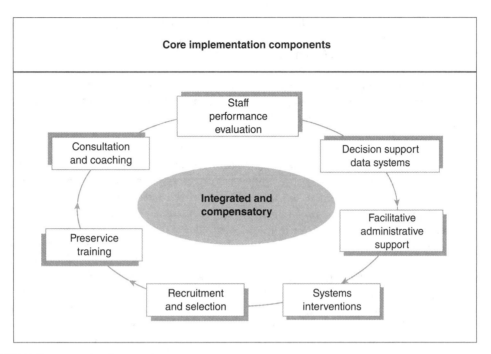

FIGURE 12-7 Fixsen core implementation components

Reproduced from Fixsen, D. L., Blase, K. A., Naoom, S. F., & Wallace, F. (2009). Core implementation components. *Research on Social Work Practice, 19*(5), 531–540.

selection, which addresses who is qualified to carry out the evidence-based practice or program. What are the methods for recruiting and selecting practitioners with those characteristics? Beyond academic qualifications or experience factors, certain practitioner characteristics are difficult to teach in training sessions, so these qualities must be part of the selection criteria (e.g., knowledge of the field, basic professional skills, common sense, sense of social justice, ethics, willingness to learn, willingness to intervene, good judgment, empathy). Some programs are purposefully designed to be very simple in order to minimize the need for careful selection (e.g., a reading tutoring program designed to be staffed by volunteers) (Baker, Gersten, & Keating 2000.) Likewise, preservice and in-service training are commonly used ways to help new program users understand how to effectively deliver this new innovation; they need to learn when, where, how, and with whom to use new approaches and new skills. Interestingly, these common training practices are considered

ineffective implementation strategies when used alone (Azocar, Cuffel, Goldman, & McCarter, 2003; Schectman, Schroth, Verme, & Voss, 2003; Stokes & Baer, 1977).

However, preservice and in-service training are efficient ways to provide knowledge of background information, theory, philosophy, and values; introduce the components and rationales of key practices; and provide opportunities to practice new skills and receive feedback in a safe training environment.

One of the most important components illuminated by Fixsen and colleagues is ongoing coaching and consultation. Most skills needed by successful practitioners can be introduced in training, but in reality are mostly learned on the job with the help of a coach (de Vries & Manfred, 2005; Joyce & Showers, 2002; Schoenwald, Sheidow, & Letourneau, 2004). A coach provides craft information along with advice, encouragement, and opportunities to practice and use skills specific to the innovation (e.g., engagement, program planning). Implementation of human service innovations requires behavior change at the practitioner, supervisory, and administrative support levels. Training and coaching are the principal ways in which behavior change is brought about for carefully selected staff in the beginning stages of implementation and throughout the life of evidence-based practices and programs.

A famous meta-analysis by Joyce and Showers (2002) summarized years of research on the effect of training and coaching of teachers in public schools (see **TABLE 12-2**). They found that training, which consisted of only theory and discussion, resulted in absolutely no transfer to the teacher's behavior in the classroom afterwards. This essentially means that none of the teachers used the new skills they ostensibly received in the training. More substantial gains were made when demonstration, practice, and feedback were added to theory and discussion in the training session, but still very few teachers (5%) used the new information in their own classroom. When on-the-job coaching was added, large gains were seen in knowledge, ability to demonstrate new skills, and actual use of the new skills in the classroom with students (95%). Joyce and Showers also noted that this level of training and coaching can only be accomplished with strong support of the school administration and the teachers themselves (reiterating points that have been made throughout this chapter).

Does Implementation Really Matter?

In Durlak and DuPre's (2008) review of over 500 studies, they found that carefully implemented programs are two to three times more effective than those that had serious implementation errors. Of course, there are lots of "buts" and caveats to this finding. It is important to have a reliable way of assessing implementation. Implementation is usually assessed by some combination of observation (live or recorded), review of records and documentation, and the report of service delivery staff and/or the program participants. Evaluating the quality of program implementation is essential if we want to understand the program outcomes. Let's say you evaluated your favorite school-based youth violence prevention program only to find that rates of fighting and weapon carrying went up in your evaluation schools, not down. The school board may ask whether it was a poorly conceived program that will never work or whether was it a promising program that was poorly implemented. How would you know the difference? If you don't measure implementation carefully, you won't know how to explain your program's failure (and you probably won't impress that school board, either).

On this same note, many programs have multiple components and implementation of some components may be more important than others. These are sometimes referred to as core

| **TABLE 12-2** The Effects of Training and Coaching of Teachers in Public Schools ||||
Component	**Knowledge (%)**	**Skill Demonstration (%)**	**Use in Class (%)**
Theory & discussion	10	5	0
Training demo	30	20	0
Practice & feedback	60	60	5
Coaching in classroom	95	95	95

Joyce, B., & Showers, B. (2002). *Student achievement through staff development* (3rd. ed.). Alexandria, VA: Association for Supervision and Curriculum Development., with permission

components (not to be confused with the "core components to implementation"), but identifying which components should be deemed "core" is a difficult task in and of itself. Furthermore, there may be a threshold effect for implementation. For instance, getting enough dosage is important, but more than enough may not provide any additional value.

When programs are not implemented with fidelity, we should all be concerned that the money invested in developing, testing, and disseminating these programs may be viewed as being wasted. Furthermore, the additional human and financial resources used to deliver the program should probably be redirected elsewhere if implementation failure threatens effective outcomes.

Fidelity and Adaptation

Program fidelity is defined as the degree of correspondence between the program as intended and the program as actually implemented. Of course, the program has already been deemed effective or at least evidence based, and there is no question that quality implementation and fidelity are necessary for optimal outcomes. However, many people, particularly those in community organizations that deliver these programs, argue that "one size does not fit all" and that programs must be adapted to fit local needs, resources, history, demographics, culture, and other contextual variables. In addition, people have a greater commitment to programs they have helped to create (or adapt), and this commitment and ownership may lead to greater enthusiasm in its delivery.

For a long time, adaptation was seen as the opposite of fidelity, if not its enemy. Gradually, both common sense and research have supported the idea that a certain amount and type of adaptation is almost unavoidable, and can be harmless or even improve the effectiveness of a program. What is critical is that adaptation should not include substantial modification or elimination of the core components of a program.

Another key concept in reaching a balance between program fidelity and adaptation is program theory. A program's theory includes the theorized (or proven) linkages (i.e., theoretical mediators) between program activities and their effects on the target population. For example, a dating violence prevention program may be based on the theory that good communication and respect will reduce the risk for violence in a dating relationship. Removing those concepts (promotion of communication skills and respect) from the program would violate its theory, but adapting the program to teach these skills in a more culturally relevant manner could be a beneficial adaptation.

The National Research Council and Institute of Medicine (2009) compared the advantages of implementing an evidence-based program "as is" versus "adapting it" to meet community needs. The "as is" approach led to a higher degree of fidelity and somewhat higher likelihood of achieving the intended impact, whereas "adaptation" was likely to create greater cultural relevance, ownership, and support from the community as well as higher levels of adoption.

Challenges to Implementation

The National Research Council and Institute of Medicine (2009) identified six challenges to appropriate implementation of prevention programs. First, funding for implementation (e.g., labor, materials, and technical assistance) is often higher than many organizations can afford. Cutting costs in these areas may result in ineffective implementation. Second, some of the most common settings for the delivery of prevention programs (e.g., schools and healthcare settings) have primary missions other than prevention. Thus, there may not be sufficient commitment to effective implementation of prevention programs. Third, implementing new programs

These program components can be likened to the "active ingredients" in a medicine—those that are responsible for the program's effects. Of course, we don't always know which components are core, so adaptation should be done with care.

requires training staff and administration in how to implement the program correctly and provide ongoing technical assistance as problems arise. If a program is adopted at many sites, this system of training and assistance must be equally expansive, and it is not common to have such resources available (National Research Council & Institute of Medicine, 2009). Fourth, the kinds of data systems that can help us target and monitor our prevention programs do not currently exist. For example, there is no integrated data system that links health care, education, and mental health services for children, but if these systems shared information more effectively, we could reduce duplication of services, track families across systems, identify children and families who are particularly vulnerable, link family need levels to services, and assess delivery and outcomes for diverse families in particular communities. Fifth, participation in prevention programs is usually voluntary. A well-designed and effective program will have limited impact if the intended target population fails to recognize its value. Even when participation begins at a reasonable level, participants often drop out if they fail to see immediate benefits, which are sometimes less evident when taking a prevention approach. Finally, some organizations are better positioned to implement new prevention programs effectively. By contrast, implementation is threatened when organizations are less flexible, have fewer resources, have fewer community partnerships, and have less experience and comfort with change (National Research Council & Institute of Medicine, 2009).

▶ Take Home Messages

- There is a large gap between public health research and everyday practice, a gap that we can close by drawing from diffusion of innovations and knowledge exchange theories, social marketing, systems thinking, and implementation science.
- Most of our energy, focus, and resources in prevention and public health are focused on developing and evaluating effective programs—dissemination and

implementation do not receive the necessary attention, resources, and research that they deserve.

- Effective prevention includes not only developing effective programs but also focusing on making sure that these programs are feasible and relevant to the practice field, and that potential users know about them.
- Effective prevention includes not only persuading users to adopt new programs, but also providing the resources (e.g., training, coaching, monitoring), and fostering partnerships between researchers and practitioners to ensure effective, sustainable implementation within the complex environments of public-health practice.
- Most evidence-based prevention programs have not been widely implemented.
- Implementation is a complex process requiring extensive attention and resources that are often unavailable.
- Fidelity to the original program model (in terms of core components and program theory) is critical to program effectiveness, but adaptation of other elements may be necessary to fit into a local setting.

▶ References

Aarons, G. A., & Sommerfeld, D. H. (2012). Leadership, innovation climate, and attitudes toward evidence-based practice during a statewide implementation. *Journal of the American Academy of Child & Adolescent Psychiatry, 51*(4), 423–431.

Allen, F. (1994). *Secret formula: How brilliant marketing and relentless salesmanship made Coca-Cola the best-known product in the world.* New York, NY: HarperBusiness.

Azocar, F., Cuffel, B., Goldman, W., & McCarter, L. (2003). The impact of evidence-based guideline dissemination for the assessment and treatment of major depression in a managed behavioral health care organization. *The Journal of Behavioral Health Services and Research, 30*(1), 109–118.

Baker, S., Gersten, R., & Keating, T. (2000). When less may be more: A 2-year longitudinal evaluation of a volunteer tutoring program requiring minimal training. *Reading Research Quarterly, 35*(4), 494–519.

Best, A., Clark, P. I., Leischow, S. J., & Trochim, W. M. (2007, April). *Greater than the sum: Systems thinking in tobacco control.* Tobacco Control Monograph No. 18. Bethesda, MD: U.S. Department of Health and Human Services,

National Institutes of Health, National Cancer Institute. NIH Pub. No. 06-6085.

Bopp, M., Saunders, R. P., & Lattimore, D. (2013, June). The tug-of-war: Fidelity versus adaptation throughout the health promotion program life cycle. *The Journal of Primary Prevention, 34*(3), 193–207.

Brownson, R. C., Colditz, G. A., & Proctor, E.K., (Eds.). (2017, December 8). *Dissemination and implementation research in health: Translating science to practice.* Oxford, UK: Oxford University Press.

Carey, G., Malbon, E., Carey, N., Joyce, A., Crammond, B., & Carey, A. (2015, December 1). Systems science and systems thinking for public health: A systematic review of the field. *BMJ Open, 5*(12), e009002.

Clancy, C. (2006). The $1.6 trillion question: If we're spending so much on healthcare, why so little improvement in quality? *MedGenMed, 8*(2), 58. Retrieved from http://www.ncbi.nlm.nih.gov/pmc/articles/PMC1785188/

Close, J. C. (2005). Prevention of falls—A time to translate evidence into practice. *Age and Ageing, 34*(2), 98–100.

Conklin, A., Hallsworth, M., Hatziandreu, E., & Grant, J. (2008). *Briefing on linkage and exchange: Facilitating diffusion of innovations in health services.* Cambridge, UK: Rand.

Dearing, J. W. (2009). Applying diffusion of innovation theory to intervention development. *Research on Social Work Practice, 19*(5), 503–518.

de Vries, K., & Manfred, F. R. (2005). Leadership group coaching in action: The zen of creating high performance teams. *The Academy of Management Executive (1993–2005), 19*(1), 61–76.

Durlak, J., & DuPre, E. (2008). Implementation matters: A review of research on the influence of implementation on program outcomes and the factors affecting implementation. *American Journal of Community Psychology, 41*(3), 327–350.

Emshoff, J. G. (2008). Researchers, practitioners, and funders: Using the framework to get us on the same page. *American Journal of Community Psychology, 41*(3–4), 393–403.

Fixsen, D. L., Blase, K. A., Naoom, S. F., & Wallace, F. (2009). Core implementation components. *Research on Social Work Practice, 19*(5), 531–540.

Fixsen, D. L., Blase, K. A., Timbers, G. D., & Wolf, M. M. (2001). In search of program implementation: 792 replications of the teaching-family model. In G. A. Bernfeld, D. P. Farrington, & A. W. Leschied (Eds.), *Offender rehabilitation in practice: Implementing and evaluating effective programs* (pp. 149–166). London, England: Wiley.

Fixsen, D. L., Naoom, S. F., Blase, K. A., Friedman, R. M., & Wallace, F. (2005). *Implementation research: A synthesis of the literature* (Vol. FMHI #231). Tampa, FL: University of South Florida, Louis de la Parte Florida Mental Health Institute, The National Implementation Research Network.

Gottfredson, D. C., & Gottfredson, G. D. (2002). Quality of school-based prevention programs: Results from a national survey. *Journal of Research in Crime and Delinquency, 39*(1), 3–35.

Green, L. W. (2008). Making research relevant: If it is an evidence-based practice, where's the practice-based evidence? *Family Practice, 25*(suppl 1), i20–i24.

Hansen, W. B. (2013, June 21). Introduction to the special issue on adaptation and fidelity. *Health Education, 113*(4), 260–263.

Institute of Medicine. (2001). *Crossing the quality chasm: A new health system for the 21st century.* Washington, DC: Author.

Joyce, B., & Showers, B. (2002). *Student achievement through staff development* (3rd. ed.). Alexandria, VA: Association for Supervision and Curriculum Development.

Kennedy, M. G., & Crosby, R. A. (2002). Prevention marketing: An emerging integrated framework. In R. J. DiClemente, R. Crosby, & M. Kegler (Eds.), *Emerging theories in health promotion research and practice: Strategies for enhancing public health* (pp. 255–284). San Francisco, CA: Jossey-Bass.

Klein, K. J., & Sorra, J. S. (1996). The challenge of innovation implementation. *Academy of Management Review, 21*, 1055–1080.

Leischow, S. J., Best, A., Trochim, W. M., Clark, P. I., Gallagher, R. S., Marcus, S. E., & Matthews, E. (2008, August 31). Systems thinking to improve the public's health. *American Journal of Preventive Medicine, 35*(2), S196–203.

Leschied, A. W., & Cunningham, A. (2002). *Seeking effective interventions for serious young offenders: Interim results of a four-year randomized study of multisystemic therapy in Ontario, Canada.* London, England: Centre for Children and Families in the Justice System.

Lize, S. E., Andrews, A. B., Whitaker, P., Shapiro, C., & Nelson, N. (2014). Exploring adaptation and fidelity in parenting program implementation: Implications for practice with families. *Journal of Family Strengths, 14*(1), 8.

Luke, D. A., & Stamatakis, K. A. (2012, April 21). Systems science methods in public health: Dynamics, networks, and agents. *Annual Review of Public Health, 33*: 357–376.

National Research Council & Institute of Medicine. (2009). *Preventing mental, emotional and behavioral disorders among young people: Progress and possibilities.* Washington, DC: The National Academies Press.

Noonan, R. (2010). *Translating "translation:" What do we know? What can we do better?* Paper presented at the expert panel meeting: Prevention of falls among older adults, Atlanta, GA.

Peters, D. H. (2014). The application of systems thinking in health: Why use systems thinking? *Health Research Policy and Systems, 12*(1), 1.

Puddy, R., Wilkins, N. J., Thigpen, S., Singer, H., & Donovan, J. (2017). Expanding the definition for evidence in child maltreatment prevention. In S. Alexander, R. Alexander, & N. Guterman (Eds.), *Prevention of child maltreatment.* St. Louis, MO: G.W. Medical Publishing.

Rogers, E. M. (1962). *Diffusion of innovation.* London, England: The Free Press.

Schectman, J. M., Schroth, W. S., Verme, D., & Voss, J. D. (2003). Randomized controlled trial of education and feedback for implementation of guidelines for acute low back pain. *Journal of General Internal Medicine, 18*(10), 773–780.

Schoenwald, S. K., Sheidow, A. J., & Letourneau, E. J. (2004). Toward effective quality assurance in evidence-based practice: Links between expert consultation, therapist fidelity, and child outcomes. *Journal of Clinical Child Adolescent Psychology, 33*(1), 94–104.

Senge, P. M. (1990). *The fifth discipline: The art and practice of the learning organization.* New York, NY: Doubleday.

Sorian, R., & Baugh, T. (2002). Power of information: Closing the gap between research and policy. *Health Affairs, 21*(2), 264–273.

Soumerai, S. B., & Avorn, J. (1990). Principles of educational outreach ('academic detailing') to improve clinical decision making. *Journal of the American Medical Association, 263*(4), 549–556.

Stokes, T. F., & Baer, D. M. (1977). An implicit technology of generalization. *Journal of Applied Behavior Analysis, 10,* 349–367.

Vakola, M. (2013, March 1). Multilevel readiness to organizational change: A conceptual approach. *Journal of Change Management, 13*(1): 96–109.

Wandersman, A., Duffy, J., Flaspohler, P., Noonan, R., Lubell, K., Stillman, L., & Saul, J. (2008). Bridging the gap between prevention research and practice: The interactive systems framework for dissemination and implementation. *American Journal of Community Psychology, 41*(3), 171–181.

Warhop, B. (2006). Atlanta Magazine.

Washington State Institute for Public Policy. (2005). *Washington state's implementation of functional family therapy for juvenile offenders: Preliminary findings (Vol. No. 02-08-1201).* Olympia, WA: Washington State Institute for Public Policy.

Weinrich, N. K. (1999). *Hands-on social marketing: A step-by-step guide.* Thousand Oaks, CA: Sage.

Weisz, J. R., Ng, M. Y., & Bearman, S. K. (2014). Odd couple? Reenvisioning the relation between science and practice in the dissemination-implementation era. *Clinical Psychological Science, 2,* 58–74.

Wilkins, N. J., Myers, L., Kuehl, T., Bauman, A., & Hertz, M. (2017). Connecting the Dots: State health department approaches to addressing shared risk and protective factors across multiple forms of violence. *Journal of Public Health Management and Practice, 24,* S32–S41.

Wiseman, S. H., Chinman, M., Ebener, P. A., Hunter, S. B., Imm, P., & Wandersman, A. (2007). *Getting to outcomes: 10 steps for achieving results-based accountability.* Santa Monica, CA: RAND Corporation.

Section Opener: © lzf/Shutterstock; © Henrik Sorensen/Getty Images; © MeskPhotography/Shutterstock; © Hero Images/Getty Images
Chapter Opener: © Hero Images/Getty Images; © lzf/Shutterstock; © Henrik Sorensen/Getty Images; © MeskPhotography/Shutterstock

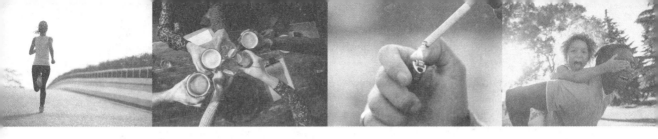

CHAPTER 13

Learning to Combine Theories: An Introduction to Intervention Mapping

Richard A. Crosby, Ralph J. DiClemente, and Laura F. Salazar

Perfection is achieved, not only when there is nothing more to add, but when there is nothing left to take away.

—**Antonie de Saint Exupery**

▶ Introduction

Throughout the preceding chapters of this book it appears that theories are commonly used in isolation rather than in a complementary fashion. Although this theoretical orthodoxy is far from ideal, an unfortunate number of researchers and practitioners limit themselves to this paradigm. As you will recall from reading Chapter 3 (the PRECEDE–PROCEED model of health-promotion planning), theory is best conceived as a critical yet subservient aspect of program planning and implementation. Theory is critical because it serves as a lynchpin, first identifying personal and/or external determinants, then informing intervention activities and guiding implementation.

Program planning, in essence, can be viewed as a large tapestry where theory and its associated constructs are main threads. Another main thread would be the empirically derived determinants and methods. Intervention Mapping provides guidance for creating this tapestry and binds the identified theoretical and empirical determinants of behavior change with a practical approach (e.g., empirically derived practice) to fostering conditions that produce enduring change. This change is achieved by using theory and previous research to identify and alter determinants that foster long-term adoption of health-protective behaviors.

A useful framework for understanding the entire process of program planning, including the use of multiple theories combined synergistically, is known as Intervention Mapping (Batholomew et al., 2016). Intervention mapping is a framework to guide assessment, program planning, implementation, and evaluation. These four terms are frequently referred to in health-promotion practice as being the backbone of prevention science. A popular six-step planning model called Intervention Mapping is a useful framework, presented in **FIGURE 13-1**, that incorporates these four terms: Assessment is part of Step 1, planning is a part of steps 2–4, implementation is Step 5, and evaluation is Step 6. This seemingly linear framework may be more iterative in actual practice in that some steps may be revisited several times throughout the process. Theory can be used during each step illustrating its place within intervention mapping.

Thus, throughout this chapter we will refer to various principles and techniques used in Intervention Mapping. More importantly, however, we will emphasize the value, and associated precautions, of strategically combining theories, theoretical constructs, and evidence-based practices.

LEARNING OBJECTIVES

1. Identify and describe the six steps of the Intervention Mapping process.
2. Identify the requirements and conditions of combining theories to achieve a more ecological approach to health-promotion practice.
3. Describe the process of prioritizing determinants, selected from across all levels of ecological influence, for intervention mapping.
4. Distinguish between methods and strategies, as applied to program planning.
5. Identify common theoretical constructs that can be used in isolation from theory.

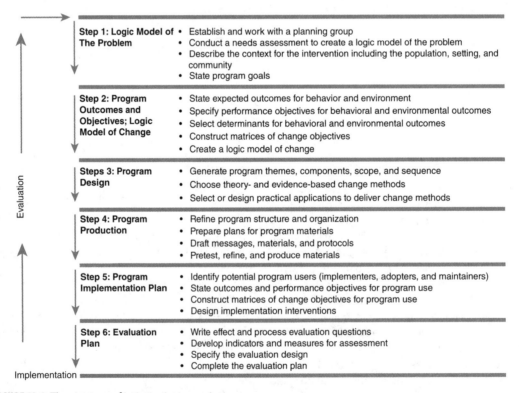

FIGURE 13-1 The six steps of intervention mapping

Reproduced from Kok G. A practical guide to effective behavior change: how to apply theory- and evidence-based behavior change methods in an intervention. The European Health Psychologist 2014;16:156-183.

▸ Understanding the Intervention Mapping Framework

Intervention Mapping (IM) is a complete process—one that begins with a **contextual analysis** of the health problem at-hand and concludes with evaluation. IM involves six steps; however, its primary and unique contribution to program planning lies within the "heart" of the model. At its heart, the IM specifies that change can and should occur at two or more of four levels: (1) interpersonal, (2) organizational, (3) community, and (4) policy. Within each level, the IM encourages theory selection, thereby creating an inherent and determinant-driven combination of multiple theories. For instance, if the overall health issue is obesity in a community, identified determinants of a reduced caloric intake might be self-efficacy to prepare good-tasting low-calorie foods (individual-level), social and cultural norms relative to food (family- and community-levels), and availability, acceptability, accessibility, and affordability of fresh vegetables (community and organizational levels). Each identified determinant is then linked to one or more program objectives targeted to each of the stated levels. Changing social norms, for example, may be linked to several program objectives at multiple levels, such as avoiding the consumption of high-fat and high-caloric foods among individuals, families and their friends, and among the community.

In addition to the four levels (i.e., interpersonal, organizational, community, and policy) IM guides program planning through the previously mentioned six steps. Each step is vital and thus warrants further elaboration. Because a primary goal of this chapter is to provide you with the information needed to effectively combine theories to enhance program effects, much of this chapter will focus on Step 3 of the model (as this is the step where theory selection occurs).

Step 1: Assessment of the Problem

Understanding how people interact with their immediate and distal environments is a necessary starting point for planning directed by the IM. Thus, the initial step of IM involves formally making assessments of the problem within the context of the interpersonal, organizational, community, and policy environments. The best way to do this is by creating a logic model of the problem itself (note: this is very different than a logic model of how the problem will be addressed though intervention). To enhance the accuracy of this logic model, we suggest that you form and convene a local advisory group, that is, people within the target population who are fluent in the problem, its causes, and its possible solutions. A logic model of the problem will identify likely antecedents of the risk and protective behaviors that apply to the condition, disease, or outcome being addressed. **FIGURE 13-2** displays an example of such a logic model.

Step 2: Prioritizing Determinants for Intervention Mapping

You will recall from Chapters 2 and 11 that the concept of an ecological approach to health promotion involves intervention at multiple levels of influence on any one given health behavior, with levels of influence including the individual, family, relational, community/peers, and societal structures. We suggest that any challenging health behavior problem must be addressed using an ecological approach. Indeed, completing the first step will produce a profile of determinants that resemble a socio-ecological–based description of the problem. Once the profile of determinants has been completed, in Step 2, you will create matrices that link these different levels of determinants to corresponding program objectives. Then, each matrix will be ranked in terms of changeability and level of impact.

We wish to emphasize the importance of carefully constructing a matrix of changeability and impact, as doing so optimizes your efforts and prevents you from potentially pursuing goals with

Determinants   **Intervention points**

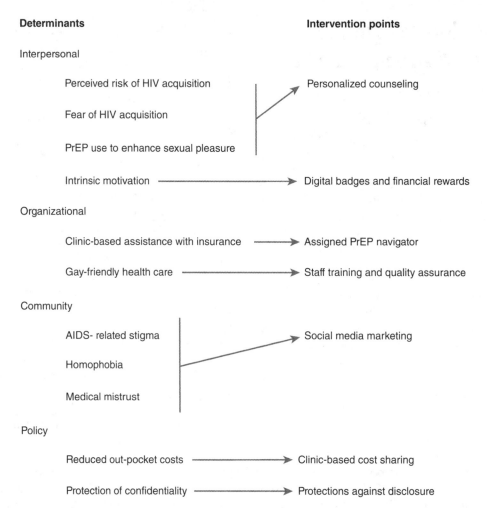

Interpersonal

    Perceived risk of HIV acquisition   Personalized counseling

    Fear of HIV acquisition

    PrEP use to enhance sexual pleasure

    Intrinsic motivation   Digital badges and financial rewards

Organizational

    Clinic-based assistance with insurance   Assigned PrEP navigator

    Gay-friendly health care   Staff training and quality assurance

Community

    AIDS- related stigma   Social media marketing

    Homophobia

    Medical mistrust

Policy

    Reduced out-pocket costs   Clinic-based cost sharing

    Protection of confidentiality   Protections against disclosure

FIGURE 13-2 Logic model of adherence to pre-exposure prophylaxis among young black males having sex with males

little chance of success. Consider, for instance, the health behavior of daily sweetened beverage consumption (an identified leading cause in the United States of obesity and diabetes). **FIGURE 13-3** displays a hypothetical profile of how this behavior might appear when sorted into four levels of influence.

As shown in Figure 13-3, the assessment indicated that only about 10% of the total cause for the daily consumption of sweetened beverage is attributed to individual-level determinants. Thus, an immediate implication for program planning is that theoretical constructs emphasizing the individual-level (e.g., perceived threat from health

belief model, decisional-balance from trans-theoretical model, or behavioral skills from the information–motivation–behavioral skills model) are unlikely to be as effective as other theoretical constructs from higher level theories given the obtained profile of influences. It is clear from the profile that societal influences are the lion's share of the cause; thus, theoretical constructs such as "availability/accessibility" from Cohen's structural model of health behavior (see Chapter 11), can more effectively affect change in the societal-level determinants. For example, the first U.S. city to pass a sugar-sweetened beverage tax (Berkeley, CA), directly affected the availability/accessibility

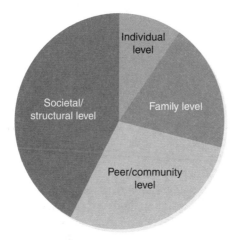

FIGURE 13-3 Hypothetical distribution of determinants to sweetened beverage consumption

scale through this form of intervention at the societal level (Falbe et al., 2016). The challenge in this example is that enacting policy change requires the use of additional strategies such as advocacy to gain the political support and commitment needed to effectively leverage change such as a new tax. **BOX 13-1** provides a description of the hard-fought success in passing a sweetened beverage tax in Philadelphia, PA. As described in Box 13-1, political "give and take" is required to make this level of intervention a public health reality.

The hypothetical distribution of determinants shown in Figure 13-3 suggests that about 50% of the daily sweetened beverage consumption can be attributed to a combination of family and community factors. As can easily be envisioned then, theories such as Diffusion of Innovations or approaches such as Social Marketing could potentially be used to promote the daily consumption of replacement beverages such as vitamin water or other healthy water-based choices. As indicated, this planning step requires that the "changeability-impact" matrix be used as a guide for prioritizing the determinants that will become the objectives of the public health program. Once these priorities have been set, the process

of the product by increasing its price. The concept of price elasticity is key here and suggests that people will buy less of a product as the price goes up. Evidence from research on the Berkeley, CA tax found a 21% decrease in the consumption of sugar-sweetened beverages in Berkeley, compared to a 4% increase in a comparison city and strongly supports behavior change can occur on a massive

---

BOX 13-1 Sweetened Beverage Tax as a Public Health Intervention

In June of 2016, the city of Philadelphia, PA passed a tax of 1.5 cents per ounce on all sugar-sweetened or artificially sweetened soft drinks sold within the municipality. Philadelphia was the only second large U.S. municipality to win this victory for public health (with Berkeley, CA being the first in 2014). Ironically, political and public support for this law was garnered by the expressed intent to burden the well-off sweetened beverage industry in favor of creating revenue earmarked for popular government-sponsored programs such as prekindergarten. In cities that tried but failed to pass this type of legislation, a more health-focused approach had been used (perhaps leading people to conclude that the government was playing too large of a role in their health-related decisions). Opposition to the tax was led by the soft drink industry and their teamsters union, spending approximately $5,000,000 in efforts to persuade a "no" vote from Philadelphia residents. The Health Commissioner for Philadelphia plans to evaluate the immediate effect of the tax on sales of sweetened beverage and the long-term effects on obesity.

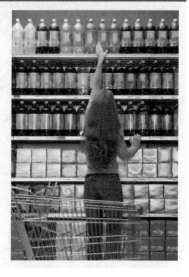

Data from Philadelphia finds winning strategy for soda tax, and other cities notice. New York Times, June 17th, 2016. Page A21. Photo credit: © FangXiaNuo/Getty Images

of selecting theories, theoretical constructs, and empirically derived practices can be conducted that will inform the methods and strategies of the program. The goal of this process is to build an effective and comprehensive program that is constructed from the blueprint of the assessment and planning process. It is at this juncture that you will develop the logic model that will ultimately guide the entire process of program implementation and evaluation. **FIGURE 13-4** provides an example of a comprehensive logic model applied to the task of integrating mental health services into chronic disease prevention. As shown, the flow begins with program inputs and then proceeds to program activities. The program activities, in turn, lead to short-term (sometimes called immediate), mid-term, and long-term outcomes.

Step 3: Program Design

Once the determinants are identified and linked to program activities and outcome objectives, the next step is to use theory and empirically derived practices to assist in the selection of **methods** and **strategies** that will become the program. A method is the program activity that will be used to leverage change in a given identified determinant. Method selection is perhaps the most vital step in the entire IM process,

> An eloquent property of IM in that empirically derived practices are valued equally along with theory-derived selection of methods.

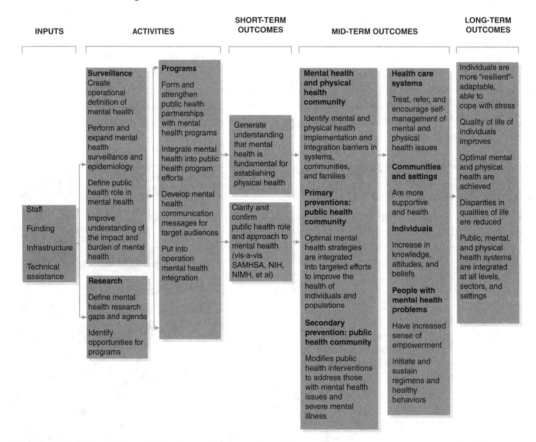

FIGURE 13-4 Draft of a logic model for integrating mental health into chronic disease prevention and health promotion

Reproduced from Centers for Disease Control: Preventing Chronic Disease. A Logic Model for the Integration of Mental Health Into Chronic Disease Prevention and Health Promotion
James Lando, MD, MPH, corresponding author Sheree Marshall Williams, PhD, MSc, Stephanie Sturgis, and Branalyn Williams, MPH. Prev Chronic Dis. 2006 Apr; 3(2): A61

as it culminates in the development of the intervention plans and thus the program as it is delivered to a community or population. Methods commonly used in IM (Kok, 2014) include modeling (from social cognitive theory), acting as a facilitating agent (a construct from Diffusion of Innovations theory), consciousness raising (from the Transtheoretical model), cue altering (from social cognitive theory), planning coping resources (an aspect of a theory known as *conversation of resources*), participatory problem solving (from a framework known as *community capacity*), and organization diagnosis and feedback (from theories of mobilizing organization change, described by Butterfoss, Kegler, & Francisco, 2008). To conveniently orchestrate the entire process of method selection, the IM divides these methods into the previously listed four categories (i.e., interpersonal, organizational, community, and policy).

BOX 13-2 provides an example of a multi-level intervention program that was developed using IM. As you can see in this example, taking place in the Netherlands, the planning process identified ten methods of leveraging change pertaining to four program objectives. Examination of these 10 selected methods is instructive as it can be readily seen that many are derived from theories you may

have already learned about in this textbook; however, it is also the case that some of these selected methods stem from empirically derived practice rather than theory per se. This is an eloquent property of IM in that empirically derived practices are valued equally along with theory-derived selection of methods.

Another aspect of step three involves using selected methods of change in the context of various **applications**. As you may have garnered from reading Box 13-2, a method is a theory-based (or empirically derived) way of altering a determinant of health behavior. The next step after methods selection is the selection of the application procedure, thus allowing the method to be translated into a program-based action. This process is known as the intervention strategy. For instance, using social reinforcement is a method for increasing adherence to a daily exercise routine. But, how do we use it in this context? It is at this juncture in program planning that theory per se leaves off and the wisdom of the planning group begins. (The challenge is to select strategies that optimize the value of the method.) Consider, for example, the following possibilities relative to enhancing exercise adherence:

BOX 13-2 Multi-Level Intervention Program That Was Developed Using IM

In response to the obesity epidemic occurring among teenagers in the Netherlands, Dutch program planners diligently followed the principles of IM to develop a multi-level, school-based program designed specifically to address four key objectives:

- Reduced time spent viewing television and using computers
- Reduced intake of sugar-sweetened beverages
- Reduced intake of snack foods
- Increased engagement in vigorous physical activity

Drawing on multiple theories and empirically derived practices, the planners identified nine selected methods of change: (1) passive learning, (2) active processing of information, self-monitoring, and feedback, (3) guided practice, (4) social modeling, (5) breaking automatic stimulus-response relationships, (6) goal setting, (7) reinforcement, (8) association of attitude objects with positive stimuli, and (9) environmental changes. The long-term effects of the program included a reduction in adipose tissue (as measured by skin-fold thickness) in females and a reduction on the consumption of sugar-sweetened beverages in both females and males.

Data from Singh, A. S., Chin, A., Paw, M. J. M., Kremers, S. P. J., Visscher, T. L. S., Brug, J., & van Mechelen, W. (2006). Design of the Dutch Obesity Intervention in Teenagers: A systematic development, implementation, and evaluation of a school-based intervention aimed at the prevention of excessive weight gain in adolescents. *BMC Public Health, 6*, 340. DOI: 10.1186/1471-2458-6-304; Singh, A. S., Chin, A., Paw, M. J. M., Kremers, S. P. J., Visscher, T. L. S., Brug, J., & van Mechelen, W. (2009). Dutch Obesity Intervention in Teenagers: Effectiveness of a school-based program on body composition and behavior. *Archives of Pediatrics and Adolescent Medicine, 163*, 309–317.

- Social reinforcement can be vicariously experienced through the use of video presentations touting the social benefits of daily exercise.
- Organized athletic events (for runners, bicyclists, swimmers, etc.) can become a focal point for the social rewards of being in-shape and thus able to compete—all participants should be provided with a shared token of this social recognition (e.g., race t-shirts)
- Small "work-out clubs" (sponsored by the program) can become miniature support groups to provide members with a sense of social belonging and praise for their daily adherence to established routines.
- Exercise "milestones" such as running a full marathon, cycling 100 miles in a single day, or swimming the width/length of a local lake can be socially recognized achievements that are publicized in local media and in social media.

As you can easily envision just from considering these four possibilities, the number of strategy options for any one method is almost infinite. From a practical standpoint, you can rely on a combination of past empirically derived practices, constraints related to budget and resources, and input from other stakeholders such as a community advisory group assisting with intervention development. **BOX 13-3** provides an example of a multi-level, and multi-theory, intervention program that was designed in conjunction with a planning model and with a community advisory group. Although "methods" were not specified using the IM terminology, the program was highly focused on the methods of raising awareness and providing information. The applications spanned an impressive array of options ranging from events held at churches to individual-based counseling conducted in women's homes. Because healthcare providers were also a target of the intervention, the methods and applications relevant to this aspect of the program are also described in the article cited in Box 13-3.

A key aspect of Step 3 is the careful and parsimonious use of theory to achieve the desired changes in the identified antecedents. This step requires that you have a command of the available theories that are available, and it requires caution in the process of combining these theories.

Requirements and Conditions for Combining Theory

Without question, changing health behaviors for protracted periods of time, across entire populations, is a daunting task—one that frequently fails despite the best-laid plans. Similar to being on a long journey in unknown lands, the public health profession needs a guide for the pending journey to success. The ultimate "guide" in this case is not

---

BOX 13-3 An Example of Using the Six Steps of Intervention Mapping

In response to elevated rates of smoking, sedentary living, and intake of fatty foods among persons living with HIV (PLHIV), a web-based intervention program was designed for this population, using the IM framework (Cote et al., 2017). The planning group followed each of the six IM steps to create an effective approach to this problem. Their first step was to conduct an extensive literature review on the problem and its determinants. One outgrowth of this review was selecting the theory of planned behavior as a lens for conceptualizing the problem and the possible solutions. Next, the planning group identified and prioritized program outcomes in the context of a matrix of change (see Figure 13.2). In the third step, the program planning group selected tailoring, modeling, and feedback reinforcement as their primary strategies. Additionally, they identified behavioral belief selection and persuasive communication as strategies to change attitudes. Strategies for enhancing perceived behavioral control (a construct from the theory of planned behavior) were also selected. In Step 4, the program was constructed to consist of three 50-minute components. In turn, each component comprised seven interactive web-based sessions, lasting 5–10 minutes each. Program implementation (Step 5) occurred in the context of a randomized, controlled trial.

Cote et al., 2017

a person, but a logic model. Indeed, a centerpiece of IM is a carefully developed and thorough logic model. Figure 13.2 provides an example of a logic model that was used to prevent mental illness (primarily depression) at the community level. As with most logic models, your desired endpoint or program objective is the fulcrum for planning. Planning, in turn, begins with two most vital steps: (1) program inputs and (2) program activities. Inputs refer to resources, materials, and staff needs, whereas activities refer to tangible events such as meetings, trainings, and ultimately intervention methods and monitoring for fidelity. A different type of monitoring then occurs that records short-term, intermediate, and long-term outcomes of the activities.

A primary requirement for combining theories is that the program logic model can be traced to show how each theory selected maps onto the various activities shown. For instance, an activity shown in Figure 13.4 is to "develop mental health communication messages." For this action, the Elaboration Likelihood Model (see Chapter 8) might be an excellent theory for achieving this objective. Adding complementary theories to the logic model is desirable if they are relevant to the program activities and serve the objectives that are required to achieve the endpoint. For instance, another activity displayed in the logic model shown in Figure 13.4 involves strengthening public health partnerships. In this case, using a theory that promotes coalition building (e.g., Butterfoss & Kegler, 2009) and maintenance among health agencies may be useful.

A second requirement for combining theories is that they align with the IM process. Alignment implies that the theories are relevant to the intervention activities and their corresponding objectives as shown in the logic model developed to guide behavior change. Although alignment seems somewhat obvious, it is important because a tendency exists for researchers to employ only the most established theories in health behavior rather than the full range of possibilities (Painter, Borba, Hynes, Mays, & Glanz, 2008). Thus, the consummate public health professionals strive to expand their range of theoretical approaches to a stated health problem. An Intervention Mapping approach begins with the problem then defines questions related to that problem and

finally selects the most appropriate theories to answer these questions. An example involves the prevention of opioid abuse, an emerging public health priority. To address this issue the

> *A second requirement for combining theories is that they align with the IM process.*

research questions would be centered on the social determinants (e.g., prescribing practices of physicians) and how can these be changed. Thus, a theory such as the Structural Model of Behavior (see Chapter 11) may be applied to identify the most relevant determinants whereas social cognitive theory (see Chapter 7) could be applied to enhance knowledge among physicians regarding opioid abuse and encourage more stringent prescribing practices. Additionally, physicians can provide information to patients about the potential for opioid dependency.

A third requirement involves the accurate interpretation and application of theory. Theory is frequently misapplied and thus misused (Crosby and Noar, 2010). Using theories correctly is vital for two reasons: (1) the theoretical constructs can only be helpful if the full meaning of these constructs is translated into actionable program components, and (2) when combining theories the addition of a second, third, or even fourth theory may unknowingly (based on incorrect application or interpretation of the theory) be redundant with a previously selected theory.

In addition to these aforementioned requirements, several conditions should always be met when combining theories. First, the health behavior(s) being targeted by the intervention must be sufficiently complex to warrant the decision to combine theories. A second condition is that no single theory adequately addresses the problem nor provides a suitable solution. Pulling constructs from multiple theories to inform intervention strategies may be labor intensive from a planning perspective; thus, we caution you to be strategic and include the most relevant constructs that are likely to affect program objectives or facilitate meeting the goals of the public health program.

Theoretical Constructs Used Separately from Theory

Earlier in this textbook (Chapter 2, Table 2.2) you learned that several elements (i.e., theoretical constructs) are essentially used in multiple theories. Indeed, a common practice in health promotion has been to adopt one or two constructs from a theory and then predicate intervention planning on hypothesized mediators of change stemming from these constructs. Although scholars working in academia who specialize in behavioral and social sciences theory may vigorously object, we suggest that the primary goal is always "what works for health promotion" rather than what works to protect the field of theory. In fact, the "what works" approach that we advocate here is also quite capable of adding to the field of theory if a paradigm of fluidity is adopted. Theories should indeed be fluid when evaluated over time—this is the essence of true scholarship and program evaluation. When deviations from commonly accepted application of theory occur, and the results are positive for the health-promotion program, the field does indeed move forward. In the spirit of this fluidity, we suggest here that you become familiar with key theoretical constructs as they appear at all levels of an ecological approach. **TABLE 13-1** provides an illustration of the point that key theoretical constructs exist across the span of ecological influences. This is shown by our selection of five constructs for each of four selected levels of influence. The listing of key theoretical constructs is thus arranged by level of influence within an ecological model.

As shown in Table 13-1 it is clear that selecting a host of constructs across all level of influence is indeed possible. Again, this approach would "defy" theory and thus it is similar to a performer walking a high-wire without a safety net underneath. The figurative safety net, however, is Intervention Mapping.

IM asserts that each and every applicable level of an ecological model must be addressed to achieve optimal program effectiveness. The selection of constructs (from a listing such as that shown in Table 13-1) across these levels should be *a priori* for the planning group—a group comprising persons within the community for which the intervention program is intended for implementation.

We suggest that this process be considered as a logical conclusion to an extensive community needs assessment (CNA). Indeed, Step 1 of the IM process, conducting a thorough CAN, is vital to program success. **TABLE 13-2** displays key principles of conducting a community needs assessment. By selecting the methods of change based on the guidance offered by the selected constructs, an intervention can be tailored for a specific health behavior implemented with a pre-determined population.

The principles displayed in Table 13-2 are, in many ways, the essence of public health practiced at the community level. Thus, program planning and community engagement are linked. As you will recall from reading the chapter on the PRECED–PROCEED model (Chapter 3), the great advantage of conducting a community needs assessment, in the context of an engaged community, involves sustainability and ease of translation from planning to practice. Thinking back to Box 13-3 in this chapter, it is well worth noting that the project described was one based on substantial levels of community engagement and thus a highly detailed CNA.

> *Conducting a thorough CAN, is vital to program success.*

Step 4: Program Construction

Having completed the planning process, your next step is to construct the intervention program from start to finish. This is somewhat anti-climactic in comparison to the work required in Step 3, but equally important. Methods and strategies must be clearly articulated, with ample detail so as to ensure a high degree of program fidelity. Fidelity (defined as the degree to which a program is implemented as planned) is a primary concern in planning public health programs; thus, it is imperative at this stage in your work to lay a strong foundation for achieving consistently high levels of fidelity.

Step 5: Program Implementation

Perhaps the most vital aspect of program implementation is training those people who will conduct the various facets of the planned interventions. This

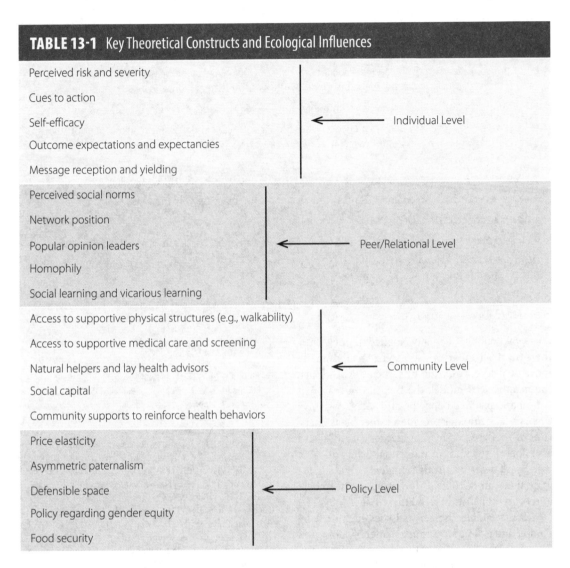

TABLE 13-1 Key Theoretical Constructs and Ecological Influences

Perceived risk and severity	
Cues to action	
Self-efficacy	← Individual Level
Outcome expectations and expectancies	
Message reception and yielding	
Perceived social norms	
Network position	
Popular opinion leaders	← Peer/Relational Level
Homophily	
Social learning and vicarious learning	
Access to supportive physical structures (e.g., walkability)	
Access to supportive medical care and screening	
Natural helpers and lay health advisors	← Community Level
Social capital	
Community supports to reinforce health behaviors	
Price elasticity	
Asymmetric paternalism	
Defensible space	← Policy Level
Policy regarding gender equity	
Food security	

training should be viewed as an investment in the ultimate success of the program. Training, however, is not a one-time investment; instead, it requires follow-up monitoring of performance with corrective feedback being provided on a systematic basis. This ongoing monitoring crates a quality assurance process and serves as a form of process evaluation.

Step 6: Program Evaluation

This final step of IM is one that you will learn about in great detail in Chapter 14. For now, the main take-home message is that carefully conducted evaluation will provide a "diagnosis" of your overall assessment, planning, and implementation process. The logic model of change (from Step 3) will serve as the ultimate guide to the entire evaluation.

▶ Take Home Messages

A review study published by Painter and colleagues (Painter et al., 2008) is instructive as to the state of theory and how it must change to better serve health-promotion practice. The authors obtained and reviewed 193 journal articles reporting investigations or interventions of health behavior. Of the 193, only 69 used at least one theory. Of

TABLE 13-2 Suggested Principles of a Community Needs Assessment
■ Form multi-sectorial collaborations that support shared ownership of all phases of community health improvement, including assessment, planning, investment, implementation, and evaluation
■ Ensure proactive, broad, and diverse community engagement to improve results
■ Use a definition of community that encompasses both a significant enough area to allow for population-wide interventions and measurable results, and includes a targeted focus to address disparities among subpopulations
■ Strive for maximum transparency to improve community engagement and accountability
■ Use evidence-based interventions and encourage innovative practices with thorough evaluation
■ Conduct ongoing evaluation to inform a continuous improvement process
■ Use only the highest quality data pooled from, and shared among, diverse public and private sources
Centers for Disease Control and Prevention and Rosenbaum S. Principles to Consider for the Implementation of a Community Health Needs Assessment Process

Data from Centers for Disease Control and Prevention and Rosenbaum S. Principles to Consider for the Implementation of a Community Health Needs Assessment Process. The George Washington School of Public Health.

these 69, only 15 actually applied theory. Further, most all theories used were located at the individual-level (e.g., the transtheoretical model, the health belief model, the theories of reasoned action and planned behavior, and social cognitive theory). The findings provide a rather bleak snapshot of "being stuck in an a theoretical rut"—and also "being stuck in an individual-level rut." The principles described in this chapter provide guidance that can help health-promotion researchers and practitioners transcend these issues.

Transcending these two issues identified by Painter and colleagues is thus a matter of adopting a different overall method of theory application—one that perhaps relies on the wise, CNA-directed selection of constructs and the use of principles such as those associated with the practice of IM. Perhaps even more critical to success in the future of health promotion, program planning must be guided by a framework that clearly prescribes the use of theories and/or theoretical constructs that span the full range of an ecological model. The field of public health can clearly benefit from theory; however, this benefit will only materialize if theory is viewed as ever-changing and thus evolving to meet the needs of various intervention challenges, across diverse cultures and within the socio-political context of nations throughout the world.

▶ References

Batholomew Eldridge, L. K., Markham, C. M., Ruiter, R. A. C., Fernandez, M. E., Kok, G., & Parcel, G. S. (2016). *Planning health promotion programs: An intervention mapping approach*. San Francisco, CA: Jossey-Bass.

Butterfoss, F. D., Kegler, M. C., & Francisco, V. T. (2008). Mobilizing organizational for health promotion: Theories of organizational change. In K. Glanz, B. K. Rimer, & K. Viswanath. (Eds.), *Health behavior and health education: Theory, research, and practice*. San Francisco, CA: Jossey-Bass Wiley.

Cote, J., Rouleau, G., Thouvenut, V. I., Boucoiran, I., & Pokmandy, A. (2017). From VIH-TAVIE™ to TAVIE-WOMAN™: Development of a web-based virtual nursing intervention to meet the specific needs of women living with HIV. *Journal of the Internatioal Society for Telemedicine and eHealth, 5*, e3.

Crosby, R. A., & Noar, S. M. (2010). Theory development in health promotion: Are we there yet? *Journal of Behavioral Medicine, 33*, 259–263.

Falbe, J., Thompson, H. R., Becker, C. M., Rojas, N., McCulloch, C. E., & Madsen, K. A. (2016). Impact of the Berkley excise Tax on sugar-sweetened beverages. *American Journal Public Health, 106*, 1865–1871.

Kok, G. (2014). A practical guide to effective behavior change: how to apply theory- and evidence-based behavior change methods in an intervention. *The European Health Psychologist, 16*, 156–183.

Painter, J. E., Borba, C. P. C., Hynes, M., Mays, D., & Glanz, K. (2008). The use of theory in health behavior research from 2000 to 2005: A systematic review. *Annals of Behavioral Medicine, 35*, 358–362.

Chapter Opener: © lzf/Shutterstock; © Henrik Sorensen/Getty Images; © MeskPhotography/Shutterstock; © Hero Images/Getty Images

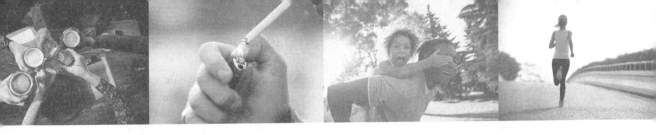

CHAPTER 14

Measurement and Design Related to Theoretically Based Health Promotion, Research, and Practice

Laura F. Salazar, Ralph J. DiClemente, and Richard A. Crosby

There is a measure in all things.

—**Horace**, *Satires*

PREVIEW

Theories are useful in that they advance our understanding of the specific individual and environmental factors that greatly influence various health behaviors. But, theories must be applied. Application of theory greatly depends on having sound measurement instruments for the theoretical constructs and factors.

OBJECTIVES

1. Have an overview of the history of measurement for intangibles.
2. Understand the importance of measurement to the field of health promotion.
3. Define measurement as used in health-promotion research and practice.
4. Describe the different types of measurement tools used in theory testing and application.
5. Compare and contrast scales and indexes.
6. List the standards used to gauge whether measures are reliable and valid.
7. Describe the appropriate research designs and statistical methods for theory testing.

▶ Introduction

A scientific discipline or field will advance when research provides new evidence that either supports newly conceived ideas or disconfirms previously held views. General relativity and quantum mechanics are but two examples from the field of physics that propelled the discipline light years forward in terms of understanding the universe on both the largest and the smallest of scales. However, the theories of relativity and quantum mechanics could only be widely accepted within the field given the existence of accompanying scientific evidence, which, when these ideas were first conceptualized and introduced, was somewhat problematic, as sophisticated measurement tools were not available to test these theories.

Over the years, however, physicists were able to conduct studies and make observations that allowed them to test predictions based on these ideas. Eventually, support for relativity and quantum mechanics was provided. In fact, physicists were hugely successful in confirming with remarkable accuracy all possible predictions. Thus, we now accept these ideas as foundational theories of modern physics. Yet if physicists had been unable to make scientific observations using accurate and precise instruments to measure such phenomena as radar reflections from planets, radial velocity, or the quark-gluon sea, then these theories could have remained ideas or hypotheses at best or, at worst, they might have been sucked into the proverbial black hole.

Of course, the main thrusts that propelled the field forward were the development of good theory and the invention of powerful new technology. Physicists and other scientists developed more sophisticated devices and techniques that in turn allowed for the accurate and precise measurement of the phenomena under investigation. Of course, innovative technological developments in measurement have continued. For example, in 2017, the Nobel Prize in physics was awarded to scientists Rainer Weiss, Barry C. Barish, and Kip S. Thorne for their work on measuring gravitational waves, which were first theorized by Albert Einstein a hundred years ago and are thousands of times smaller than an atomic nucleus. Up until now, gravitational waves had eluded capture. Using gigantic laser interferometers, the scientists were able to capture and measure gravitational waves stemming from a collision of two black holes over 1.3 billion years ago.

Just as physicists understandably are very serious about measurement, health-promotion researchers and practitioners should be equally as serious. The theories described in this textbook are only as relevant as the tools available with which to measure the theories' constructs. Without the proper measurement tools, we can never be certain as to whether certain theories should be supported, confirmed, or swept into the theory dust bin.

Although the measurement tools we use in health-promotion research and practice are qualitatively different from the sophisticated devices used by physicists, there are similarities. For example, we hold our measurement tools up to similar standards (e.g., physics is concerned with accuracy and precision, while health promotion is concerned with validity and reliability). We also acknowledge that *how* we measure attitudes, beliefs, traits, and behavior has serious implications for advancing the field. Just like physicists who attempt to measure particles or phenomena that are seemingly intangible (e.g., a gravitational wave), healtromotion researchers also attempt to measure properties or characteristics of individuals, systems, and communities that are seemingly intangible, such as perceptions, attitudes, or norms (see **BOX 14-1** for an example). In these respects, we face challenges similar to those that physicists face when conducting research, but acknowledge that while we are not trying to uncover the mysteries of the universe, we are trying to understand and change health behavior. We will leave it up to you to decide which challenge is more difficult.

This chapter provides an overview of the basic principles of measurement and how these principles apply to health-promotion research and practice. We describe the different types of measurement tools and the processes involved in the development of those tools. We explain the standards to which our measurement tools must

BOX 14-1 Example of a Measurement Tool Used in the Social Sciences

Couple Efficacy to Reduce HIV Threat Scale

Using the following scale, with (1) being not at all confident to (5) being very confident, please indicate how confident you are that you and your partner can work together when it comes to …

1.	Using condoms when having sex with each other	1	2	3	4	5
2.	Limiting the number of other sex partners	1	2	3	4	5
3.	Deciding whether to have sex outside the relationship	1	2	3	4	5
4.	Using condoms when having sex outside the relationship	1	2	3	4	5
5.	Getting tested regularly for STDs and/or HIV	1	2	3	4	5
6.	Deciding who will be the top and who will be the bottom when having sex with each other	1	2	3	4	5
7.	Being sexually faithful to each other	1	2	3	4	5

adhere and how we gauge whether they "measure up." We provide the appropriate statistical analyses for measures with varying properties. Finally, we articulate the research designs used to test applicability of the theoretical constructs to particular health behaviors.

▶ Key Concepts

The Importance of Measurement

Many of us take for granted the many procedures and processes we use on a daily basis that help order our day. For example, when the alarm clock goes off in the morning, we don't give much thought to how the clock measures time or even to how the system for measuring time was developed; rather, we tend to focus only on what time it is (and whether we are late!). If we are traveling somewhere, then we may gauge the distance (either in miles or kilometers, depending on where you live) and subsequently calculate when we will arrive at our destination based on our speed; however, we don't give much

thought to how the procedures were developed to measure velocity. Virtually every moment of our day involves some type of measurement, whether it is how many calories we consume, how much we weigh, what size pants we wear, how tall we are, how old we are, how intelligent we think we are, what level of education we have achieved, how much money we make, etc. The list is infinite, but it alludes to the importance of measurement in our lives and that "things" such as time, weight, length, height, age, grades, intelligence, cost, and salary are measured in certain ways using different **metrics**, or standards of measurement.

Measurement helps to order our lives because it uses rules to assign numbers to events and objects and characteristics of those events and objects such that relationships of the numbers reflect relationships of the events and objects (Stevens, 1946). Measurement creates order out of chaos and helps us to make sense of our physical world. However, the rules must be devised in such a way that they can be applied systematically; otherwise, there is no standardization or order.

> *Measurement creates order out of chaos and helps us to make sense of our physical world.*

Extending this logic to the discipline of public health research and practice, we can extrapolate that measurement is also an important aspect of our understanding and influencing of health behaviors through research and programs. A fundamental challenge involves measuring intangibles (i.e., nonphysical entities that are nonetheless believed to exist). Self-efficacy, for example, is a fairly robust element in most of the individual-level behavioral theories. It is worth bearing in mind that self-efficacy exists theoretically and thus is considered a **construct** (i.e., a theoretical entity). Self-efficacy was theorized to better explain human behavior. This is not to imply that the construct of self-efficacy is not real, only that it is not tangible. Indeed, the philosophical tradition of constructivism posits that reality is largely created through perception. In essence, it is quite useful to define a given theoretical concept, such as self-efficacy, so that everyone can hold a shared understanding of the otherwise mysterious entity. Having the ability to measure and create relationships among constructs, such as individuals' self-efficacy to exercise, quality of care at a certain public hospital, or social norms surrounding binge drinking on college campuses, is essential to the field.

As is the case with measurement of tangible physical properties, rules must be devised so that quantification of the characteristic by a particular measuring tool is a standardized process, which is the only way we can make sense of our comparisons. In these next sections, in order to obtain an understanding of the process of measurement, we provide a brief history of how measurement systems were developed for intangibles important to health-promotion research and practice.

History of Measurement of Intangibles

Relatively speaking, it has been only recently (i.e., in the past 150 years or so) that procedures for measuring certain intangible human characteristics or psychological processes such as intelligence, personality traits, perceptions, and attitudes were developed. Prior to the late 19th century, psychology was a branch of philosophy where psychological processes were not studied using the same rigorous scientific methods as the natural sciences. It wasn't until Wilhelm Wundt founded the first psychological lab in 1879 to study psychological processes through objective experimental methods that psychology began to emerge as a scientific and experimental discipline (Zusne, 1975). Thus, up to this point, standardized measurement tools to assess psychological processes had not been developed, as they were not needed. **FIGURE 14-1** provides a timeline of some of the historical moments from this period that propelled the field forward.

Beginning in the mid-19th century, psychologists became more interested in developing tests to measure psychological processes and mental abilities. In 1869, Sir Francis Galton, a British scientist and cousin of Charles Darwin, published his ideas about intelligence in a book titled *Hereditary Genius*, in which he articulated his observations that "eminent" men, who were considered "illustrious" by society's standards of education, occupation, or achievement also had eminent and illustrious ancestors (Galton, 1869). Galton developed ways in which he thought he could measure intelligence through the senses. His tests involved visual acuity, auditory acuity, tactile sensitivity, and reaction time. Although his methods were flawed (by modern standards), he nonetheless understood that he needed a way to analyze his data and to specifically examine the interrelationships. His work paved the way for the development of the correlation statistical measure, which was subsequently developed by his student, Karl Pearson—for whom the widely used Pearson product–moment correlation coefficient is named. Galton has been credited with founding the study of measurement of individuals and is referred to as the father of **psychometrics**. Psychometrics is the field of study concerned with the theory and technique of educational and psychological measurement, which includes the

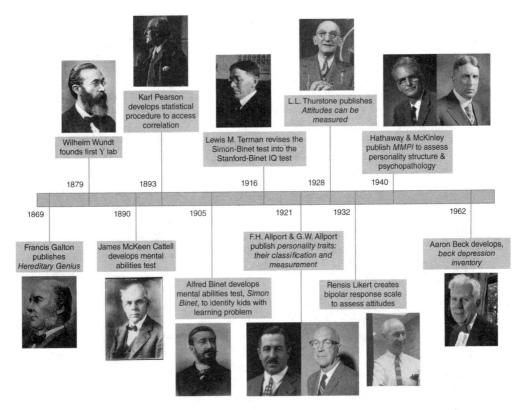

FIGURE 14-1 Timeline of history of measurement for intangibles

Top row, left to right: © INTERFOTO/Alamy Images, © Courtesy of the National Library of Medicine, © Courtesy of the National Library of Medicine, © George Skadding /Time Life Pictures/Getty Images, © University of Minnesota Archives, Courtesy of Library of Congress, Prints & Photographs Division, Harris & Ewing Collection [reproduction number LC-H25-65869-E]. Bottom row, left to right: © Courtesy of the National Library of Medicine, © The Granger Collection, New York, © Courtesy of the National Library of Medicine, © Syracuse University Archives, © Bill Ingraham/AP Photos, © Institute for Social Research/University of Michigan, © Leif Skoogfors/Corbis Historical/Getty Images.

measurement of knowledge, abilities, attitudes, and personality traits. Thus, as the father of this burgeoning field, Galton's work served as a springboard for other psychologists interested in measuring mental abilities.

One such psychologist was James McKeen Cattell. Cattell took Galton's work and expanded it to create 10 mental tests to be administered to the general public. His 10 tests used a range of anthropometric tests such as the strength of a person's hand squeeze, hand movements, reaction times for sound and for naming colors, judgments of time, etc. Unfortunately, data collected using Cattell's mental abilities test failed to find a significant correlation (using the Pearson correlation) with academic grades among college students. Nevertheless, his work was significant in that it set the stage for new and improved tests, such as Alfred Binet's, which would attempt to capture higher-level mental abilities (Zusne, 1975).

In France, Alfred Binet developed a test (Simon–Binet test) for measuring children's mental abilities. The original purpose of the test was to help educational authorities distinguish children who needed remedial attention. Interestingly, Binet himself argued that his test should not be used as a general measure of intelligence, and he issued a caveat to educators and psychologists as he feared that the use of his test would have implications for children whose test scores could be used to label them as intellectually inferior, and thereby affect their life and livelihood. He indicated that the complex and varied nature of intellectual qualities precludes the ability to accurately measure the construct of intelligence in the same way as linear surfaces are measured (i.e., with a single score measurement) (Gould, 1981). An original test item is provided in **FIGURE 14-2**. When viewing this picture, children were asked "which face is prettier" from each pair of faces.

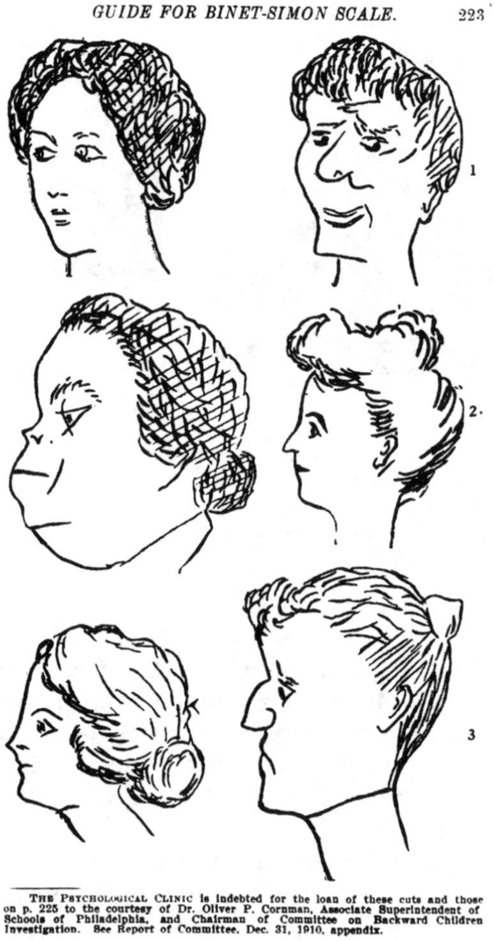

GUIDE FOR BINET-SIMON SCALE.   223

THE PSYCHOLOGICAL CLINIC is indebted for the loan of these cuts and those on p. 225 to the courtesy of Dr. Oliver P. Cornman, Associate Superintendent of Schools of Philadelphia, and Chairman of Committee on Backward Children Investigation. See Report of Committee. Dec. 31, 1910, appendix.

FIGURE 14-2 Test item from the original Simon—Binet Intelligence test

Reproduced from the article "A Practical Guide for Administering the Binet-Simon Scale for Measuring Intelligence" by J. W. Wallace Wallin in the March 1911 issue of the journal *The Psychological Clinic* (volume 5 number 1).

Unfortunately, educators and psychologists did not heed Binet's wishes for how his intelligence test was to be used. Lewis M. Terman, a cognitive psychology professor at Stanford University, worked on revising the Simon–Binet Scale. His final product, published in 1916 as the *Stanford Revision of the Binet–Simon Scale of Intelligence* (also known as the Stanford–Binet), became the standard intelligence test in the United States for the next several decades (Linden & Linden, 1968). The Stanford–Binet and other popular intelligence measures are still used today in a wide range of applications, some of which are considered controversial.

Over the course of the 20th century, other psychologists developed measurement tools for other psychological processes and constructs. For example, Allport and Allport in 1921 developed a tool to distinguish personality traits (Allport & Allport, 1921). In 1928, L. L. Thurstone challenged the position that attitudes could not be measured with the publication of his article, "Attitudes Can Be Measured" (Thurstone, 1928). Thurstone used three attitudinal scales—pacifism–militarism, prohibition, and attitude toward the church—to illustrate the process. Each scale encompassed a series of statements that represented a range of attitudes on a continuum going from positive to neutral to negative and for which respondents would indicate their agreement or disagreement with each statement.

Building off of Thurstone's work, Likert (1932) developed a less cumbersome technique to measure attitudes where statements did not have to be categorized *a priori*, but rather positive, neutral, or negative attitude was captured in the response options following each statement. The bipolar response options typically ranged from "strongly agree" to "strongly disagree" on a five-point scale. Likert's technique is probably the most common form of scale measurement used in the social sciences today. Examples of different Likert response scales are provided in **BOX 14-2**.

As the saying goes, necessity is the mother of invention. Thus, as psychology and other social science disciplines progressed, so did the need for measurement tools to advance the field. In 1940,

BOX 14-2   Common Likert-Type Response Scales Used in the Social Sciences

Level of Agreement—5 point
1—Strongly disagree
2—Somewhat disagree
3—Neither agree nor disagree
4—Somewhat agree
5—Strongly agree

Level of Importance—7 point
1—Not at all important
2—Low importance
3—Slightly important
4—Neutral
5—Moderately important
6—Very important
7—Extremely important

Frequency of Use—5 point
1—Never
2—Almost never
3—Occasionally/Sometimes
4—Almost every time
5—Every time

Likelihood—5 point
1—Extremely unlikely
2—Unlikely
3—Neutral
4—Likely
5—Extremely likely

Level of Concern—5 point
1—Not at all concerned
2—Slightly concerned
3—Somewhat concerned
4—Moderately concerned
5—Extremely concerned

Frequency—5 point
1—Never
2—Rarely
3—Sometimes
4—Often
5—Always

Knowledge of Action—7 point
1—Never true
2—Rarely true
3—Infrequently true
4—Neutral
5—Sometimes true
6—Usually true
7—Always true

Level of Satisfaction—5 point
1—Not at all satisfied
2—Slightly satisfied
3—Moderately satisfied
4—Very satisfied
5—Extremely satisfied

The Minnesota Multiphasic Personality Inventory (the MMPI), one of the most frequently used personality tests in the mental health fields, was developed by Hathaway and McKinley (1940) to help identify personal, social, and behavioral problems in psychiatric patients. The test helps provide relevant information to aid in problem identification, diagnosis, and treatment planning for the patient and is used widely in a variety of contexts including legal cases such as child custody and criminal defense. The test has also been used as a screening instrument for certain professions, especially high-risk jobs and to evaluate the effectiveness of treatment programs, including substance abuse programs. The MMPI has been

revised and updated over the years with the most recent version, MMPI-2-RF in 2008.

In 1962, Dr. Aaron Beck developed the Beck Depression Inventory to assist clinicians in their assessments of major depressive disorders. As the 20th century progressed, many other scales, too numerous to document, were developed. Coinciding with this development were technological and statistical advancements. For example, more sophisticated statistical techniques to determine that these measurement tools met certain standards were developed and the widespread adoption of the personal computer allowed for the implementation and ease of using these statistical techniques (DiIorio, 2005).

From Constructs to Variables

At the crux of many of the public health theories described in this textbook are various psychological constructs, such as attitudes, as well as knowledge, abilities, and, of course, behavior. For example, attitudes form the basis of the theory of reasoned action and self-efficacy is at the core of social cognitive theory. However, before we can develop appropriate measurements for these constructs, it is important to consider several aspects of these constructs and how these aspects will affect the way in which you are able to measure them.

First of all, it is important to acknowledge that some of these constructs manifest in individuals (e.g., attitudes), some are specific to systems (e.g., accessibility to health care), while still others are attributes of communities (e.g., social capital). Also, when thinking about how to develop a particular measure, you must think about how that measure will be administered (e.g., face-to-face interview, computer-assisted interview, or self-administered questionnaire), to whom or what the measure will be administered and generalized, and what sources of information are available for developing that measure.

The "to whom or what" aspect associated with measurement is referred to as the **level of analysis**. The level of analysis, simply put, indicates the socioecological level at which findings will be applied. For example, studies that examined depression (an individual-level characteristic) among female clinical patients would be at the individual level of analysis if the findings were applied only to the sample, whereas other studies that examined depression among teens living in the United States would be at the societal level of analysis. For understanding level of analysis, it is important to differentiate between what is being measured, who is being measured, and what conclusions will be drawn. For example, "neighborhood cohesion" is not an individual-level construct, but can be viewed as a community-level construct; however, some studies measure neighborhood cohesion by administering a measurement tool (e.g., a questionnaire) to groups of individuals residing in a particular community and then discussing the results in terms of the neighborhood. It is not necessarily inappropriate to aggregate to the larger group, but rather we make this point as something to consider when you develop your tools to measure certain constructs and the conclusions you can draw based on those tools. The level of analysis is an important consideration when developing appropriate measurement tools because of the implications for your methodology.

> *The level of analysis, simply put, indicates the socioecological level at which findings will be applied.*

Secondly, because much of what we do in public health research and practice is to examine how individuals, systems, and communities differ, we are interested in measuring constructs and behaviors that can take on more than one value. For example, if the construct of "attitudes toward exercising" could have only one value (e.g., "positive"), then this would mean that "attitudes toward exercising" would be classified as a **constant**. In contrast, a measure that can take on more than one value is classified as a **variable**.

Types of Variables

In general, variables can be classified into one of two types: **qualitative** and **quantitative**. When there is variability in kind (e.g., rural versus urban community, male versus female students, married versus single), the variable is qualitative; when there is variability in degree (e.g., weight, height, low versus high confidence, low versus high scholastic aptitude, lower versus higher depressive symptomatology), the variable is quantitative. **FIGURE 14-3** presents the comparison of data types using the example of "first-year graduate students."

Qualitative variables generally do not involve a system of classification that is ordered. Quantitative variables, on the other hand, do involve an ordering of the values or categories as they represent differing amounts, frequencies, or degrees. Because of these and other distinctions, the metrics used in measuring each type of variable also differ.

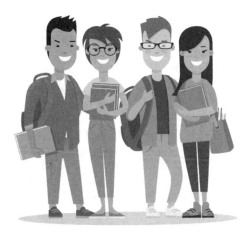

First-year graduate students

Qualitative data	Quantitative data

• Environmentalists
• Highly intelligent
• Outgoing
• Civic minded
• Politically involved
• Racial/ethnic diversity
	• N=650 students
	• n=300 males; n=350 females
	• Mean GPA=3.9
	• Mean age=22.8 years
	• 17% black/african american
	• 48% white/caucasian
	• 10% latino
	• 15% asian
	• 6% american indian/alaska
	  native
	• 4% native hawaiian/other
	  pacific Islander

FIGURE 14-3 Qualitative versus quantitative data
© Sentavio / Shutterstock

TABLE 14-1 Variable Examples and Statistical Tests Associated with Four Metrics

Metric	Applied Variable Examples	Statistical Tests
Nominal	Sex, race/ethnicity, marital status, HIV status	Frequency counts, mode, phi coefficient, Cramér's V, chi-square
Ordinal	High school standing, socioeconomic status, birth order, attitude scales, self-efficacy scales	Same as nominal, but also median, percentiles, Kendall's tau, or Spearman's rank
Interval	Temperature in Fahrenheit or Celsius	Same as ordinal, but also mean, standard deviation, range, Pearson product–moment correlation, ANOVA, regression
Ratio	Yearly income, temperature in Kelvin, age, HIV incidence, HIV knowledge test	Same as interval, but also geometric and harmonic means

Stevens (1946) first proposed a system of classification for metrics used to measure intangibles in the social sciences. His system identified four metrics (nominal, ordinal, interval, and ratio) and delineated the rules associated with each. Qualitative variables use a nominal metric, whereas quantitative variables use ordinal, interval, and ratio. This system is still widely used today and conveys specific information about these different metrics, such as the nature of the object being measured and the type of statistical analysis that can be performed. **TABLE 14-1** presents these metrics along with example variables and appropriate statistical tests used when analyzing these variables.

Metrics of Measurement in Health Promotion

Nominal

By definition, qualitative variables differ in kind; thus, the metric used for qualitative variables is called **nominal** (i.e., existing in name or form

When developing a nominal measure, an important consideration is that each category must be mutually exclusive, so that assignment to one and only one category is possible.

only). Nominal variables *classify* whatever object or characteristic it is that you are measuring into groups or categories based on all the different types of that characteristic. As such, nominal variables are sometimes referred to as categorical. As stated previously, there is no ranking or ordering of the categories, but there must be at least two categories, indicating that the variable is dichotomous. For example, if we were evaluating a health-promotion program and the design called for only two conditions (e.g., experimental and control), then a dichotomous nominal variable would be used to designate the assigned condition of each participant in the evaluation. When developing a nominal measure, an important consideration is that each category must be mutually exclusive, so that assignment to one and only one category is possible.

For example, a variable that measures a person's sex, a biological characteristic, would have only two categories, male and female, and people would be assigned to one or the other. Of course, depending on the nature of the research, some variables are more complicated and necessitate more categories. In fact, you must create as many categories as are necessary to capture all of the different "kinds." Having as many categories as are necessary speaks to the second important aspect of nominal measurements, namely that the categories must also be exhaustive.

To illustrate this idea, if we were recruiting people to participate in a smoking cessation health-promotion program, then we could create a nominal variable that would be used to screen people. Ostensibly, this "smoking" variable could have two mutually exclusive categories to measure whether or not people would qualify for entrance into the program: smoker and nonsmoker. However, perhaps this program is tailored specifically to smokers who have tried to quit at some point, rather than smokers who have never tried to quit.

Thus, the dichotomous variable we created would not have exhaustive categories in the sense that we did not capture all of the instances of smoking that apply. We should have three categories for our smoking variable: current smoker who has never tried to quit, current smoker who has tried to quit, and nonsmoker.

Once the nominal variable has been created, to be viewed as a measure (recall that measurement involves the assignment of numbers), we must also assign a numeric value to the different categories. As the categories do not represent ordering of values or differences in degree, arbitrary numbers are fine. The important thing to consider is that whatever rule is created, it must be applied consistently. Thus, if you assign a value of "0" to represent smokers who have tried to quit, a value of "1" to represent smokers who have never tried to quit, and a value of "2" to represent nonsmokers, then people who fall into each of these behavioral categories must be assigned the corresponding value. With this metric, you can clearly see that "2" does not represent higher levels of smoking in comparison to "0" and "1," only that those who have a "2" assigned to them are qualitatively different from those who have a "0" or a "1."

Statistics that are allowable with nominal measures include determining the frequency or number of cases assigned to each category and corresponding percentages. Calculating the mode is acceptable, meaning that we can determine which category has the most assigned to it. Furthermore, using contingency methods, you can examine whether two nominal variables are related using the contingency correlation coefficient, *phi* coefficient or Cramér's V. You could also test whether distributions across categories are significantly different from what is expected using the chi-square statistic.

For example, suppose you want to determine whether the distribution of males differs significantly from the distribution of females in terms of smoking. In a hypothetical research study involving 625 people, using a popular statistical software package for the social sciences (SPSS; Chicago, IL), you could create two nominal variables, each having two categories: one that represents sex (male and female) and one that represents smoking (smoker and non-smoker). You could then create a 2 × 2 contingency table that cross-tabulates the number of males/females by whether they are smokers or not. This table is shown in **FIGURE 14-4**. You could then calculate the chi-square statistic based on these counts. As indicated by the significant chi-square in this example, you conclude that, based on the overall percentage of smokers (23.2%) in your sample, there are significantly more females (27.2%) who smoke than males (19.6%). Furthermore, you could determine whether there is a relationship between sex and smoking by examining the appropriate correlation coefficients for these data.

As shown in the correlational measures table, under the nominal by nominal category, the correlation between sex and smoking is 0.09 for all three appropriate coefficients and is significant. Finally, for more sophisticated multivariate analyses, if the dependent variable is a dichotomous nominal variable (e.g., have the disease versus do not have the disease), then you could perform a logistic regression.

Ordinal

An **ordinal** measurement is the metric used for variables whose assigned values differ by degree and are ordered in some fashion. Ordinal metrics are used in everyday life to rank myriad things such as birth order, pain level, and marathon race results (e.g., 1st place, 2nd place), to name a few. Assigned values represent a hierarchal ordering that is based on some rationale, for instance 1st, 2nd, 3rd; low, medium, high; and strongly disagree to strongly agree. However, differences among the represented levels of the characteristic may not be equal and it is this latter criterion that defines an ordinal metric.

Take, for example, a characteristic that is used quite frequently within health-promotion research and practice: self-efficacy. Self-efficacy is typically measured using an ordinal metric by presenting statements theoretically related to the characteristic, followed by potential responses, of which the latter represent various levels of self-efficacy. An item from a self-efficacy measure could be the

following statement: "I can solve most problems if I invest the necessary effort." The presentation of this statement is followed by asking respondents to pick the best response from the following responses: 1 (definitely not true), 2 (somewhat untrue), 3 (neither untrue nor true), 4 (somewhat true), and 5 (exactly true). Because equal distance between these five ordered response options cannot be ascertained, this example constitutes using an ordinal metric for measuring self-efficacy.

As indicated, the numeric values are assigned in such a way that the numbers reflect the ordered relation defined on the variable. For example, a value of "5" equates with greater self-efficacy than the lower possible values. Comparisons of "greater than" or "less than" can be made and are meaningful; however, it is uncertain whether exact differences between the assigned numeric values are analogous to exact differences in the characteristic being measured. Thus, you cannot say that the difference in self-efficacy levels between someone who responded "exactly true" to the preceding statement and someone who responded "somewhat true" is the exact same difference in self-efficacy as for someone who indicated "neither true or untrue" and someone who responded "somewhat untrue."

Appropriate statistics for ordinal measures are the same as for nominal; however, we may also calculate the median, meaning we could rank order the values and determine the score at which half of the scores fall below and half fall above. The median is also referred to as the 50th percentile; we could also calculate other percentiles such as quartiles (25th) and deciles (10th). Calculating the median is very useful in public health research and practice, for example, knowing the 50th percentile score among a sample of elementary school students on a measure of behavioral nutrition (i.e., measures good eating behaviors with ranks of low, medium, and high).

Also, to determine the correspondence between two ordinal variables, say, for example, our measure of behavioral nutrition and a measure of socioeconomic status, we could calculate a rank–order

The median is also referred to as the 50th percentile.

Sex * Smoking-Status Cross-tabulation

			Smoking status at baseline		Total
			No	Yes	
Sex	Male	Count	263	64	327
		Percentage within sex	80.4%	19.6%	100.0%
	Female	Count	217	81	298
		Percentage within sex	72.8%	27.2%	100.0%
Total		Count	480	145	625
		Percentage within sex	76.8%	23.2%	100.0%

Chi-Square Tests

	Value	df	Asymp.Sig. (2-sided)	Exact Sig. (2-sided)	Exact Sig. (1-sided)
Pearson Chi-Square	5.067(b)	1	.024		
Continuity Correction(a)	4.649	1	.031		
Likelihood Ratio	5.067	1			
Fisher's Exact Test				.029	.016
Linear-by-Linear Association	5.059	1	.024		
N of Valid Cases	625		.025		

a. Computed only for a 2x2 table.
b. 0 cells (0%) have expected count less than 5. The minimum expected count is 69.14.

Correlational Measures

		Value	Asymp. Std. Error(a)	Approx. T(b)	Approx. Sig.
Nominal by Nominal	Phi	.090			.024
	Cramér's V	.090			.024
	Contingency Coefficient	.090			.024
Interval by Interval	Pearson's R	.090	.040	2.257	.024(c)
Ordinal by Ordinal	Spearman Correlation	.090	.040	2.257	.024(c)
N of Valid Cases		625			

a. Not assuming the null hypothesis.
b. Using the asymptotic standard error assuming the null hypothesis.
c. Based on normal approximation.

FIGURE 14-4 SPSS output: Contingency table, chi-square statistical test to show difference in distribution of sexes across smoking status

correlation coefficient such as Kendall's tau or Spearman's rank. In this example, a significant positive correlation would indicate that a higher level of behavioral nutrition was related to higher socioeconomic status.

Interval

An **interval** metric is similar to ordinal in that there is a ranking of values that is meaningful; however, interval metrics differ significantly from ordinal metrics in that the difference between possible values is consistent and is known to be equal. Therefore, the interval between values is interpretable in that differences among assigned numeric values represent to the same degree exact differences in the characteristic being measured. Thus, we are able to say that the difference between interval 1 and interval 3 is the same difference as between interval 4 and interval 6, and that these differences correspond to similar differences in the characteristic. Also, an important aspect of interval measurements is that there is no true zero point for the characteristic, meaning that a score of zero is only arbitrary; a zero value does not equate with a true absence of the characteristic being measured.

Common interval measures that you may be familiar with are Fahrenheit and Celsius, which measure heat energy or temperature. Heat energy represents the amount of molecular activity in a body or object. Using these measures we can say that the reduction in molecular activity that occurs when going from 80°F to 40°F represents the exact same reduction in amount of molecular activity as going from 160°F to 120°F. However, because there is still molecular activity at 0°F and at 0°C, you cannot say that a temperature of 0° equates with a complete lack of molecular activity. More important, because 0° is an arbitrary point on both measures, you cannot make ratio comparisons. Thus, you cannot say that 80° (Fahrenheit or Celsius) is twice as hot as 40°.

In terms of public health research and practice, true interval measures are rare, as many of the constructs are intangible and we cannot determine anything more than the rank ordering of the data. It would be virtually impossible to know with certainty that the difference in the numbers assigned to each of the levels of a construct, such as attitudes toward exercising, reflect the true difference between any two levels. It is important to note that you may see examples of interval measurements in public health research and practice. Many researchers apply equal intervals to the various levels mainly for statistical analysis purposes; however, in reality these measurements should be classified as ordinal. For example, the Health Utilities Index (HUI) has been used to measure health-related quality of life in clinical studies (Furlong, Feeny, Torrance, & Barr, 2001). The HUI defines health status in terms of capacity rather than performance and has either 14 or 40 items, depending on the version. The HUI has been called an interval metric because ostensibly the numbers used to represent the varying degrees of health-related quality of life equate with equal intervals; however, is it correct to say that a score of 25 on the HUI as compared to a score of 20 represents the same difference in health-related quality of life as the difference between 15 points and 10 points? It is not entirely correct to make this assumption, as it cannot be verified in the same way as levels of molecular activity.

Although the HUI is a measure of an intangible construct similar to other health-promotion constructs such as self-efficacy and attitudes toward exercising, and should therefore be classified as ordinal; it has been classified as interval where equal intervals are assumed. The HUI is but one example; this type of misclassification of ordinal as interval is frequently done in health-promotion research as well as other social science disciplines. Thus, an important caveat is that caution should be used when drawing

An important aspect of interval measurements is that there is no true zero point for the characteristic, meaning that a score of zero is only arbitrary.

conclusions on ordinal measurements when performing statistical analyses meant for true interval scales.

Descriptive statistics for interval measures include the mode and the median; however, we can also calculate an arithmetic mean and standard deviation. Assessing correlation between interval scales can be performed using rank–order correlations as well as the Pearson product–moment correlation. Many more sophisticated analyses can also be performed such as Analysis of Variance (ANOVA), linear regression, and advanced correlational analyses such as path analysis.

Ratio

A **ratio** metric has the same properties as an interval metric, such as having an ordered continuum and differences between intervals that are equal and reflect proportionally similar differences in the actual levels of the characteristic. The main difference is that a ratio metric has a true zero point. As stated previously, a value of zero means there is a complete lack or absence of the characteristic being measured. Common ratio metrics are duration in seconds, age, weight, height, and temperature in degrees Kelvin. Do you recall that 0°F did not equate with a lack of molecular activity? In contrast to the Fahrenheit and Celsius measures, the Kelvin measure has a true zero point, meaning that at 0 K (i.e., −460°F) there is a complete lack of molecular activity.

There is a definite advantage of being able to use a ratio metric for a particular construct in that you can make meaningful proportional comparisons. For example, 60 years old is twice as old as 30 years old; 200 lbs. is twice as heavy as 100 lbs.; and 3 feet is half as tall as 6 feet. These types of relational comparisons cannot be made with any of the other described metrics.

Ratio measures relative to health promotion are simply counting the number of individuals, objects, or events related to a particular disease or underlying health behavior. Many times

A ratio metric has a true zero point.

it is important to know how many individuals manifest a certain disease at a given point in time. In the field of epidemiology, it is very useful to be able to say that there are three times as many individuals infected with "disease X" in 2017 as there were in 2010 so that resources can be directed to combating the disease. One specific public health issue that has garnered a lot of attention in recent years is obesity. Because of surveillance studies, it has been shown that the prevalence of obese children ages 12–19 years has nearly tripled since 1980 increasing from 5.5% to 17.2% in 2014 (Ogden, Carroll, Fryar, & Flegal, 2015). In addition to counting individuals with diseases or health issues, it is also important to count the number of risk behaviors (e.g., sexual risk behavior, exercise behavior, nutritional behavior) in which individuals engage. These numbers are quite useful for documenting behavioral trends over time. See **FIGURE 14-5** for an example from the Centers for Disease Control and Prevention.

Another example of a ratio measure would be a knowledge test. Knowledge has been identified as necessary, but not sufficient, to affect behavioral change (O'Leary, 2001). Knowledge of the risks and benefits of engaging in a certain behavior serves as the precondition for change (Bandura, 2004). Thus, knowledge of various health issues is an important construct to assess. Health-promotion practitioners can use knowledge tests to first identify at-risk populations who possess low levels of knowledge, and subsequently these populations could be targeted with health-promotion programs.

In addition, knowledge tests are needed to further evaluate these programs. A measure of knowledge of HIV, for example, would hold great utility in health-promotion research and practice. A measure of HIV knowledge should typically include multiple test items that cover all of the content relevant to the various aspects of the virus, such as how it is transmitted and how it is treated. Scores could be assigned proportionally based on how many items were answered correctly. Given that higher scores would reflect greater knowledge, the difference between a score of 90% and 100% is the same

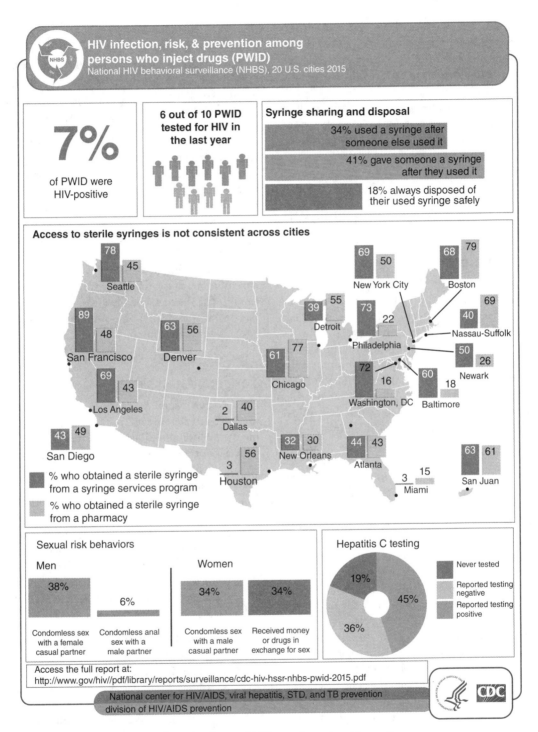

FIGURE 14-5 Surveillance example from the Centers for Disease Control and Prevention

Reproduced from Centers for Disease Control and Prevention. HIV Infection, Risk, Prevention, and Testing Behaviors among Persons Who Inject Drugs—National HIV Behavioral Surveillance: Injection Drug Use, 20 U.S. Cities, 2015. HIV Surveillance Special Report 18. http://www.cdc.gov/hiv/library/reports/hivsurveillance.html. Published September 2017.

as the difference between 75% and 85%; differences in actual scores would reflect a proportionately similar difference in true knowledge, and so knowledge can be classified as a ratio variable.

Statistical analyses using ratio scales include all of the previously mentioned analyses for the lower level scales; however, the geometric and harmonic means can also be calculated.

Developing Measurement Tools for Theoretical Constructs

Definitions

Now that you have a foundation for understanding some of the main issues involved in measurement in general and in measurement of health-promotion constructs specifically, we can begin to guide you through the process of developing measurement tools to capture the theoretical constructs. To begin, DiIorio (2005) suggests we first define the theoretical construct in general terms, referred to as the **theoretical definition**. For the theoretical definition, we need only turn to the original theory and the author. The measurement of attitudes serves as a good example at this juncture. In general, attitudes are typically thought of as consisting of three components: cognitive, affective, and behavioral. The cognitive component refers to the ideas, opinions, or knowledge related to the object; affective refers to the emotions or feelings related to the object; and behavioral refers to the action or reaction to the object. With this in mind and referring back to the theory of reasoned action, Ajzen and Fishbein (1980) provided the following theoretical definition: "Attitudes toward the health behavior are the underlying beliefs related to what will happen if the behavior is performed (i.e., cognitive) and the personal evaluation of that outcome (affective)." Once this definition is applied to a specific health behavior (e.g., getting the flu vaccine), then the **operational definition** can be stated.

An operational definition is simply the way in which the construct will be measured in a particular study (DiIorio, 2005). As noted previously, abstract concepts that are developed or adopted for use in a theory are correctly referred to as constructs. For each specific construct, an operational definition is required. For example, an operational definition could be: "attitudes toward the flu vaccine will be measured using the scale developed by Montano." Of course, this particular operational definition depends on the existence of a measurement tool. If a tool exists, then we would simply state the name of the measurement tool as our operational definition; however, if a tool does not exist, then one must be developed.

> *An operational definition is simply the way in which the construct will be measured in a particular study.*

Concept Analysis

How do we begin to develop a measurement tool? The development of adequate measurement tools for theoretical constructs can begin with a **concept analysis**. A concept analysis is an involved, six-step process that provides an in-depth and thorough understanding of the construct. Providing an extensive description of the six-step process is beyond the scope of this chapter; for more information about this process, we refer you to DiIorio (2005), who writes extensively on the topic. Engaging in these six steps prior to writing the items that will eventually constitute the measurement scale will greatly enhance the process:

1. Identify definitions and uses of the concept
2. Identify critical attributes
3. Identify similar and different concepts
4. Identify dimensions of the concept
5. Identify antecedents and consequences of the concept
6. Write a model case

Scales

One important aspect of the construct to be measured and one that would be gleaned from performing a concept analysis is whether the construct is a unitary construct, meaning that the construct comprises one dimension, or whether the construct is a multidimensional construct. Attitudes toward the flu vaccine would be considered a unitary construct. Other examples are global self-esteem, general self-efficacy, and depression. However, a construct such as intelligence has multiple dimensions, such as the capacity to reason, plan, think abstractly, comprehend ideas, use language, and learn.

A second important aspect of the construct is whether the questions or items are distinct **effect indicators**. Effect indicators signify that the questions or items designed to measure the construct infer some "effect" or influence on a directly observable behavior (Streiner, 2003). For example, depression, which is a theoretical construct that is not directly observable, can be measured with items that assess the various observable behaviors purported to be associated with being depressed, such as not being able to get out of bed, not being able to laugh, or not being able to sleep or eat. Theoretically, the level of depression a person has essentially "affects" their responses to the items on the depression measure. The more depressed you are, the more likely you would respond that you experienced many of the purported behaviors associated with being depressed. Effect indicators of a construct are deemed a scale. Specifically, "a scale is a measure that is composed of theoretically correlated items that are measuring the same construct" (Streiner, 2003, p. 217). Thus, the items of a scale should all be highly inter correlated. Examples of other scales include the Rosenberg Self-Esteem Scale (Rosenberg, 1989), and self-efficacy to refuse sexual intercourse scale (Cecil & Pinkerton, 1998).

Indexes

Alternatively, if the construct you are measuring is not directly observable but involves items that are **causal indicators**, you would call your measure an **index** instead of a scale (Streiner, 2003). For example, quality of life is considered a construct that is not directly observable. Items that measure quality of life should correspond to tangible behaviors, traits, or outcomes that theoretically *represent* aspects of quality of life, such as having the ability to walk without difficulty, dress without difficulty, hear or see without difficulty, and be free from pain. However, in contrast to scale items, responses to these causal items "cause" or define the value of quality of life. In other words, a person who responds "yes" to the aforementioned items would have a much higher quality of life than someone who responded "no." The items in an index typically are heterogeneous although they could be and may not necessarily be correlated with each other, unlike the items for a scale. Other examples of an index would be the Apgar test for newborns, tests that assess level of physical functionality and stressful life events, and knowledge tests.

The distinctions between causal indicator items, which measure an index, and effect indicators using a scale are illustrated in **FIGURE 14-6**. As shown, in the scale example (depression), the arrows move away from the depression construct to the observable items, indicating that the level of depression essentially "affects" the responses to those items, whereas in the index example (stressful life events), responses to the items "cause" or define the level of stressful life events. Thus, in the index example, the arrows move from the observable items to the construct.

Item Wording Considerations

Whether your theoretical construct is unitary or multidimensional, or it is considered a scale or an index, there are several important considerations when developing the items. These issues involve trying to standardize the items in terms of time referents and behaviors and provide sufficient context so that accurate interpretation of responses is possible.

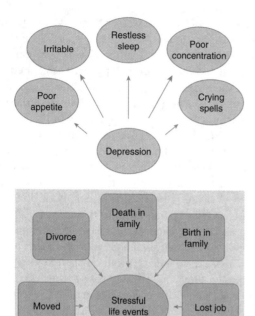

FIGURE 14-6 Observable items as effect indicators for a scale measuring depression and observable items as causal indicators for an index measuring stressful life events

The first consideration involves providing a **behavioral anchor**. For example, the construct of perceived susceptibility from the health belief model (Chapter 5) is defined as one's subjective perception of the risk of contracting a health condition given a particular behavioral context. Thus, when assessing the likelihood of getting HIV or lung cancer, for instance, it is important to provide a conditional behavioral anchor (e.g., "if you had sexual intercourse with a casual sex partner and did not use a condom" and "if you quit smoking soon") rather than ask the question in absolute terms, as such: What is the likelihood of you contracting HIV?

Another issue relates to the principle of correspondence and is relevant to measurement of theoretical constructs, especially intentions, normative beliefs, and attitudes. The premise of this principle is that health behavior typically has four defining components: action, target, time, and context, which should be specified. These four components essentially combine to define the health behavior. **TABLE 14-2** presents examples of how these components, once specified, define four different health behaviors. The table also provides a corresponding sample item to

| **TABLE 14-2** Principle of Correspondence's Four Defining Components |||||
Action	**Target**	**Context**	**Time**	**Item**
Get	Mammogram	Women's health clinic	Next 6 months	How likely are you to get a mammogram at the women's health clinic in the next 6 months?
Use	Sunscreen	While exercising outside	Always	Using sunscreen every time while running is beneficial.
Take	Blood pressure medication	Unspecified	Daily	My wife thinks it is important that I take my blood pressure medicine every day.
Perform	Breast self-exam	Shower	Weekly	Performing a breast self-exam in the shower once a week is unnecessary.

measure relevant theoretical constructs. Changing any one component would result in a completely different health behavior. Thus, from the principle-of-correspondence perspective, "using sunscreen every time I go for a run" is a different health behavior than "using sunscreen when I am at the pool."

There may be some health behaviors where specifying all four components is not necessary. For example, as shown in Table 14-2, the behavior "taking blood pressure medication daily," does not have context specified. However, regardless of how the health behavior is defined in terms of components, the items constructed to measure the theoretical constructs must also specify the components in the same way. For example, we can define the following health behavior as "getting (action) a colonoscopy (target) in the next 6 months (time) at Dr. Gastroenterologist's office (context)." We are interested in measuring attitudes, intentions, and normative beliefs related to this behavior. Thus, one attitudinal item could be, "Getting a colonoscopy in the next 6 months at Dr. G's office" is worthless/useful; one intentional item could be, "I intend to get a colonoscopy in the next 6 months at Dr. G's office" strongly disagree/ strongly agree; and one normative belief item could be, "My wife thinks that I [should/should not] get a colonoscopy in the next 6 months at Dr. G's office."

Reliability and Validity

In physics, precision and accuracy of measurement instruments are imperative. Precision refers to how much confidence you are willing to put into your measurement; in other words, high precision means that you are very confident that an additional measurement would produce a value very close to the previous measurements. Accuracy refers to the degree of conformity of a measured value to its true value. A measurement that is highly accurate means that there is virtually no error and it is a very close representation of the actual value. An analogy used frequently to illustrate these concepts is a target, with the measurement tool being the arrows. The closer the arrow is to hitting the bull's-eye, the more accurate; however, even if subsequent arrows do not hit very close to the bull's-eye, the arrows can still cluster together. The more tightly clustered together the arrows are, the more precise.

A measurement that is highly accurate means that there is virtually no error and it is a very close representation of the actual value.

Thus, you can have a measurement tool that is precise, but not necessarily accurate. One example is a scale that measures weight. It may provide the same measurement every time you stand on it; however, the measurement it provides could be off by a few pounds. In this instance, your scale would be precise, but not accurate.

In health-promotion research, we too have standards for gauging our measurement tools. Analogous to precision and accuracy are the properties of reliability and validity. **Reliability** of a measure indicates the extent to which the scale or index consistently measures the same way each time it is used under the same condition with the *same subjects*. **Validity** refers to the extent to which the scale or index measures what it is supposed to measure. As is true in physics, a measurement used in health promotion could be highly reliable, yet not be a valid measure of the construct.

There are several ways of estimating the reliability of a measure. First, reliability could be established by administering the index or the scale to a sample at two points in time and looking for a relatively strong correlation in scores for Time (1) and Time (2). This is known as **test-retest reliability**. An underlying assumption to test-retest reliability is that the construct being measured is stable; therefore, a reliable measure should produce approximately the same score at Time (2) that it did at Time (1) for each person in the sample.

Reliability can also be estimated through a statistical procedure calculating the inter-item correlations composing the measure. This statistical technique is especially appropriate for establishing the reliability of a scale versus an index because scale items should be highly correlated with each other. This is not true for all indexes, however, where the items may be heterogeneous. Therefore, for indexes, computing inter-item correlations is not an appropriate technique for estimating reliability (Streiner, 2003). Calculating the inter-item correlations is called assessing **internal reliability**.

We can determine the intercorrelations among items on a scale by employing a specific statistical procedure that yields the statistic Cronbach's alpha (α). An advantage of this method is that only one administration of the scale is necessary. The formula for Cronbach's alpha utilizes a variance–covariance matrix of the items along with the total number of items. The resulting statistic represents the ratio of the sum of the inter-item covariances to the variance of the total scores. Thus, Cronbach's alpha has a potential range of 0–1, with higher scores representing greater inter-item reliability. In health-promotion research, α equal to 0.70 or higher is sufficient evidence of reliability. Extremely high alpha would suggest that there may be redundancy among some of the indicators and perhaps the scale could be reduced to fewer items. Conversely, a low alpha indicates that some of the items are not representative of the construct, that there are too few items, or that the response options are too restrictive (e.g., having three potential responses versus five or seven).

Reliability can also be estimated using a technique called the **split-half** method. This analytic procedure begins with dividing the scale into two parallel forms of the measure. For example, a 10-item scale would be randomly divided into two 5-item measures. These two shortened forms would then be administered to a sample. The correlation between scores for the two halves is calculated and then used in a formula (i.e., the Spearman Brown) to estimate the reliability of the total measure (Ghiselli, Campbell, & Zedeck, 1981). Similar to inter-item reliability, this method is appropriate only for scales that are measuring the same unitary construct and not appropriate for indexes, as splitting the index into parts would not be meaningful.

As mentioned previously, validity refers to the degree to which a measurement tool measures what it is supposed to measure. Let's say, for instance, that you have developed an instrument to measure the construct "attitudes toward flu vaccine." Your scale comprises 10 items and you administered your scale twice to a sample of 100 adults. You calculated the test–retest reliability coefficient (0.75) and you estimated its internal reliability to be $\alpha = 0.85$. Thus, you determined that your scale is reliable. But, is it valid?

Although a measurement tool that is reliable does not necessarily have to be valid, the reverse is not true. In other words, for a measurement tool to be valid, it must be reliable; thus, reliability is necessary to achieve validity, although there are also other requirements. Validity can be established through the application of several different techniques that get at these other requirements. In **TABLE 14-3**, we describe most types of validity; however, we will also discuss several of these in more detail.

Two of the most elementary techniques are **face validity** and **content validity**. Both techniques employ a **jury of experts** (a panel of professionals who possess expertise with respect to the construct(s) under consideration). Face validity is judged by asking the jury, "Does the index or scale appear to measure the construct?"

Content validity, on the other hand, goes a bit further and can be assessed for both scales and indexes, but judgments made regarding the items differ. Scales assume that there is a universe of potential items from which to draw a sample that represents the unitary construct, whereas items composing an index should be viewed more as a census of items and are dependent on the underlying theory of the construct and prior research (Streiner, 2003). Thus, for scales, to determine content validity, you would want to ask, "Do the items adequately represent the 'universe' of all possible indicators relevant for the construct?" For indexes, you would want to

For a measurement tool to be valid, it must be reliable.

TABLE 14-3 Types of Validity

Type of Validity	Description
Face	Experts decide if the scale "appears" to measure the construct.
Content	Experts decide if the items of a scale are relevant and representative of the range of possible items to measure the construct.
Construct	The degree to which scale items measure the theoretical construct and relate to other measures as hypothesized by the theory.
Convergent	One aspect of construct validity that indicates the degree to which the scale measure correlates with other measures of the same construct.
Divergent	One aspect of construct validity that indicates the degree to which the scale measure does not correlate with other measures that it should not be related to.
Criterion related	The degree to which the scale measure correlates with an outcome to which, by definition, it should be related.
Predictive	A type of criterion-related validity that assesses the degree to which the scale measure "predicts" scores on a criterion measure assessed later in time.
Concurrent	A type of criterion-related validity that assesses the degree to which the scale measure correlates with a measure that has previously been validated. The two measures may be for the same construct or for different, but presumably related, constructs.

ask, "Do the items represent a census of items underlying the construct?"

Another related form of validity that is especially important for theoretical constructs is **construct validity**. As its name suggests, construct validity refers to the ability of a measure to perform the way in which the underlying theory hypothesizes. There are several ways to assess construct validity; one way is to show that the scale measure has **convergent validity**. For instance, to determine construct validity of a newly developed measure of attitudes toward the flu vaccine, we would turn to the theory of reasoned action, which hypothesizes that attitudes toward the flu vaccine are related to intentions to get the flu vaccine. To determine this relationship, we would administer our attitudes scale along with a measure of intentions to get the flu vaccine and calculate the correlation between these two scales. If they were, in fact, positively correlated such that positive attitudes are related to intentions to get the vaccine, then this would provide evidence of construct validity and would indicate that the scale is a valid measure of attitudes.

Another method of establishing validity involves comparing the assessed construct to a tangible measure such as a behavior (e.g., eating a low-fat diet, exercising, using condoms, receiving the flu vaccine) or outcome (e.g., losing weight, increasing aerobic capacity and muscle mass, reducing incidence of infection with sexually transmitted diseases, and reducing incidence of influenza). Known as **criterion-related validity**, this method is predicated on the basic question: Is the construct statistically associated with the expected criterion measure? For example, the theoretical construct of subjective norms (from the theory of reasoned action and the theory of planned behavior) toward the use of seat belts would ideally be expected to have a significant relationship with the actual use of seat belts. Thus, if the scale assessing this construct is indeed valid, then a statistically significant relationship with seat belt use would provide evidence of criterion-related validity. There are two ways to establish criterion-related validity (see Table 14-3).

Another method or technique for determining construct validity is called **factor analysis**. Factor analysis is a statistical technique for assessing the underlying dimensions of a construct, if in fact they exist, and for refining the measure. Factor analysis is commonly used in the development stage of a new measure. Before a new measure is adopted and accepted widely, it should be subjected to rigorous evaluations of its reliability and validity. Factor analysis is yet one more tool in the psychometric toolbox for assessing whether a measure is indeed valid.

Although many of the theoretical constructs in health-promotion research can be considered unitary constructs, they may still encompass several underlying dimensions. For instance, intelligence is considered a unitary abstract construct; however, there are many dimensions to intelligence, such as verbal ability, mathematical ability, and spatial ability. A valid measure of intelligence should comprise items representing each theoretical dimension of intelligence. Factor analysis allows us to statistically show with data that the items corresponding to each theoretical dimension or "factor" are more strongly correlated with each other than with items from other dimensions (DiIorio, 2005). The correlations between items and their underlying factor are called **factor loadings**.

Conducting a factor analysis in this situation would be referred to as an **exploratory factor analysis** and is very useful in the early stages of scale development. An exploratory factor analysis is data driven in that it will reveal whether items cluster together to form a factor and will

reveal any underlying dimensions of the construct that may not have been specified *a priori*. At this stage, factor analysis is also useful for weeding out items that are weak—meaning that certain items may not correlate strongly with other items and fail to load significantly onto any one factor. Because health-promotion research is theory based, it typically involves the administration of questionnaires that comprise multiple measurement scales or indexes. Being able to reduce the number of items of any one scale or index without compromising validity or reliability is a distinct advantage.

Applying Theory to Health Behaviors

Understanding Health Behaviors

As mentioned in the beginning of this chapter, a discipline advances when new evidence is collected to either support or disconfirm previously held or new views. The evidence, however, is only as good as the measurement tools used to gather it. Now that you have a foundation for what is involved in measurement of theoretical constructs, we will take it a step further and illustrate how to conduct theoretically derived basic research that can help the field advance. The objective is to provide an overview of the process so that you can apply the various theoretical perspectives to a specific health issue by incorporating what you have learned about measurement.

Imagine that you are interested in HIV/AIDS prevention. You feel passionately about working with young people and would like to understand the antecedents to condom use among adolescents aged 14–18 years. You decide that the theory of planned behavior is the theoretical perspective that you would like to use to frame your research, although there are other theories that would apply to this issue. Before you can obtain funding for implementation of a health-promotion program that will target the theoretical constructs, you need to collect data that support the application of the theory to one specific health behavior: condom use among adolescents.

The nature of this research is **observational**, meaning that the variables involved will be observed as they exist in nature—no manipulation of variables will occur (as opposed to **experimental research**). Thus; the research design used can be **cross-sectional**, **successive independent samples**, or **longitudinal**. A cross-sectional design is one in which measurement is conducted at a single time point; this design precludes the ability to establish the temporal order of relationships implied by the theory, and so causality cannot be ascertained. Successive independent samples is a design that incorporates multiple cross-sectional studies over successive time points using an independent sample for each time point. This design is an improvement over cross-sectional designs; however, it has similar limitations and is best for documenting trends in knowledge, attitudes, beliefs, or behaviors. A longitudinal design follows the same sample over a period of time and conducts measurements more than once; thus, temporal ordering of certain occurrences can be assessed, but causality is still precluded. Longitudinal designs are very costly and subject to attrition. Thus, for the purposes of your research, although a longitudinal design is most appropriate, given your resources and time limits, a cross-sectional design can still provide the necessary information.

Now that you have chosen an appropriate research design and you have worked out other logistical issues, such as gaining access to your sample and recruiting your sample, you begin to construct your questionnaire. Fortunately, your review of the existing research literature reveals that previous psychometric work has been conducted with your target population. You are able to locate measures of the theoretical constructs that have been used previously and these measures have published psychometric data, so you can determine that they are reliable, valid, and are relevant to your target population.

You review the measures and ascertain that all items constituting each measure are on an ordinal scale; however, you rationalize that if individual items are summed and a total score is calculated for each measure, then you can treat the ordinal variables as interval. You are then able to calculate means and standard deviations and perform correlational analyses. In addition to the measurement of the theoretical variables, you also create an item that measures actual condom-use behavior using a ratio scale (e.g., "In the past 3 months, how many times did you use a condom when you had sex?").

Once the data are collected, you are faced with the statistical analysis. You may recall from Chapter 5 that it is possible that something such as "thinking about statistics" can evoke fear in some (see **FIGURE 14-7**); however, if the process is broken down into several simple steps, it is much less scary.

First, you must perform a reliability analysis of the scale measures to ensure adequate reliability. Then, calculate descriptive statistics (means, standard deviations, and other measures of central tendency) and examine the data for violations of normality. The best approach for your data would be to conduct a multivariate analysis where

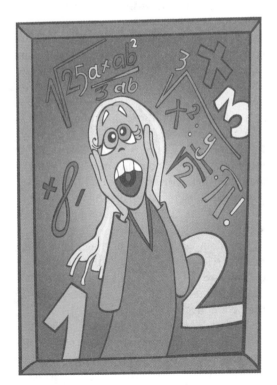

FIGURE 14-7 Fear of statistics
© Igor Zakowski/Shutterstock

you can assess the specified relationships among the theoretical constructs.

Referring back to your chosen theory, it is helpful to first specify the role of each of the constructs. Attitudes, subjective norms, perceived control, and intentions are all deemed predictor variables because they are hypothesized to cause or precede the specified outcome, which, in this example, is the health behavior "condom use." The theory also asserts that attitudes, subjective norms, and perceived control predict intentions. Intentions, in turn are related to actual behavior. Consequently, because intentions come between the other theoretical constructs and the behavioral outcome, intentions are deemed a mediating variable.

The main outcome variable, condom use, is measured using a ratio scale; thus, one possibility would be to use linear regression to analyze the data. The mediating variable, intentions, is viewed as an interval variable as well; thus, linear regression is also appropriate when testing intentions as the outcome. The first equation would entail regressing intentions on the three predictor variables: attitudes, subjective norms, and perceived control. If the variables account for a significant amount of variance (known and represented as R2), then there is partial support for the theory. Also, the regression weights will determine which of the predictors contributed to predicting condom-use intention. This is an important step because, although collectively the set of predictors may be related to condom intentions, it is possible that not all of the individual predictors are significant in the equation. The predictors that are significant should be targeted by the health-promotion program. The second regression equation would entail regressing condom-use behavior on intentions. A significant relation would provide the other piece of evidence to confirm the utility of applying this theory to the understanding of adolescents and their condom-use behaviors.

An excellent example of this type of observational research was conducted by Malek, Umberger, Makrides, and ShaoJia (2017). In their study, they examined the theory of planned behavior (TPB) in predicting intentions to

consume a healthy diet during pregnancy and actual food consumption behavior. The study described the measures for the TPB constructs in terms of number of items, the wording for the items (can be examined for face and content validity), the response format (e.g., Likert-type), how the scale was scored, and the internal reliability estimate for each scale (i.e., Cronbach's alpha). Their measures had satisfactory reliability and they appeared to be valid measures. Their analyses centered on identifying the significant theoretical variables and the amount of variance accounted for by the theoretical variables. They found that attitudes, subjective norms, and perceived behavior control were significant predictors of intentions to use condoms. Furthermore, the TPB variables accounted for a significant proportion of variance (66%) in healthy eating behavioral intentions. In the model that assessed actual food consumption, they found that the TPB constructs collectively explained only 3.4% of total variance in adherence to food group recommendations. The authors nonetheless suggested that their study provided support for TPB in explaining healthy eating intentions among this population and can serve as a starting point for a future health-promotion intervention.

Alternatively, a second, more complicated but advantageous way to analyze your data would be to perform a path analysis using structural equation modeling (SEM) techniques. Path analysis is a technique to assess the direct causal contribution of one variable to another and, by using SEM techniques, the full model can be considered as a system of equations that can estimate the coefficients directly. You begin by specifying your model and using a covariance matrix as input. In this example, the model is the articulation of the theory of planned behavior as applied to health eating behavior. To illustrate, the model is shown in **FIGURE 14-8**.

Attitudes, subjective norms, and perceived control are deemed **exogenous variables**, which are analogous to predictor or independent variables; intentions hold a dual role of being both an exogenous and an **endogenous variable**, and as such are also deemed a **mediator** variable. Endogenous variables correspond to criterion,

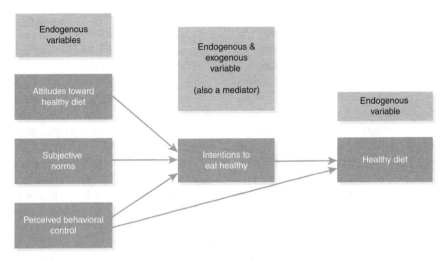

FIGURE 14-8 Path model of the theory of planned behavior as applied to healthy diet among pregnant women

dependent, or outcome variables depending on the research design (i.e., observational or experimental). Healthy diet, the behavioral variable, is also an endogenous variable. As shown in Figure 14-8, the exogenous variables are hypothesized to have direct effects on intentions and indirect effects on eating healthy through intentions, while intentions directly affect healthy diet behavior. Perceived behavioral control is also hypothesized to affect healthy diet directly. Statistical estimates are made for each path and are interpreted as regression coefficients. Estimates of both the direct and indirect effects, as well as their significance, are calculated in addition to indicators of model fit.

When it comes to determining the appropriateness of applying a particular theory to a specified behavior within a specified population, path analysis using SEM is a much more thorough and sophisticated approach than regular multiple linear regression. SEM can identify how well your theoretical model fits your data, in this instance it can determine the significance of an indirect effect, and it can calculate the amount of variance accounted for by your model while it pinpoints which paths are significant. It does of course have its limitations; however, for observational research that implies causality, this is the recommended approach. In fact, Record (2017) used this approach to test the applicability

of TPB constructs to predict compliance with tobacco-free policies on college campuses (i.e., not smoking on campus). She found the model to be a good fit to the data. All three TPB constructs, attitudes, subjective norms, and perceived behavioral control, were significant predictors of intentions to comply with the policy. Moreover, intentions and perceived behavioral control showed significant direct effects on compliance with the policy.

Intervening with Health Behaviors

Once enough evidence has been generated toward understanding a particular health behavior among a specific population, it may be an appropriate time to intervene. Continuing with the example of complying with tobacco-free policies on college campuses, you could use previous observational and, if available, other intervention research, combined with your own observational research, to develop a preventive intervention that would target compliance. You would create a program that would incorporate activities to target those theoretical mediating factors that were found to be significant direct and/or indirect predictors of not smoking on campus and that are also modifiable. Your intervention could be tested for its effectiveness using either an **experimental** or **quasi-experimental**

design. Experimental designs entail the manipulation of a variable and randomization to test the effects of the manipulation on some outcome; quasi-experimental designs approximate experimental designs, but do not use randomization. Thus, in this instance, manipulation of the variable would mean the implementation of a health-promotion program and the outcomes of interest would be both the theoretical mediators and the health behavior. For example, Cameron et al., (2015) developed, implemented, and tested an online theory-based intervention to promote healthy lifestyle behaviors (avoiding smoking, exercise, fruit and vegetable intake and avoiding alcohol use) in new university students in the United Kingdom. Theory-based messages were developed to encourage adequate fruit and vegetable intake and regular exercise, and to discourage binge drinking and smoking. The messages were developed on the basis of formative work and were designed to target several theoretical mediators such as beliefs, subjective norms, and perceived behavioral control to engage in each of the four behaviors. To determine whether this intervention was effective in changing the targeted theoretical mediators, the following measures were implemented in a questionnaire:

> Single-item measures of social cognitive variables for each behaviour were included. Intentions (e.g., 'Do you intend to avoid smoking at university?') were measured at all three time points. Affective attitudes (e.g., 'Smoking at university would be... unpleasant/pleasant'), cognitive attitudes (e.g., 'Smoking at university would be... harmful/beneficial'), subjective norms (e.g., 'Most people who are important to me think I should/should not smoke at university'), descriptive norms (e.g., 'Most students will avoid smoking at university'), self-efficacy (e.g., 'If I wanted, I could easily avoid smoking at university'), perceived control (e.g., 'How much control do you have over whether or not you avoid smoking at university?'), and

> planning (e.g., 'To what extent do you have a clear plan of how to avoid smoking at university?') were assessed at the 1- and 6-month follow-ups.

(Cameron et al., 2017)

The results of their randomized controlled trial (a type of experimental design) indicated that the intervention had a nonsignificant effect on the primary outcomes. However, secondary analyses revealed that the intervention had significant effects on having smoked since attending university (lower number of intervention participants who smoked since starting university) and alcohol use as measured by a biomarker (lower level of alcohol use among intervention participants). Thus, in this example, based on the findings, using theory as the framework for an intervention approach to encourage healthy lifestyle behaviors was somewhat effective in modifying two of the measured outcomes, but perhaps needs to be more specific to one behavioral outcome to be more effective.

In sum, measurement of theoretical constructs used in health-promotion research and practice is relatively younger than and qualitatively different from measurement in the physical sciences; nonetheless, there are similar standards (i.e., precision–reliability and accuracy–validity) and both must overcome the challenge of measuring intangibles. Moreover, in both fields, there is an ever-growing need for new measures. In fact, as a whole, the field of health promotion is deficient in standardized measures that can be used widely. This may be because each theoretical construct can be applied to myriad health behaviors and to diverse populations, necessitating a different measure specific to each behavior and sometimes specific to each population. Thus, the challenge for the field is to continue to work toward developing valid and reliable measures of the many theoretical constructs used in public health research and practice and to perform psychometric evaluations of those measures with diverse populations. Furthermore, accessibility to standardized measures poses a challenge. There is an urgent need to develop a repository of valid and reliable measures such as the one created by the National Cancer

> *The challenge for the field is to continue to work toward developing valid and reliable measures of the many theoretical constructs used in public health research and practice.*

Institute (2008). Such a repository serves "to advance theory-based basic and intervention research by providing common definitions, measures, and language; increase consistency in applying many of these theoretical constructs; allow researchers to more easily incorporate theory testing and development into research; and allow applied researchers and students to make comparisons of major theoretical elements" (National Cancer Institute, 2008). Ultimately, valid and reliable measures are the cornerstone to public health research and practice. Practically speaking, without good measures, all of the theories described in this textbook would be of no real use. It would be impossible to gain a better understanding of behavior, to determine the antecedents to health behavior, to understand how to change behavior, or to evaluate which intervention activities worked when attempting to change behavior.

- Research findings should serve as the framework for designing interventions to affect the theoretical mediators of interest, and ultimately the desired health behaviors.
- Evaluation research must then be conducted to determine the effectiveness of the intervention approach in achieving goals.
- The measures are the *means* to test the theories and the measures will ultimately represent *the outcomes* of interest.
- If the measures employed are unreliable, not valid, or are inappropriate for the population, then the results may not reflect the true state of affairs.
- Good measurement is critical to the advancement of the field, as it determines what the target of our efforts will be and whether our efforts are truly having an impact.

▸ Take Home Messages

- Developing valid and reliable measures is not for the faint of heart and involves deciding what the metric will be, the level of analysis that will be administered, the mode of delivery (e.g., face-to-face interview format, paper and pencil survey), and whether it is an index or a scale.
- All newly developed measures should be put through rigorous psychometric evaluations to determine reliability and validity using diverse samples and several layers of statistical analyses.
- Once adequate measures have been devised and are available for implementation, then the next step should be conducting research that tests the theoretical constructs across different health behaviors, situations, and populations.

▸ References

Ajzen, I., & Fishbein, M. (Eds.). (1980). *Understanding attitudes and predicting social behavior*. Englewood Cliffs, NJ: Prentice-Hall.

Allport, F. H., & Allport, G. W. (1921). Personality traits: Their classification and measurement. *Journal of Abnormal and Social Psychology, 16*, 6–40.

Bandura, A. (2004). Health promotion by social cognitive means. *Health Education & Behavior, 31*, 143–164.

Cameron, D., Epton, T., Norman, P., Sheeran, P., Harris, P. R., Webb, T. L., … Shah, I. (2015). A theory-based online health behaviour intervention for new university students (U@Uni:LifeGuide): Results from a repeat randomized controlled trial. *Trials, 16*, 555. http://doi.org.ezproxy.gsu.edu/10.1186/s13063-015-1092-4

Cecil, H., & Pinkerton, S. D. (1998). Reliability and validity of a self-efficacy instrument for protective sexual behaviors. *Journal of American College Health, 47*, 113–121.

DiIorio, C. (2005). *Measurement in health behavior*. San Francisco, CA: Jossey-Bass.

Furlong, W. J., Feeny, D. H., Torrance, G. W., & Barr, R. D. (2001). The health utilities index (HUIReg.) system for assessing health-related quality of life in clinical studies. *Annals of Medicine, 33*, 375–384.

Galton, F. (1869). *Hereditary genius: An inquiry into its laws and consequences*. London, England: Macmillan.

Ghiselli, E. E., Campbell, J. P., & Zedeck, S. (1981). *Measurement theory for the behavioral sciences*. San Francisco, CA: Freeman.

Gould, S. J. (1981). *The mismeasure of man*. New York, NY: W. W. Norton.

Hathaway, S. R., & McKinley, J. C. (1940). A multiphasic personality schedule (Minnesota): I. Construction of the schedule. *Journal of Psychology: Interdisciplinary and Applied, 10*, 249–254.

Likert, R. (1932). A technique for the measurement of attitudes. *Archives of Psychology, 140*, 1–55.

Linden, K. W., & Linden, J. D. (1968). *Modern mental measurement: A historical perspective.* Boston, MA: Houghton Mifflin.

Malek, L., Umberger, W. J., Makrides, M., & ShaoJia, Z. (2017). Predicting healthy eating intention and adherence to dietary recommendations during pregnancy in Australia using the theory of planned behaviour. *Appetite, 116*, 431–441. doi:10.1016/j.appet.2017.05.028

National Cancer Institute. (2008). *Health behavior constructs: Theory, measurement and research.* Retrieved from http://dccps.cancer.gov/brp/constructs/aboutproject.html

Ogden, C. L., Carroll, M. D., Fryar, C. D., & Flegal, K. M. (2015). Prevalence of obesity among adults and youth: United States, 2011–2014. *NCHS Data Brief, 219*, 1–8.

O'Leary, A. (2001). Social–cognitive theory mediators of behavior change in the National Institute of Mental Health multisite HIV prevention trial. *Health Psychology, 20*, 369–376.

Record, R. A. (2017). Tobacco-free policy compliance behaviors among college students: A theory of planned behavior perspective. *Journal of Health Communication, 22*(7), 562–567. doi:10.1080/10810730.2017.1318984

Rosenberg, M. (1989). *Society and the adolescent self-image* (rev ed.). Middletown, CT: Wesleyan University Press.

Stevens, S. S. (1946). On the theory of scales of measurement. *Science, 103*, 677–680.

Streiner, D. L. (2003). Being inconsistent about consistency: When coefficient alpha does and doesn't matter. *Journal of Personality Assessment, 80*, 217–222.

Thurstone, L. L. (1928). Attitudes can be measured. *American Journal of Sociology, 33*, 529–554.

Zusne, L. (1975). *Names in the history of psychology: A biographical sourcebook.* New York, NY: Wiley.

Chapter Opener: © Henrik Sorensen/Getty Images; © MeskPhotography/Shutterstock; © Hero Images/Getty Images; © lzf/Shutterstock

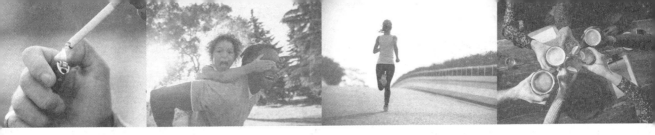

CHAPTER 15

Evaluating Theory-Based Public Health Programs: Linking Principles to Practice

Ralph J. DiClemente, Richard A. Crosby, and Laura F. Salazar

It's kind of fun to do the impossible.

—**Walt Disney**

PREVIEW

Public health promotion efforts have the potential to transform environments and social contexts, individual's attitudes, behaviors, perceptions, and, ultimately, affect rates of morbidity and early mortality, especially when appropriate theories are used. When determining whether health-promotion interventions work, we cannot rely on hope; instead, we must rely on the empirical evaluation of each and every step that constitutes the health-promotion effort. Although this evaluation effort can be labor intensive, the work is vital to the continuation and dissemination of effective programs. As a professional, one of your upmost obligations is to always determine whether your work in public health has been effective, and if so, to what degree. Indeed, as Walt Disney noted, "It's kind of fun to do the impossible"—the challenge for your work then lies in assessing the success of a program.

OBJECTIVES

1. Understand the role of evaluation research in theory-driven health-promotion programs.
2. Identify key steps in the evaluation research.
3. Distinguish between various types of evaluation research.
4. Describe the role of evaluation research during the process of program planning.
5. Understand methods of increasing the rigor and utility of evaluation research.

▶ Introduction

In the Middle Ages, it was both flawed assumptions and Biblical dogma that promoted the idea that the sun revolved around the Earth. The Earth was the center of the known universe—how could it be otherwise? This was the belief accepted by many during this time. Overturning preconceived notions about the natural world, which were based on Biblical dogma or common sense, was a daunting challenge fraught with personal peril. Consider the consequences experienced by Galileo (i.e., excommunication from the Catholic Church and imprisonment).

Throughout the ages, historical records are replete with preconceptions based on anecdote or "common sense," which have subsequently been relegated to the dustbin of empiricism. Indeed, it is axiomatic that the only real truth about "common sense" is that it is woefully uncommon. In the modern era, we have come to understand the importance of questioning our current knowledge. An analysis of how we come by our knowledge applies to determining whether health-promotion programs make a difference in enhancing health and reducing the risk of disease morbidity and mortality. Everything we know about the world is, for the most part, obtained through careful observation, meticulous documentation, and rigorous scientific methods. Thus, it stands to reason that health-promotion efforts should also be subjected to these same methods.

Much of the field of public health revolves around the development, implementation, and evaluation of programs designed to modify personal and environmental risk factors associated with adverse chronic (e.g., heart disease, diabetes, or cancer) and acute (e.g., injury, influenza, or sexually transmitted infections) health outcomes. Often, these risk factors are behaviors such as smoking; eating foods high in saturated fats, trans fats, and cholesterol; unprotected sexual intercourse; and drinking while driving. The ultimate goal of health-promotion programs is to eliminate or reduce these health-risk behaviors and encourage the adoption and maintenance of health-promoting behaviors. The elimination or reduction in health-risk behaviors may subsequently result in reductions in morbidity and early mortality; yet, without an evaluation of the health-promotion program, we cannot be sure of its impact and whether it was successful in achieving targeted outcomes.

Although the development and implementation of innovative health-promotion programs are at the core of the field, so too is the need to systematically evaluate health-promotion programs. In many ways, program evaluation can be viewed as the lifeblood of any health-promotion program. Program evaluation is the systematic application of scientific methods to assess the design, implementation, improvement, or outcomes of a program (Rossi & Freeman, 1993). The term "program" may include any organized action, such as media campaigns, service provision, educational services, public policies, and research projects (Centers for Disease Control and Prevention [CDC], 1999).

Program evaluation requires rigorous methodological strategies to assess whether programs are actually effective in promoting the desired changes in health-risk behaviors (i.e., eliminating or reducing them). Without appropriate research designs and strategies, it is difficult to evaluate whether health-promotion programs are meeting their stated objectives of modifying health-risk and health-protective behaviors.

A good way to begin thinking about program evaluation is to be reminded about phases five through eight in the PRECEDE–PROCEED model that was presented in Chapter 3. Recall that the key aspect of implementation (phase 5) is process evaluation (phase 6), which is also known as quality assurance. Further, impact evaluation (phase 7) shows the intermediate effect of a program with the final phase, outcome evaluation (phase 8), examining whether the program had a long-term effect on reducing incidence of disease or premature mortality. In addition, in our current cost-constrained environment, there is an increasing emphasis on program accountability and the need for demonstrated programmatic efficacy. Thus, outcome evaluations that demonstrate programmatic efficacy are critical to justify the continued expenditure of fiscal and social

Outcome evaluations that demonstrate programmatic efficacy are critical to justify the continued expenditure of fiscal and social resources to support the existence and expansion of health-promotion programs.

resources to support the existence and expansion of health-promotion programs and for informing public health policy.

Assessment of programmatic efficacy is critical to identifying evidence-based interventions and, thus, indispensable for advancing the science of health promotion. Clearly, program evaluation as a core concept is central to the field; however, what research designs and methods are appropriate to optimize program evaluation is not as clear. Although seemingly simple in theory, how best to conduct rigorous program evaluations to assess programmatic efficacy is, in fact, not simple in practice. Indeed, program evaluation can be a daunting challenge, often confusing new, as well as established, researchers and practitioners in the field.

This chapter provides an overview of program evaluation and the methods used to evaluate health-promotion programs. The chapter also provides students and professionals with an understanding of the knowledge base: an array of methods and diverse skills useful in evaluating the efficacy of health-promotion programs. In addition, we recognize that for some readers this may be their initial exposure to program evaluation or research methods, whereas others may have ample exposure and experience in the evaluation of health-promotion programs. To bridge the chasm between those with limited exposure and experience and those with considerable exposure and experience, we briefly describe the logic of scientific research (Crosby, DiClemente, & Salazar, 2006). Some readers may find this redundant, whereas others will be newly exposed to these concepts. In either case, we feel confident that both new and experienced program evaluators will glean some value from this synoptic review. Finally, to assist you

in acquiring these fundamental concepts, we illustrate program evaluation methods and concepts from our own research as well as that of others.

Before we begin in earnest, we need to explicitly address the unorthodoxy of including a program evaluation chapter in a theory book. Certainly it's not typical—just examine the table of contents from a random sample of theory books and chances are none include a chapter on program evaluation. This examination then begs the question: Why a chapter on program evaluation?

As you will see, we recognize the integration between theory and evaluation; they are braided, intimately related, and inseparable. From our perspective, designing, implementing, and evaluating a health-promotion program is inextricably tied to the underlying theoretical framework or models that informed the design and implementation of the health-promotion program. This chapter takes a holistic view of health promotion, one that sees the inherent value in linking different aspects of health-promotion theory, practice, and research. Program evaluation represents the "research" aspect of this triad. Developing program evaluation research objectives first involves identifying the theoretical constructs that should be measured. These theoretical constructs are the hypothesized determinants, personal and environmental, that are expected to change as a function of exposure to the health-promotion program. A brief illustration may help elucidate this point (see **BOX 15-1**).

The question posed in Box 15.1 typifies the challenges faced by person engaged in program evaluation. Fortunately, theory can be employed to aid you in meeting this challenge. There are almost an infinite number of constructs that could reasonably be included in the evaluation assessment. However, if you are familiar with the underlying theory guiding the development of the motivational DVD, then it is easier to identify the constructs that should be assessed as you develop your evaluation instrument. The same theoretical constructs that are hypothesized to mediate medication adherence in the health-promotion

---

BOX 15-1 What to Measure in an Evaluation of a Type 2 Diabetes Program

Let's say that a local clinic has asked you to evaluate a new health-promotion program that has the expressed goal of increasing medication adherence among adults with type 2 diabetes. Clearly, this is an important topic that warrants a careful and rigorous evaluation. The program involves exposure to a theory-based motivational DVD that encourages medication adherence. The theory underlying the DVD (the new health-promotion program) and a meticulous review of the empirical literature suggests that targeting key psychosocial determinants, such as enhancing perceived peer norms about medication adherence, increasing perceived self-efficacy to take their medication, increasing adults' knowledge about the benefits of regular medication use and the health threats associated with sporadic adherence, and changing beliefs and attitudes about the benefits of medication use will be an effective approach. In this example, the underlying theory has delineated key determinants, corroborated by a thorough review of the empirical literature, that are hypothesized to be associated with medication adherence; the DVD was developed to target these determinants.

Let's assume that you decide to implement a randomized controlled trial design and you randomly sample and randomize 200 adults attending the clinic using a 1:1 allocation ratio to the (1) usual care condition, or (2) the usual care condition plus the motivational DVD. You propose a pre-post-test design, with baseline data collected before random assignment to the study conditions and follow-up data collected 6 months after program exposure.

A key question: Which constructs do you include in the pretest and posttest assessments?

Program evaluation is never divorced from the underlying intervention theory and is, indeed, inextricably dependent on it.

program are the same ones that need to be targeted for inclusion in any assessment measuring program efficacy. Thus, when we use the term "program evaluation," we are really implying theory-driven program evaluation. Program evaluation is never divorced from the underlying intervention theory and is, indeed, inextricably dependent on it.

integrity intrinsic in the evaluation process. Ultimately, there is only one scientific method, which forms the basis for guiding careful and deliberate observation, meticulous documentation, and rigorous evaluation present in both research and program evaluation.

Evaluation Is Theory Driven

Perhaps the key assumption in theory-driven health-promotion evaluation is that theory was used to design the health-promotion program, and therefore, theory will guide the evaluation objectives. In health promotion, the different theories used to explain and change health behaviors assert that there are a variety of influences that affect disease acquisition and health: (1) personal cognitions, (2) the social network, and (3) the physical environment.

Let's assume that you have been asked to evaluate an exercise promotion program for older, sedentary adults. We know that lifestyle factors, such as lack of physical activity, may increase the risk of an adverse health outcome (e.g., heart attack). In this case, older adults' attitudes toward exercise, knowledge of the benefits of exercise, knowledge of the different types of exercises, perceived

▶ Key Concepts

Is Program Evaluation the Same as Research?

An overarching misperception is that research, with its strict methodology and statistical analysis, is rigorous, while program evaluation is a second-class science. This perception, however, is false and unjustly underestimates the scientific

ability to exercise, belief that exercising will offer some health-promotion benefit, and perceptions of exercise as normative among similar older adults in their community are all personal cognitions that may affect their willingness to exercise. Likewise, having a social network of friends who do not reinforce exercise as a health-promoting behavior may impede one's willingness to engage in exercise. And, finally, residing in a community that has limited access to golf courses, parks, running trails, or safe walking trails/areas may also militate the likelihood that a person will increase their physical activity.

From an ecological perspective, we now understand, at least in a cursory manner, the diverse array of factors (individual, social, and environmental) that may affect an individual's exercise behavior. As such, the exercise health-promotion program will be theory based in that it will target those factors identified theoretically as being associated with exercise behavior. Theory-driven evaluation assumes that changes to the personal cognitions, social networks, and/or physical environment will result in changes in exercise behavior. A graphical depiction of a health-promotion program is a **logic model**, which we present in **FIGURE 15-1**. Logic models are useful and should always be used to guide the program evaluation.

As shown in the figure, participation (exposure) in the health-promotion program is expected to produce changes in several hypothesized mediators such as personal cognitions, social network, and/or the physical environment, which, in turn, should result in a change to the health-promoting behavior (i.e., an increase in physical activity). Thus, one assumption in public health practice and research is that there is a direct, linear relationship between exposure to the program, its effect on hypothesized mediators, corresponding changes in the health-promoting behavior (i.e., exercise), and ultimately the outcome (i.e., reduced risk of a heart attack). In the logic model, we assume that increasing exercise will translate to health benefits, such as a reduction in heart disease.

Program Planning Is the Starting Point of Evaluation

Contrary to popular belief, evaluation should not be an afterthought. Instead, the evaluation process should be *a priori* versus *posteriori*; that is, it should begin at the initial stage of program planning. Program planning begins with stating the goals and objectives of the program. Program goals are broad statements describing what the program (intervention) is designed to accomplish. For example, a program addressing intentional injury may have a goal to reduce the number of deaths due to handguns, or a program on unintentional injuries may have a goal of limiting or delaying the involvement of youth in motor vehicle crashes. **Program objectives** are specific aims needed to accomplish **program goals**. Objectives should be SMART; the acronym "SMART" is a helpful mnemonic device in which each letter represents a key aspect of appropriately constructed objectives.

SMART objectives, as noted in **BOX 15-2**, should include all of the following: the time period for expected changes, the specific direction of change that is expected, and how the change will be measured. In addition, objectives must be realistic and appropriate for the target population, precise in defining the behavior to be changed,

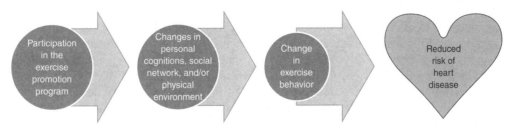

FIGURE 15-1 Logic model of a healthy heart program

BOX 15-2 Characteristics of Program Objectives

SMART objectives are:
S = Specific
M = Measurable
A = Appropriate
R = Realistic
T = Time bound

---

and measurable in terms of health outcomes (Green & Kreuter, 2005).

To achieve an effective alignment between the program objectives and the specific needs of the target audience, a thorough assessment of the needs of the targeted community should occur first. A **community needs assessment** is a data-gathering process that can be time consuming but is nonetheless essential to program planning. The assessment may involve simple data-gathering activities, such as determining the number of publicly available community recreation facilities (both indoor and outdoor) that exist within the defined geographic regions of the community. The data gathering, however, becomes a bit more complex when you expand efforts to determine, for example, how many people use each facility, how frequently they use each facility, or the barriers to using the facilities. The needs assessment may then also include a determination of what types of new facilities community members would like to see built so as to increase their physical activity levels or how improvements to the community could be made to enhance walkability and be more user friendly for cyclists.

Every needs assessment will have quite different goals and, thus, it is the task of the needs assessor to decide what should be measured when taking this type of inventory. The guiding principle, however, is to always gauge what community members think in addition to existing services, structures, laws, policies, etc. We encourage you to learn more about community needs assessments by reading *A Practical Guide to Needs Assessment* by Sleezer, Russ, and Gupta (2014).

A final note about program planning is warranted at this juncture: it is critically important that you develop a detailed evaluation plan *before* the program is implemented. In general terms, evaluation of a health-promotion program involves a determination of whether the specific goals and stated objectives of the program have been met. This typically involves assessing whether the health-promotion program reached its target audience, whether it was implemented with fidelity, and comparing applicable measures of psychosocial mediators (see Chapter 14 regarding measurement) and health behaviors before and after exposure to the health-promotion program. By planning for the evaluation during the program planning phase, we can anticipate exactly what should be evaluated while conducting the needs assessment and while developing the specific program objectives. Subsequently, relevant data can be collected at every step to inform the evaluation. Conversely, if the evaluation plan comes into the picture after the fact, then a critical opportunity is missed for collecting and analyzing data in accordance with the specified goals and stated objectives of the program. The true impact of a program may not be fully detectable without building in a thorough and theory-driven evaluation during the program planning phase.

> *The true impact of a program may not be fully detectable without building in a thorough and theory-driven evaluation during the program planning phase.*

Integrate Evaluation Questions into Program Objectives

Part of a successful impact or outcome evaluation is a clear statement of measurable objectives from which relevant measurements and subsequent comparisons can be drawn. Therefore, sound evaluation questions should be developed based on objectives constructed early in the planning process. For example, with regard to adolescent norms regarding reckless or drunk driving, an objective might be to increase by 50% the proportion of high school students who hold unfavorable attitudes toward reckless or drunk driving. Evaluation questions might include, "Does the target audience think driving drunk is frowned upon or altogether unacceptable?" This question could be used to develop specific survey questions in the assessment and evaluation plan, such as, "Do you approve or disapprove of people who drive while drunk?" Similar questions could also be developed for an objective related to a behavioral outcome. If the objective is to decrease by 30% the number of targeted high school students who drive a vehicle under the influence of alcohol, then the specific survey question used in the evaluation plan might be, "During the past 30 days, how many times did you drive a car or other vehicle when you had been drinking alcohol?"

Develop a Comprehensive Evaluation Framework

A sound evaluation plan needs to have a framework: a plan for evaluating implementation objectives (process evaluation), a plan for evaluating impact objectives, targeted health outcomes (outcome evaluation), and procedures for managing and monitoring the assessment or evaluation. An evaluation framework helps to organize the evaluation process, to identify what to evaluate, to formulate questions to be answered in the evaluation, and the time frame for the evaluation.

A plan for evaluating the dosage and fidelity of the planned program (process evaluation) typically involves identifying the type of information needed, such as the number of sessions participants attended, quality control checks of activities, the sources of that information (e.g., sign-in sheets by session or independent raters of activities), the time frame for collecting the information, and the methods for collecting the information. A plan for conducting impact and outcome evaluations often focuses on number of participants to ensure adequate statistical power to detect program effects, participation rates, theoretically derived assessment instruments, how data will be collected, the number of data collection points, the research design (i.e., pre-post comparison group design) and specifies *a priori* applicable methods for data analysis. Procedures for managing and monitoring the evaluation include training staff to collect all sources of data in a reliable and valid manner, and developing a timeline for collecting, analyzing, and reporting findings.

Differentiate Between Types of Evaluation

There are two methods for categorizing evaluations in the literature. The first is based on when an evaluation is conducted. If the evaluation is conducted before the program begins, then it is known as formative evaluation. If the evaluation occurs after the program ends, then it is known as summative evaluation. The latter method is based on which objectives the evaluation is attempting to measure (process, impact, and outcome). Of note, although process evaluation can occur in both program development and implementation phases, impact and outcome evaluation occurs only in the program implementation phase.

> *Although process evaluation can occur in both program development and implementation phases, impact and outcome evaluation occurs only in the program implementation phase.*

Formative Versus Summative Evaluation

The term "formative" means to assist in the formation of new information, while the term "summative" means the summing up of the effects of a program. The two terms are used often in the health-promotion literature. Although different, both are important to the design and evaluation of a program. Formative evaluation is designed to produce data and information used to improve a health-promotion program during the developmental phase and document the feasibility of program implementation (Windsor, Clark, Boyd, & Goodman, 2003). Although the methods used to conduct a formative evaluation are similar to those used in conducting a needs assessment, the purpose is different. A formative evaluation addresses short-term objectives and is used often in pilot testing or field testing of programs (Windsor et al., 2003). Formative evaluation provides a method to study activities undertaken during the design and initial testing of the program to guide the process (Rossi & Freeman, 1993). Typically, formative evaluation is qualitative in nature and is often conducted using small groups of people to pretest various components of the program during its developmental stages. Depending on the goals of the formative evaluation, the methods for formative evaluation can be one or more of the following: observation, in-depth interviews, surveys, focus groups, analysis, reports, and dialogue with participants (Crosby et al., 2006). Formative evaluation is an important tool for ensuring program success. Although it is challenging to conduct formative evaluations with limited time and tight budgets, it is critical for a health-promotion program to achieve its objectives more effectively.

In contrast to formative evaluation, summative evaluation is designed to produce data and information on the program's efficacy or effectiveness (its ability to do what it was designed to do) during its implementation phase. Summative evaluation is considered a method of judging the worth of a program after the program is developed and implemented. It is typically quantitative in nature, using numerical scores to assess participants' achievement (e.g., behavior change or health status change).

Process, Impact, and Outcome Evaluation

There are three important areas often referred to in summative evaluation. These three areas provide a comprehensive approach to measuring what is happening in the program because each has a different purpose. Also, each evaluation area is considered important; however, their contributing level of importance may vary. We depict these three evaluation areas in a pyramid of importance as shown in **FIGURE 15-2**.

Process evaluation focuses on how a program was implemented and operates. It is designed to document the degree to which the intervention program was implemented as intended by assessing how much of the intervention was provided (dosage), to whom, when (timing), and by whom. It answers the question, "Was the intervention put into place as planned, and what alterations were required for implementation?" In clinical terms, a process evaluation can be called a quality assurance review. Process evaluation is often conducted prior to program implementation and can help with improving the program before a full-scale implementation; however, if conducted during implementation, process evaluation can reveal pertinent information that will answer questions during the impact or outcome evaluation. Thus, process evaluation is extremely valuable throughout the entire lifecycle of a program.

Impact evaluation assesses whether exposure to the health-promotion program resulted in some measurable change. Often, impact evaluation comprises measurement of the theoretical mediators and related health behaviors. However, we purposefully differentiate the two types of measures. Clearly, determining the impact of participation in a health-promotion program on relevant health behaviors is vitally important and directly relevant to assessing the value or worth of the program. Often, however, program evaluators are confronted with severely limited fiscal resources and time constraints. Thus, it may not

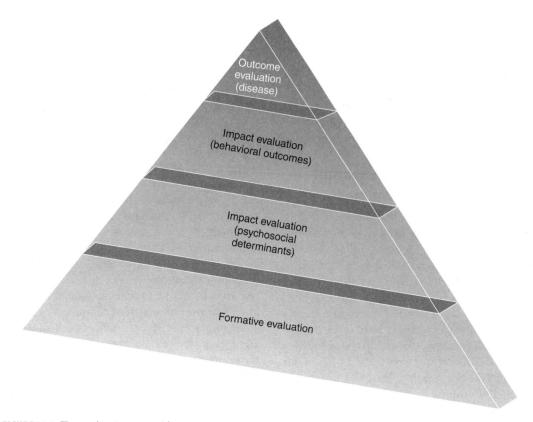

FIGURE 15-2 The evaluation pyramid

be feasible to assess behavior changes as a function of program participation. In these instances, evaluators will often assess changes in the theoretically derived determinants associated with relevant health or risk behaviors—when framed in a logic model, these determinants are considered the mediators of health and risk behaviors (see Chapter 2). Referring back to the logic model (see Figure 15-1), you see that changes in attitudes, knowledge, beliefs, and perceived norms are hypothesized to be associated with subsequent changes in relevant health or risk behaviors. Thus, it is through the manipulation (changing) of these mediators that you can promote change in relevant health and risk behaviors associated with disease outcomes. In our ongoing example, we can evaluate whether participation in an exercise enhancement program leads to changes in knowledge of and attitudes toward exercise, perceived norms about exercise, and beliefs that engaging in exercise behaviors will be heart healthy.

As shown in Figure 15-2, the second component of an impact evaluation assesses changes in actual health behaviors. Continuing with our example, we assume that changing the risk of a heart attack requires modifying behavioral risk factors predictive of them—in this case, increasing physical activity or conversely, reducing sedentary lifestyle behaviors (refer back to the logic model in shown in Figure 15-1). If one objective of the exercise enhancement program is to increase exercise behavior, then this behavior becomes an important outcome for assessing program impact. Following our logic model, we assume that exposure to the exercise enhancement program results in favorable changes in relevant mediators (personal cognition, social networks, or physical environment), which will theoretically translate into increased physical activity. Thus, comparing measurement of physical activity prior to participation in the exercise enhancement program (pre-test) and after participation (post-test) will yield a quantitative assessment of the program's impact on this key behavior. One side note; using a representative sample of the community for your evaluation study would further strengthen the confidence in your results.

Outcome Evaluation (Assessing Change in Health Outcomes)

In an outcome evaluation, we are interested in assessing whether participation in the health-promotion program resulted not only in health-protective changes in the mediators and relevant health behaviors; however, it is of utmost interest to know whether there is also a demonstrable change in the targeted health outcome. As health-promotion practitioners and researchers, it is the health outcomes that we are trying to affect through development of and participation in our programs. The changes in disease acquisition represent the so-called hard outcomes of program evaluation. Although eminently desirable, most program evaluations do not include "hard" disease measures as an outcome because some disease outcomes manifest over long periods of time (e.g., heart disease or lung cancer) or because the rate of some disease outcomes, although problematic from a public health perspective, are too low to detect changes in the population served (e.g., HIV infection). Including disease outcomes in this level of program evaluation would require suitably large sample sizes followed over extended periods of time to ascertain whether program participation actually resulted in a lower incidence of disease.

Continuing with our example, participation in the exercise enhancement program is considered vital to reduce the risk of a heart attack. Thus, we conduct our impact evaluation and observe statistically significant changes in health behaviors for individuals exposed to the program (e.g., increases in physical activity relevant to a comparison group) and in the mediators hypothesized to be related to these health behaviors. These outcomes can be readily obtained with a relatively limited sample size and a modest follow-up period, especially given that both sets of impact measures can be assessed using scales or indexes (e.g., number of hours engaged in vigorous physical activity per week) that permit the use of quantitative analytic methods. To assess actual health status as a result of program participation would require a very large sample followed over many years to observe differences in the incidence of heart attack; unfortunately, program evaluations do not typically have the resources to recruit an adequate sample or to follow them over an extended follow-up period to assess monitoring the occurrence of a disease endpoint. However, one alternative could be whether the exercise program produced a clinically meaningful decline in a biologically assessed risk factor for heart attacks, such as serum cholesterol level, blood pressure, or obesity levels. Thus, as we will describe in the next section, one quest of outcome evaluation is to identify valid markers of altered physiology, suggesting a meaningful delay in the onset of disease.

> *One quest of outcome evaluation is to identify valid markers of altered physiology, suggesting a meaningful delay in the onset of disease.*

All Evaluation Data Are Not Created Equal

As we discussed previously, there are few program evaluations in which a measured endpoint is an actual health or disease. This is, in fact, not an atypical situation in program evaluation. However, in the past decade, we maintain that there has been a biological revolution, so to speak. We are becoming increasingly aware of biological risk indicators (i.e., disease markers such as C-reactive protein as a marker for high risk of myocardial infarction) for disease and how to measure these indicators in increasingly noninvasive ways. This has led to the possibility of selecting surrogate biological endpoints in the absence of actual disease endpoints. There has been great interest recently in using surrogate endpoints, which are laboratory measurements or physical signs used as a substitute for a clinically meaningful endpoint that measures directly how a person feels, functions, or survives, such as changes in cholesterol level, blood pressure, A1c levels for diabetics, or decreased viral load measures for evaluating treatments for HIV/AIDS. Changes induced by the health-promotion program on a surrogate endpoint are hypothesized to reflect changes in a clinically meaningful endpoint (i.e., actual disease progression).

Continuing again with our example, suppose we are unable to measure disease status (i.e., heart attack incidence) among adult men as the outcome for our evaluation endpoint. However, increasing physical activity (exercise) is hypothesized to lead to improvement in a host of health indicators; in particular, lower levels of LDL cholesterol. Following our logic model, we assume that increased physical activity (vigorous exercise) may result in lowering high LDL levels, which in turn may lead to an improvement in disease outcome (i.e., lower risk of heart attack). Thus, in the absence of actual measurement of disease outcomes, we can ascertain changes in LDL levels relatively simply and inexpensively as a proxy or surrogate marker for the disease outcome. Thus, surrogate markers (proxy markers) provide an objective and quantifiable biological measure that is in the hypothesized pathway between relevant health behavior and the disease outcome.

▶ A Step-by-Step Guide to Effective Evaluation

Whatever you do, do it well. Do it so well that when people see you do it they will want to come back see you do it again and they will want to bring others and show them how well you do what you do.

—Walt Disney

The term "rigor" indicates a high level of quality in all elements of a research study. It is a prized aspect of evaluation research. Rigor can be conceptualized on a continuum—it exists (or fails to exist) in varying degrees. Although no evaluation is perfect, evaluation research can have a high degree of rigor. Here we invoke an important principle of program evaluation: as rigor increases, confidence in the findings increases. Consequently, studies with greater rigor may have a greater likelihood of the findings being utilized by program planners and policy experts and, thus, have a greater likelihood of substantively impacting public health policy and health-promotion practice.

Scientific rigor, like ancient Rome, is built brick-by-brick. Fortunately, there are well-established guidelines based on many years of applying the scientific method. Although some of these guidelines may appear tedious, they are all essential. Following the steps to scientific rigor sequentially is equally important. In this next section of the chapter, we build upon what you have learned already and provide an overview of the process for enhancing rigor in evaluation research.

The Nine-Step Stairway to Effective Evaluation

Step 1: Defining the research population. Because "population" is a broad term that can be defined in many different ways, it is up to the evaluation researcher to specify the parameters that describe the target population. Often, the population parameters are already defined by the organization for which an evaluation is being conducted. For example, a local Boys & Girls Club would like assistance in evaluating the efficacy of a new program designed to increase the consumption of fruits and vegetables among low-income youth, ages 14–18 years, who are utilizing their facilities. In this case, the target population is well parameterized (i.e., age of participants, their socioeconomic status (SES) level, and where they will be

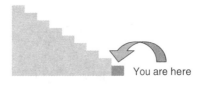

You are here

recruited have been clearly defined). On the other hand, researchers may implement and assess new and innovative health-promotion programs among new populations. Selection of the target population can be based on a number of factors, including using the results of a needs assessment of the targeted community and population and the known **epidemiology** (i.e., the scientific discipline studying the distribution of disease in human populations) of the disease or health-risk behavior under consideration.

Step 2: Identifying stakeholders and collaborators. The second step, and perhaps one of the most important, involves a thorough and inclusive identification of all parties involved with the program and those who will be affected by the evaluation. We cannot emphasize enough the importance of this step. Whether the evaluator is internal or external to the organization implementing the program does not matter.

Taking the time to put forth a concerted effort to identify all relevant parties will ensure that the evaluation runs smoothly and will be as rigorous as possible. Input from stakeholders is critical to the success of the evaluation. If all relevant stakeholders are not identified and are either inadvertently or intentionally precluded from the planning process, then there is a good likelihood that the evaluation will be a failure. In fact, one of the authors conducted a program evaluation of a dating violence prevention program developed by a community-based organization (CBO) that was implemented in a juvenile justice system. The program was tailored for African-American, male, adjudicated adolescents; however, one secondary goal was for the program representative to try and surreptitiously affect the attitudes and norms of the system personnel. After a year of planning the evaluation with the CBO, the evaluation was started. Unfortunately, after several months, we noticed a significant drop in the number of adolescents being referred to the program. The program representative made some inquiries. He was able to ascertain that the probation officers were upset because we did not consult with them about the evaluation, nor did we inform them that we were doing an evaluation; they indicated that because we were using an experimental design where some adolescents would be randomized into a wait-list control group, they decided not to make any more referrals. They did not want any of the youths to miss out on much-needed service programs during this critical period of probation. Fortunately, damage control was possible. A meeting with all the probation officers was convened to rectify the situation. A compromise was reached where the wait-list period was significantly shortened to 2 weeks versus 3 months and referrals resumed. This story highlights how including pertinent stakeholders in the process is critical for a successful and productive program evaluation. Thus, develop a plan for incorporating this important step, and be open-minded and willing to compromise to accommodate the needs and issues of all relevant parties when designing the evaluation. The take-home message here is that collaboration is key: collaborate, and then collaborate, and finally collaborate even more!

Step 3: Defining the evaluation objective. This third step is the linchpin for the remainder of the research process. As a rule, narrow and precisely defined goals are far more amenable to rigorous research designs than broadly defined goals and vague questions. At times, new evaluators propose goals and research questions that are too broad to be addressed with ample scientific rigor. Specificity should be the goal here. An effective strategy to avoid the pitfall of ambiguity is to thoroughly review the relevant empirical literature for previous evaluation studies. This can be a time-consuming process, but it is nonetheless time well spent. Engaging in a meticulous review

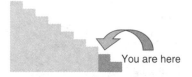
You are here

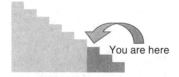
You are here

of the empirical literature will inevitably yield different methodological paths that other evaluation researchers have trodden to address their goals. For new evaluators, an understanding of what research has already been undertaken represents an important opportunity to build on and extend the evaluation literature and to utilize new methodological approaches to reaching the evaluation objective. Stated explicitly, this is a critical step that cannot be overlooked—there are no shortcuts.

Once the literature review is complete, an evaluation objective can be articulated. As we stated previously, the evaluation objective is a general statement that conveys the purpose of the planned study in precise terms. For example, "To determine the efficacy of providing behavioral interventions for youth who have recently begun to use tobacco" is an evaluation objective for an agency desiring to evaluate an innovative peer-led program designed to reduce cigarette smoking among new users; however, this objective lacks precision and specificity. We cannot stress enough the importance of defining your evaluation objective in precise and specific terms (using the SMART acronym, previously presented in this chapter). In this example, samples of a few appropriate evaluation objectives could be:

- Will a newly developed 12-hour small-group peer-led cigarette smoking cessation program promote tobacco cessation among a greater percent of youth as compared to youth who receive no program at all?
- Will a newly developed 12-hour small-group peer-led cigarette smoking cessation program promote tobacco cessation among a greater percent of youth as compared to the agency's current smoking cessation program?

Thus, the evaluation objective should provide targeted and pertinent information that ensures that the evaluation efforts are accurately directed.

Step 4: Selecting a research design that meets the evaluation objective. The choice of research designs ranges from simple studies of a single group to complex studies of entire communities. The guiding principle in making the selection of an evaluation design is "balance and practicality." For example, if the program was implemented within an entire community, then a quasi-experimental design versus a true experimental design is appropriate. Also, the amount of resources available will dictate the design. If resources are limited, then it may not be possible to collect data in a control community and a simple, one group, pre-post-test design may be all that is feasible. This point warrants a bit more discussion from the perspective of the program evaluator. Often the program evaluator does not have a great deal of latitude in selecting the most rigorous design. As noted, there may be fiscal constraints, time constraints, resource constraints, and agency or community constraints, all of which may restrict the application of the most appropriate design. As a result, program evaluators may feel dejected and demoralized, knowing that the design they would prefer to implement cannot be implemented. Remember, you are not the final arbiter in this process; you are engaged to assist an organization, community, or agency in meeting their needs and, of course, these institutions operate under different statutes, policies, and procedures that can impact both design selection and implementation. You need to be able to develop the most appropriate evaluation design within the confines specified by the agency. As Mick Jagger used to say, "You can't always get what you want. . . but sometimes you get what you need." Be flexible, be responsive, and be able to adjust your proposed design based on continued dialogue with agency representatives so that it is suitable, implementable, and feasible.

Step 5: Selecting variables for measurement. The immediate goal when selecting variables is

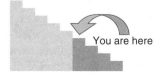
You are here

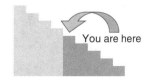
You are here

to be absolutely sure that every relevant **variable** is identified. A variable is anything that varies, meaning it can assume a range of values.

The evaluation objective, the literature review, and the needs assessment are all valuable in informing the selection of variables. In our example above of the diabetes medication adherence program, the underlying theory driving the program posits that the program should be efficacious by targeting participants' family environment, as social support is an environmental influence of individual behavior. Thus, it is incumbent upon the evaluators to measure participants' perceived level of family support in addition to other theory-derived critical variables.

The way in which the variables are measured is equally important. Like research, measurement is a carefully calibrated process. It involves identifying appropriate measures, or adapting existing measures to your unique research question, or, in some cases, creating new measures.

Step 6: Selecting the sampling procedure. There are numerous sampling procedures that can be used in evaluation research.

Sampling exists across a continuum of complexity and rigor. The sampling procedure employed is one of the most critical determinants of **external validity**. External validity refers to the ability to generalize study findings to the population of individuals with similar characteristics represented in the study sample. It should be noted, however, that not all research studies require a sampling procedure that yields high external validity. For example, a program evaluation specifically for a community agency concerned with their particular clients most likely does not need high external validity, whereas an evaluation of a newly created program designed to prevent drunk driving of teens will require a high level of external validity before it can be used in communities beyond the one in which it was tested.

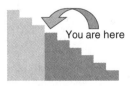

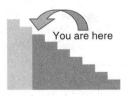

Step 7: Implementing the research plan. A basic requirement of **internal validity** is consistency in the implementation of all study protocols. Internal validity implies that the study is not confounded by design, measurement, or poor implementation of study procedures. Protocols explicitly spell out key procedures, such as the sampling procedure to be used, how participants will be assigned to intervention conditions, when and where assessments will occur, who will provide the assessments, whether assessors will be blind to participants' study condition, what participants will be told or not told about the research study, and how reticent participants will be enticed to return for follow-up assessments. Because protocols are generally quite detailed, subtle departures from these detailed plans can be a common problem. Over time, however, this "drift" can amount to substantial changes in the way late-entry participants are treated as compared with those enrolling earlier in the study.

As an example of drift, consider the study of enhancing diabetes medication adherence outlined earlier in this chapter. The protocol specifies that adults will be randomly assigned to either: (1) the motivational DVD plus usual care, or (2) the no-treatment usual care condition only. Further, assume that the protocol states that random assignment will be achieved by drawing colored marbles from an opaque container. Blue marbles signify assignment to the motivational DVD condition and green marbles signify assignment to the no-treatment usual care condition. As the study begins, 100 blue and 100 green marbles are placed in the container. A dedicated research assistant has been charged with the implementation of this procedure. In the first 3 months of the study, the research assistant performs flawlessly. Subsequently, however, the assistant learns that some adults are benefiting from participating in the motivational DVD condition. This knowledge

Drift can be averted by vigilant monitoring through quality assurance procedures and prompt corrective feedback.

could be inadvertently shared with the research assistant by participants returning to the clinic for subsequent medical testing (to monitor blood glucose levels) and care. This perception leads the assistant to invite some adults (those with symptoms and signs of severe diabetes that may indicate nonadherence to medication and who blindly pulled a green marble) to return the marble and "draw again." Though well intentioned, this deviation from the random assignment protocol, repeated over time, may create a systematic bias with respect to the composition of adults assigned to the study conditions. Other common forms of drift include departure from the planned intervention, deviations in how assessments are administered, and departure from sampling protocols. Fortunately, drift can be averted by vigilant monitoring through quality assurance procedures and prompt corrective feedback.

Step 8: Analyzing the data. Once all the assessments have been conducted, a data set can be established. The data set consists of the variables measured for each participant. The data set is, of course, what will be analyzed to answer the research questions that were formulated in Step 3. It may be very helpful to have a systematic plan for how to create a consistent and logical data set. For example, you should consider how you should code missing values, how to handle skip patterns, and so on. Knowing ahead of time how you will handle some of your data issues will ensure you create a coherent and accurate data set. Thus, after checking

the data for logical inconsistencies (called "cleaning") and handling other data issues, the evaluation process becomes dependent on the analytic skills of the evaluation team. Parsimony is important at this step—the goal is *not* to perform a sophisticated analysis; instead, the goal is to perform an analysis that meets the evaluation objectives.

In the diabetes medication adherence vignette, a parsimonious analysis would be to simply compare the mean percentage of the participants' prescribed medication taken as recommended in the past week in each group, assessed at a designated point in time after the interventions have been completed. Suppose the mean percentages are 85.3% for the DVD plus usual care condition and 57.1% for the usual care condition. The means can be compared using simple statistical tests. Analyses, however, can become quite complex when considering logically occurring questions such as: (1) Do program effects differ based on the gender of the participant?, and (2) Do effects differ based on the age of the participant? Of course, these questions are vitally important and each requires a more detailed and complex statistical analysis.

Step 9: Communicating the findings. Evaluation research warrants communicating the findings to stakeholders, interested participants, or, in the case of funded evaluations, the funding agency. In certain instances the evaluation findings may also be communicated to policymakers. Indeed, this step holds the potential for enhancing the likelihood that the program's benefits may extend beyond those who participated in the study to affect the health of many through the adoption of the program by other agencies and organizations. Or, if unfavorable, then this step can provide evidence to stop the implementation of ineffective programs. Your evaluation

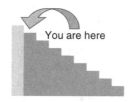
You are here

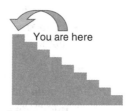
You are here

report should be constructed carefully with great attention to detail. You might also want to prepare a presentation and/or news release, in close conjunction with agency representatives, depending on the outcomes.

▶ Making the Evaluation Even Better

Start by doing what's necessary; then do what's possible; and suddenly you are doing the impossible.

—Francis of Assisi

Mediation Analysis: The Holy Grail of Program Evaluation

One area of evaluation research that has gained traction in the field is the use of mediation analysis to identify the pathway between the health-promotion program, its impact on hypothesized psychosocial mediators, and its effect on behavioral outcomes. Identifying and studying mediation may be particularly important for disentangling "active ingredients" of programs and allowing subsequent adaptations when programs are disseminated.

To illustrate mediation and its importance to program evaluation, we will use another example from our own research. In a study designed to reduce the incidence of sexually transmitted diseases among high-risk adolescent girls ($n = 715$), the theoretical framework underlying the intervention suggests some psychosocial variables as hypothesized mediators of the effects of the intervention on condom use and, as a consequence, on the proportion of girls in each study condition who are diagnosed with a sexually transmissible infection (STI). When we conducted our summative analysis, we identified statistically significant changes in the hypothesized psychosocial mediators (e.g., self-efficacy to use condoms), condom-use behaviors, and reductions in STD incidence (determined through laboratory assay) among girls in the health-promotion intervention

relative to girls randomly assigned to a comparison condition. The findings are indicative of an effective prevention program. However, the next step is to establish the pathway through which the program effectively changed the outcomes: determining the psychosocial variables that were affected by the intervention and which, in turn, affected condom use and led to a reduction in STI incidence.

Mediation is tested using a standard procedure described by Baron and Kenny (1986). To establish mediation, it is necessary to show that (1) the independent variable (participation in the health-promotion program) affects the outcome variable, (2) the independent variable (participation in the health-promotion program) affects the putative mediator(s), and (3) the mediator(s) has a significant effect on the outcome variable when the independent variable is controlled. Thus, we test for statistical significance of the intervention described earlier on the study's primary biological endpoint (i.e., incident STIs). We then test the effect on the potential mediators. Finally, we tested whether the potential mediators have a significant effect on STI incidence and self-reported condom use, controlling for program effects. This set of analyses indicates whether the three criteria of mediation are met. For example, if the health-promotion program effect were nonsignificant, these analyses would provide valuable information as to whether a lack of effects on mediators may account for the observed lack of significance. In addition, analyses establish whether changes in the mediators predict reduction in the proportion of participants with an incident STI and increase in condom use, even if the intervention effects are nonsignificant (see **FIGURE 15-3**).

While in-depth discussion of data analytic techniques is beyond the scope of this chapter, one statistical approach to test for mediation is path analysis. Path analysis determines the magnitude and standard errors for the coefficients a, b, and c, adjusting for any moderators that are independently associated with the process indicators at baseline. The magnitude of the indirect effect, or the difference between "c" in the absence of the process measure and after adding it to the model,

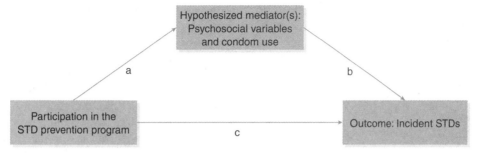

FIGURE 15-3 Analytic strategy for mediation analysis

provides an effect size for the degree of mediation for each process measure. The Sobel Test (Sobel, 1982), as specified by MacKinnon and Dwyer (1993) and MacKinnon, Lockwood, Hoffman, West, and Sheets (2002), is frequently used to test the statistical significance of the separate impact of each hypothesized mediator on the direct effect of the baseline health-promotion program by comparing adjusted and unadjusted effects of the baseline health-promotion program relative to their standard errors.

Culturally Competent Program Evaluation

> If you talk to a man in a language he understands, that goes to his head. If you talk to him in his language, that goes to his heart.
>
> —Nelson Mandela

Cultural competence is the knowledge of values, beliefs, and concepts of a given community's culture. Any effort to evaluate a health-promotion program must be firmly grounded in the culture of the target community. Ideally, an evaluator should be able to communicate and interact with individuals who are a part of the target community's culture. There are five principles that guide cultural competency in program evaluation.

An evaluator should be able to communicate and interact with individuals who are a part of the target community's culture.

- First, optimally the person conducting the evaluation should be a part of the community. The concept of "social location" applies, meaning that the evaluator should have a history of shared social experiences as a member of the community.
- Second, the evaluator should be prepared to recognize and respond to injustices observed in the community and to act as an advocate for change.
- Third, the effective evaluator should be willing and able to embrace multiple cultural perspectives. In many communities, this multicultural flexibility is required to adequately judge the value of the health-promotion program through the lens of diverse groups composing the community.
- Fourth, an in-depth understanding of the cultural norms prevalent in the target community is vital to the evaluation. Norms are a hallmark of culture in that they represent ways of thinking and viewing the world, including the beliefs that form values and guide behavior.
- Finally, the behavioral objectives of any health-promotion program should be reconciled with the cultural norms of a community. This is not to say that objectives must always be consistent with norms, as this would render many programs ineffective (e.g., tobacco reduction programs in a culture that values tobacco or sexual risk reduction programs in a culture that values sexual freedom). Instead, the consistency implies that the objectives are not squarely at odds with deeply rooted religious beliefs of highly

Finding a balance between changing prevalent health-risk behaviors and avoiding a direct challenge to cultural values can be a formidable and complex challenge.

cherished community values. We acknowledge, however, that finding a balance between changing prevalent health-risk behaviors and avoiding a direct challenge to cultural values can be a formidable and complex challenge.

Cost Evaluation Analysis in Health-Promotion Research

The increasing emphasis on cost containment, the emergence of the managed care environment, and the disproportionate increase in the cost of health care versus other expenditures over the past decade has prompted examining cost as one criterion for evaluating health-promotion programs. In a constrained fiscal environment it becomes imperative that we not only evaluate program in terms of impact (e.g., changes in behavior, attitudes, norms, and knowledge) and outcomes (e.g., changes in behavior, disease status, morbidity, mortality, and quality of life), but also assess cost-effectiveness. Such information is vitally important to program planners, policymakers, practitioners, and other persons involved in the design and implementation of health-promotion programs.

Arguably, one might question whether health-promotion programs should be held accountable to the standard that a program's economic benefits to society must outweigh its financial costs. However, whether or not one accepts that standard, the application of economic evaluation techniques is as appropriate to health promotion as they are to other health programs. For example, if two programs (e.g., interventions designed to promote smoking cessation among adolescents), using rigorous evaluation methodology yielded similar impact and outcome evaluations, but one program cost $2 to achieve smoking cessation while the other program cost $10, the

cost-effectiveness differential would favor the former program. Indeed, the former program could be markedly expanded to reach many more adolescents and still cost less than the latter program, yielding a substantial population-level benefit.

Unable to sidestep the issue of cost-effectiveness, health-promotion researchers, scientists, healthcare providers, policy analysts, and program planners need to become familiar with the theory and methods used to conduct cost-effectiveness studies. This methodology represents an entirely different perspective for many health-promotion researchers and practitioners. Most often, health-promotion researchers and practitioners have had their philosophical, theoretical, and methodological roots in the social science or health education disciplines rather than economics.

To assess cost-effectiveness, a **cost-effectiveness analysis** (CEA) can be conducted. A CEA is designed to determine the differences between two programs based on what it costs to deliver them. Stating it another way, cost-effectiveness is a method of evaluation to determine the relationship between program cost (input) and impact (output). Health economists refer to this as a ratio of cost per unit of impact. CEA can only be comparative and has little meaning when feasible alternative programs do not exist.

A CEA allows program developers and implementers to answer the question, "How much does this program cost?" For example, assume that a heart disease prevention program for the elderly has been demonstrated to be effective in reducing the risk of a heart attack. The program has a number of components, including changing the physical environment and providing physical exercises and education to produce the observed reduction in heart attacks. The program requires direct contact with the participant by a trained nurse. Assume the program has been able to demonstrate a significant difference, reducing the number of heart attacks by 20%. Including materials and staff time, it costs the program $100 for each participant, or $500 to avert one heart attack. The previous program the organization was using includes only the presentation of "heart healthy" educational materials to participants. This type of intervention is able to produce a reduction of one heart attack per hundred participants, which is obviously markedly less efficacious. It costs only $10 to produce these materials; however, it costs $1000 to reduce a heart attack. This example illustrates that the new program is cost-effective in reducing heart attacks as it cost markedly less than the current program to avert one heart attack.

Cost–benefit analysis (CBA) evaluates the relationship between program cost (input) and program health outcome. The analysis permits determination of the ratio of cost per unit of economic benefit and net economic benefit. Cost–benefit analysis can be used alone when comparable programs do not exist to determine the "value" of the program. The utility of CBA is that it can yield an absolute economic evaluation. This means the benefit is greater than the cost. CBA also allows the calculation of a standard return on investment, a calculation used often in non-healthcare settings.

We illustrate this important analytical strategy using the previous example. The new program was able to achieve 20 fewer heart attacks per 100 participants. If we assume that one fewer heart attack reduces a disabling injury, we can compute the cost for hospital care, doctor visits, medication, lost workdays, and quality of life in monetary terms. The program evaluator can compute the saving to the individual, the agency, and society of each heart attack that is averted through participation in the health-promotion program. This illustrates that the program was not only cost-effective but could be cost-beneficial. Finally, both types of analysis (CEA and CBA) are sensitive to the view of the beholder, typically one of four groups (the individual, provider, insurer or other payer, or society), and are value driven.

Conducting Cost-Effectiveness and Cost–Benefit Analyses

Conducting a cost-effectiveness or cost–benefit analysis can be as straightforward or as complex as you wish to make it. The key to conducting either is the ability to accurately monitor and capture expenditures. Cost expenditures are divided into four groups: (1) developmental costs, (2) production costs, (3) implementation costs, and (4) evaluation costs. The ability to monitor expenditures to determine categorically the different costs requires additional surveillance and data collection systems. These systems need to be structured toward the program and the specific elements of that program. The optimal time to initiate these monitoring systems is during the program development and design stages. Prospective cost assessment yields more precise and valid cost estimates than retrospective cost assessment. Attributing costs to one of these four groups allows the evaluator to have the data needed to compute the cost ratios readily available.

The optimal time to initiate these monitoring systems is during the program development and design stages.

Within the health-promotion literature, there are fewer evaluations of cost-effectiveness and cost–benefit analysis than any other type of evaluation. The majority of cost analyses have been implemented for policy and environmental interventions, such as seat belts in motor vehicles and changes in roadway design (Miller & Levy, 2000). However, given the emphasis on cost containment and the managed care environment, program evaluators will need to consider whether a cost analysis provides an important component to the planned impact and outcome evaluation.

▶ Summary

Evaluation research is an integral aspect of conducting theory-based health-promotion programs. Indeed, evaluation can and should be driven by the underlying theory used to guide the health-promotion program. The use of a logic model is essential throughout the process of program evaluation, especially with respect to the development of plans for formative and summative evaluation. Program planning and evaluation should be conducted in harmony; this is particularly vital for the critical task of developing program objectives. Great care must be taken in assessment procedures, with measurement of the outcome variable being perhaps the most critical task of the entire process. Finally, you learned in this chapter that evaluation should be culturally competent and that it may be extended to include cost-effectiveness analyses and cost–benefit analyses.

- An evaluation is a process evaluation if it assesses implementation objectives (e.g., dose and fidelity), and is an outcome evaluation if it examines the achievement of impact and outcome objectives.

▶ Take Home Messages

- No health-promotion program is perfect—not every individual exposed to a health-promotion program will adopt the appropriate health-promoting behaviors or demonstrate reductions in disease.
- Failure to adopt and maintain rigorous standards for evaluation of effective programs comes with the cost of wasting scarce resources on ineffective programs.
- Program planners and practitioners need to be directed at developing more effective programs.
- Rigorous program evaluation that identifies existing programs that demonstrate efficacy needs to be widely disseminated, adopted, and scaled-up to have optimal impact at a population level.
- Program evaluation, like program development, should be inextricably linked to theory.
- An evaluation plan should be made during program development, and program objectives and goals should be developed with their evaluability in mind.
- Program evaluations are typically categorized in one of two ways: by when the evaluation occurred and by what it attempts to measure.
- A formative evaluation is conducted before a program begins, whereas a summative evaluation is conducted after a program is completed.

▶ References

Baron, R. M., & Kenny, D. A. (1986). The moderator-mediator variable distinction in socialpsychological research: Conceptual, strategic, and statistical considerations. *Journal of Personality and Social Psychology, 51*, 1173–1182.

Centers for Disease Control and Prevention. (1999). Framework for program evaluation in public health. *MMWR Recommendations and Reports, 48*(RR11), 1–40.

Crosby, R. A., DiClemente, R. J., & Salazar, L. F. (2006). *Research methods in health promotion*. San Francisco, CA: Jossey-Bass.

Green, L. W., & Kreuter, M. W. (2005). *Health program planning: An educational and ecological approach* (4th ed.). New York, NY: McGraw-Hill.

MacKinnon, D. P., & Dwyer, J. H. (1993). Estimating mediated effects in prevention studies. *Evaluation Review, 17*, 144–158.

MacKinnon, D. P., Lockwood, C. M., Hoffman, J. M., West, S. G., & Sheets, V. (2002). A comparison of methods to test the significance of the mediated effect. *Psychological Methods, 7*, 83–104.

Miller, T. R., & Levy, D. T. (2000). Cost-outcome analysis in injury prevention and control: Eighty-four recent estimates for the United States. *Medical Care, 38*(6), 562–582.

Rossi, P. H., & Freeman, H. E. (1993). *Evaluation: A systematic approach* (5th ed.). Newbury Park, CA: Sage.

Sobel, M. E. (1982). Asymptotic intervals for indirect effects in structural equations models. In S. Leinhart (Ed.), *Sociological methodology* (pp. 290–312). San Francisco, CA: Jossey-Bass.

Sleezer, C. M., Russ, D. F., & Gupta, K. (2014). *A practical guide to needs assessment* (3rd ed.). San Francisco, CA: Wiley.

Windsor, R. A., Clark, N., Boyd, N. R., & Goodman, R. M. (2003). *Evaluation of health promotion, health education, and disease prevention programs* (3rd ed.). New York, NY: McGraw-Hill.

Chapter Opener: © MeskPhotography/Shutterstock; © Hero Images/Getty Images; © lzf/Shutterstock; © Henrik Sorensen/Getty Images

Glossary

A

action stage Stage of the transtheoretical model in which people have made specific, overt modifications in their lifestyles within the past 6 months.

adaptation Modifying a program to fit local needs, resources, history, demographics, culture, and other contextual variables.

adaptive self-endeavors The long-term formation and practice of routine health behaviors.

adoption Choosing to try something new.

alter Individuals connected to an ego who may influence the behavior of the ego.

applications Strategies will, by necessity, need to vary as a function of the population receiving the intervention – each time a new set of strategies is developed it becomes an application.

anhedonia Inability to experience pleasure.

attitude toward health behavior A primary construct in both the theory of reasoned action and the theory of planned behavior, which is composed of a person's collective evaluation of the worth or overall value of performing any given health behavior.

audience segmentation Dividing the targeted population into subgroups who have similar characteristics, preferences, and communication-related needs.

awareness knowledge Whether people do or do not know a given innovation exists.

B

backsliding Transtheoretical model of change (TMC) concept meaning that people may revert, at any time, to a previous stage. That is, individuals may "fall back" to a previous stage.

balance The extent to which two individuals who have a close relationship will share ties with a third individual to form a triadic relationship versus two individuals who do not have a close relationship.

behavior Any observable action or response of an organism, collective, or system to its environment, certain stimuli, or other inputs.

behavioral capacity A person's actual ability to perform a taskspecific behavior.

behavioral economics A hybrid field integrating principles from psychology and economics to understand individual-level values, preferences, and choices.

behavioral skills A primary construct in the information—motivation—behavioral skills (IMB) model, which includes both self-efficacy and actual ability to perform a given health behavior.

betweeness The extent to which an actor sits between others in a network.

breakpoint In demand curve analysis, the price that first suppresses consumption to zero.

bridging The connection across networks within a social system.

brokerage The lack of connection within a social network.

C

capacity building Efforts made to build the skills, motivation, and infrastructure necessary to use a scientific innovation.

causal indicators Questions or items associated with indexes that are designed to measure a construct where responses "cause" or define the value of the construct.

central route processing Evaluation of a persuasive communication message that involves active, intensive, and logical thought.

centrality The number of connections a particular node (or actor) has within a social network.

change agents People who actively attempt to promote adoption of an innovation.

changeability The likelihood that a given predisposing, reinforcing, or enabling factor can be altered by intervention efforts.

chronic diseases Conditions or health problems affecting a person for a prolonged period of time that may result in permanent residual disability (e.g., type 2 diabetes).

collective self-efficacy A group's shared belief in its ability to attain goals and accomplish desired tasks.

commodity Any product, service, or opportunity that can be traded in a formal or informal marketplace. With regard to health behaviors, this includes consumable commodities, such as food or psychoactive drugs (e.g., alcohol, tobacco, cocaine), as well as behavioral activities, such as gambling or sexual behavior.

communicable diseases See infectious diseases.

communication How network actors connect to share information and ideas within a social network and the frequency with which network actors contact one another.

communication structures Systems used for conveying information about an innovation.

community-based participatory research An approach to research that actively involves community members in all phases of the research process.

community needs assessment A data-gathering process essential to program planning.

community reinforcement approach A macrocosmic behavioral economic treatment approach that seeks to develop mutually exclusive sources of positive and negative reinforcement to compete with an undesirable behavior; typically used for treating substance use disorders.

complexity A dimension of health behavior that exists relative to skill sets and resources needed to perform a given health behavior.

concurrent validity A type of criterion-related validity that assesses the degree to which the scale measure correlates with a measure that has previously been validated. The two measures may be for the same construct, or for different, but presumably related, constructs.

confidence As used in the transtheoretical model of change, refers to the primary construct in self-efficacy and refers to individuals' belief in themselves to cope with high-risk situations without relapsing to unhealthy behaviors.

connectivity The number of nodes that would have to be removed in order for one actor to no longer be able to reach another.

consciousness raising A process of change that involves increasing awareness about the health-damaging effects of a particular behavior.

constant A measure or attribute that does not vary.

construct A theoretical or psychological concept.

construct validity The ability of a measure to perform the way in which the underlying theory hypothesizes.

contemplation stage The stage in the transtheoretical model in which people are actively thinking about changing a specific health behavior.

content knowledge Understanding and awareness of the advantages of a given health behavior.

content validity Form of validity that refers to the extent a measure represents all facets of the construct.

contingency management A microcosmic behavioral economic treatment approach that directly incentivizes protreatment behaviors, such as attendance, compliance, and, for substance use disorders, abstinence.

contingency management (also known as reinforcement management) A process of change in the transtheoretical model of change that provides consequences for taking steps in a particular direction.

convergent validity The extent to which a measure correlates with or is related to other measures designed to assess the same construct.

coping appraisal A cognitive process related to coping with a health threat that involves the perception that engaging in the protective behavior will lead to averting the threat, that the individual can confidently engage in the behavior to avert the threat, and the consideration that the costs are not too great for engaging in the behavior.

core implementation components The elements associated with effective implementation of a program, such as staff selection, in-service training, and ongoing coaching.

cost–benefit analysis An economic evaluation designed to evaluate the relationship between program cost (input) and program health (outcome).

counterconditioning A process of change in which a person substitutes healthier coping strategies for unhealthy ones.

criterion-related validity The degree to which the scale measure correlates with an outcome that to which, by definition, it should be related.

Cronbach's alpha A statistic or coefficient used to measure internal reliability that is calculated using the average interitem correlations and the number of items.

cross-sectional design A research strategy in which subjects are examined at one given point in time.

cues to action Events (internal or external), people, or things that move people to change their behavior.

D

danger control Engaging in strategies to avert a health threat.

decisional balance This process represents a "mental weighing" of the importance of the pros and cons associated with changing a specific behavior.

defensive avoidance When a person blocks further thoughts or feelings about a health threat and may also avoid exposing themselves to any further information about the topic.

delay discounting Devaluation of a reward based on its delay in time that is a behavioral economic index of impulsivity. Also referred to as capacity to delay gratification and intertemporal choice.

demand The level of actual or preferred consumption of a commodity at a single price or range of prices; commodities include behavioral outcomes as well as tangible goods.

demand curve analysis Systematic characterization of demand for a commodity from low to high prices; demand curve analysis permits multidimensional assessment of the relative value of the commodity via the topographic features of the demand curve.

density The number of actors/nodes divided by the possible number of ties. The values of density can range from 0 (nobody knows anyone) to 1 (everybody knows everybody else).

determinants Factors that influence health behavior.

diffusion The process by which a new idea (innovation) is communicated through certain channels over time among the members of a social system.

dissemination The intentional spreading of information for a specific purpose.

distal Determinants of health that are situated further back in the causal chain and are mainly in the macro-economic, political, educational, and environmental arenas, and which influence health through a number of more proximal factors.

divergent One aspect of construct validity that indicates the degree to which the scale measure does not correlate with other measures that it should not be related to.

dramatic relief A process of change used to produce increased emotional awareness or anxiety, followed by relief if appropriate action is taken.

E

effect indicators Questions or items associated with scales that are designed to measure a construct and infer some "effect" on a directly observable behavior.

ego Individuals whose behavior is being analyzed in the context of social network theory.

egocentric network analysis Using randomly selected focal nodes (individuals) to collect data on the number, nature, and characteristics of individuals who are connected to the sample of focal nodes.

elastic demand Periods of the demand curve that reflect supraproportionate decreases in consumption relative to increases in price.

elasticity In demand curve analysis, the slope of the demand curve, reflecting the relationship between price and consumption.

enabling factors Social, physical, economic, or structural elements that allow a person to enact a given health behavior; skill acquisition is also an enabling factor for many health behaviors.

enactive attainment A primary method of building a person's self-efficacy, based on guided practice often divided into subparts of a given behavior.

endogenous variable A variable in a causal or path model whose value is affected by other variables in the model.

environmental reevaluation A process of change that combines both affective and cognitive assessments of how the presence or absence of a certain health behavior affects one's social environment.

epidemiology The study of the distribution and determinants of health-related states or events (including disease), and the application of this study to the control of diseases and other health problems.

exogenous variable A variable in a causal or path model whose value is independent from the other variables in the model, but can affect other variables in the model.

expectancies The anticipated outcome of a given health behavior, combined with how much (or little) that outcome is desired.

expected net gain Weighing the perceived benefits of behavior change against the perceived barriers.

experimental design An investigation of the cause–effect relationships between variables that involves randomization, control, and manipulation on the part of the researcher.

exploratory factor analysis Type of factor analysis that is data driven and will reveal whether items cluster together to form a factor or any underlying dimensions of the construct that may not have been specified a priori.

external validity Refers to the ability to generalize study findings to the population of individuals with similar characteristics represented in the study sample.

extrinsic reinforcement A reward that is given by others for behavioral adoption of an innovation.

F

face validity Very basic form of validity in which it is determined whether the measure "appears" to measure what it is supposed to measure.

facilitating factors Internal or external factors that make the adoption of a given health behavior easier.

factor analysis Statistical technique for assessing the underlying dimensions of a construct, if in fact they exist, and for refining the measure.

factor loadings The correlations between items and their underlying factor.

fear appeal A message designed to elicit fear in an attempt to persuade an individual to pursue some predefined course of action.

fear control Engaging in coping responses that reduce fear but prevent a danger-control process from occurring.

fidelity The degree of correspondence between the program as intended and the program as actually implemented.

formative evaluation One type of evaluation that is designed to produce data and information used to improve a health promotion program during the developmental phase and document the feasibility of program implementation.

frequency The need to repeat a given health behavior on a daily, weekly, monthly, or yearly basis.

G

game theory A subdiscipline within behavioral economics that focuses on interactions between individuals in competition for resources.

goal-directed action Behaviors that are specific to a given objective, such as eating five servings of fruits or vegetables each day.

H

health A state of being indicated by the absence of disease or infirmity and encompassing complete physical, mental, and social well-being.

health behavior The actions, responses, or reactions of an individual, group, or system that prevent illness, promote health, and maintain quality of life.

helping relationships A process of change that combines caring, trust, openness, and acceptance, as well as support, for the healthy behavior change.

heuristics Experience-based techniques such as "rules of thumb," common sense, or trial and error that are used to make decisions and solve problems.

homophily The extent to which individuals within a social network form relationships with other individuals who share similar characteristics.

hypothesized mediator A factor that is influenced by a health promotion program and, in turn, influences a change in health behavior.

I

illness behavior Health behavior undertaken by individuals diagnosed with a disease to get well and manage their illness.

impact evaluation This type of evaluation asks whether the program had a direct effect on health behaviors.

implementation The execution or carrying out of a public health program.

importance The degree of correspondence between a predisposing, reinforcing, or enabling factor and actual adoption of a given health behavior.

indicated approach Public health interventions that first involve a screening process, and aim to identify individuals who exhibit early signs of developing the disease (e.g., administering a screener to identify youth who might be suicidal and then implementing appropriate intervention).

induction The direct or indirect influence that an actor has on the attitudes, beliefs, or behaviors of another person in a social network.

inelastic demand Periods of the demand curve that reflect subproportionate decreases in consumption relative to increases in price.

infectious diseases Diseases caused by pathogenic microorganisms, such as bacteria, viruses, parasites, or fungi; the diseases can be spread, directly or indirectly, from one person to another. Also referred to as communicable diseases, contagious diseases, or transmissible diseases. Influenza is an example of an infectious disease.

information The facts or knowledge shared between network actors.

inhibiting factors Internal or external factors that make the adaption of a given health behavior difficult.

innovation An idea, practice, or object that is perceived as new.

innovation–evaluation information Information that allows people to evaluate the worth of a given innovation before adoption occurs.

intensity (of demand) In demand curve analysis, demand for a commodity at zero or minimal price; also, the y-axis intercept reflecting the peak level of commodity demand.

intent As a surrogate for actual behavior, this is a way to assess whether a person has decided to adopt a given health behavior.

internal reliability Type of reliability of a measure that assesses the extent to which the measure has consistency across its items.

internal validity Refers to a study that is not confounded by design, measurement, or poor implementation of study procedures.

interval Type of measurement in which the values represent rank ordering but also reflect equal and consistent differences between values. A zero point is arbitrary, however.

intervention A planned and systematically applied program designed to produce behavior change and/or improve health outcomes.

J

jury of experts A panel of professionals who possess expertise with respect to the construct(s) under consideration.

K

knowledge Information and skills acquired through experience, observation, or education.

L

laboratory demand paradigms Human laboratory protocols that examine the relationship between consumption of a commodity and its price. These studies typically use money or effort as indices of price and examine behavior under highly controlled conditions in which price is the only variable that changes.

laggards People who are extremely slow to adopt a given innovation or innovative health practice.

law of demand The economic principle that, all other things being equal, increases in costs for a commodity will result in decreases in consumption.

level of analysis The socioecological level at which findings will be applied and conclusions drawn.

level of motivation A person's desire to adopt a given health behavior.

likelihood of action The degree of motivation a person has to engage in the health behavior.

logic model A graphical or tabular depiction of how various inputs, activities, outputs, and outcomes of a health promotion program are related.

longitudinal design A research strategy in which the same group of subjects is examined at multiple time points.

M

macro-level Examining the interactions of a large population, such as nation or civilization.

maintenance stage Stage of the transtheoretical model in which people have modified their health behavior for more than 6 months.

matching law The psychological law of allocation pertaining to behavior in a controlled environment between multiple opportunities for reinforcement that proposes that an organism's behavior over time matches the relative reinforcement available.

mavenism Having the expertise relative to a specific content area of knowledge and/or skill.

mediation analysis Identification of the pathway between the health promotion program, its impact on hypothesized psychosocial mediators, and its effect on behavioral outcomes. Identifying and studying mediation may be particularly important for disentangling active ingredients of programs and allowing subsequent adaptations when programs are disseminated.

mediator A variable that temporally "comes between" a predictor and an outcome.

method A method is the program activity that will be used to leverage change in a given identified determinant.

meso-level Examining the interactions of a population size, such as a community or town, which falls between the micro and macro levels in which the analysis may reveal connections between these two levels.

message components The theoretical building blocks of the message, such as perceived susceptibility, perceived severity, and perceived efficacy.

message tailoring Any combination of strategies and information intended to reach one specific person, based on characteristics that are unique to that person, related to the outcome of interest, and derived from an individual assessment.

message targeting The development of messages for a particular group.

metacontingencies Group-based reinforcements for a collective behavior within a community.

metric Standards or sets of measurements.

modifying factors Factors that change or influence one's perceptions related to the condition or disease, such as cultural factors, education level, past experiences, skill level, or motivation.

morbidity The number of people living with a disease in a given time period or place and expressed as a rate or proportion of persons with the disease to the total population.

mortality The number of deaths that have occurred in a given time period or place and expressed as a rate or proportion.

mutuality The reciprocal nature of relationships that involve a give and take between two entities.

N

negative reinforcement Taking away a stimulus, something valued as bad or aversive to maintain a certain behavior or response.

network A set of objects (nodes) and a mapping or description of relations between the objects/nodes.

nodes/actors Individuals who comprise a social network.

nominal Type of measurement in which the values refer to names or categories.

O

objective A quantifiable action that (when achieved) will contribute to achieving behavior change.

observational design An investigation of the possible effect of some variable of interest or treatment on an outcome with no manipulation on the part of the researcher.

operational definition A statement of the procedures or ways in which a researcher will measure the constructs or behaviors.

optimistic bias A state when people do not see themselves as being as vulnerable to the adverse consequences of health-risk behaviors as their peers who engage in the same risk behaviors.

ordinal Type of measurement in which the values represent rank ordering but do not describe relative size or degree of differences.

outcome evaluation This is a type of evaluation that asks whether the program had a direct effect on indicators of disease or actual reduction in morbidity or mortality.

outcome expectations Anticipatory outcomes of engaging in a behavior.

output maximum (O_{max}) In demand curve analysis, the maximum amount of expenditure on a commodity across prices.

P

perceived barriers Factors that a person perceives as preventing him or her from carrying out a health behavior, quitting a negative health behavior, accessing health care, or attending a program, and so on (e.g., smoking cessation program costs too much).

perceived behavioral control A collective perception of the strength of facilitating factors and inhibiting factors associated with a given health behavior.

perceived benefits A person's opinion of the value or usefulness of a new behavior in decreasing the risk of developing a disease.

perceived severity The degree to which an individual believes a condition and/or disease and its consequences are serious.

perceived susceptibility The belief regarding the probability and extent to which an individual might contract a condition and/or disease or experience a health threat.

perceived threat Theoretical construct that comprises the two constructs of perceived severity and perceived susceptibility.

perception An internally held belief.

peripheral route processing Evaluation of a persuasive communication message that is based on superficial qualities rather than cognitive processing.

personal agency A person's perception of control over his or her own behavior and the corresponding environmental conditions associated with that behavior. The capacity to exercise control over the nature and quality of one's life

persuasion The process of convincing people to adopt an attitude, opinion, idea, or action.

place The manner in which the exchange (i.e., the product reaches the consumer) happens. Places can be physical establishments or media channels.

policies Codified mandates to do something. These can be "big P" policies, such as federal regulations or "small p" such as a school policy.

positive reinforcement Giving something valued as good.

precontemplation stage The initial stage of the transtheoretical model. This is the stage in which people have no intention to take action in the foreseeable future (usually defined as within the next 6 months).

predictive A type of criterion-related validity that assesses the degree to which the scale measure "predicts" scores on a criterion measure assessed later in time.

predisposing factors Perceptions, attitudes, beliefs, and knowledge that favorably influence a person to adopt a given health behavior.

preparation stage In this stage of the transtheoretical model, people intend to adopt a new behavior in the immediate future, usually defined as within the next month. They may have already taken some steps in preparation to change their behavior.

preventive behavior Health behavior undertaken by healthy individuals to prevent the onset of disease.

price The cost to the consumer for obtaining the product, which can range from monetary, time, and effort tort, or social-psychological costs.

price maximum (P_{max}) In demand curve analysis, the price at which demand becomes elastic; also, the price at which O_{max} occurs, reflecting the transition to elastic demand.

primary prevention First level of prevention in public health that involves the use of health strategies, interventions, programs, or policies to prevent the occurrence of disease in a population before it occurs.

principles Public health principles include the emphasis on primary prevention, using data to make decisions, working across the social ecological model, population-based efforts, and evaluating our work.

principles knowledge Knowledge pertaining to the underlying method that allows the innovation to protect health and well-being.

probability discounting Devaluation of a reward based on its uncertainty that is a behavioral economic index of risk-proneness.

procedural knowledge Understanding of how to adopt a given health behavior.

processes A well-defined set of steps that should be followed to ameliorate some problem or improve programming efforts.

processes of change Processes of change are defined as essential principles that promote change. Intervention strategies that help modify a person's thinking, feeling, or behavior constitute a change process.

product A solution or package of benefits associated with the amelioration of a health-related problem. Products can range from physical products, services, or practices, to environmental changes.

program Typically behavioral change strategy that has a set of steps that should be followed. A program often has a curriculum or guide that should be implemented the same way each time.

program evaluation Application of rigorous methodological strategies to assess whether programs are actually effective in promoting the desired changes in health-risk behaviors.

program goals Broad statements describing what the program (intervention) is designed to accomplish.

program objectives Specific aims needed to accomplish program goals.

promotion The ways in which the exchange opportunity is advertised so that demand for the product occurs.

prophylaxis The prevention of disease or control of its possible spread.

prospect theory A theoretical approach to decision making that integrates perspectives from cognitive psychology and economics; according to prospect theory, preferences are not absolute, but vary based on relative gains and losses.

proximal Influences on health behavior that come from within the person's immediate environment.

psychological regulation Having control over one's own personal environment and interpersonal social milieu.

psychometrics The field of study concerned with the theory and technique of educational and psychological measurement.

purchase tasks Psychological assessments adapted from laboratory demand paradigms that characterize demand by assessing estimated consumption at an array of prices. These measures typically, but not always, use hypothetical commodities and permit greater assessment resolution, ease of administration, and applicability to typical behavior.

Q

qualitative variable A variable that has variability in kind or type.

quantitative variable A variable that has variability in degree.

quasi-experimental design An investigation of the cause–effect relationships between variables that involves control and manipulation, but not randomization.

R

ratio Type of measurement in which the values represent rank ordering, differences between intervals are equal and reflect proportionally similar differences in the actual levels of the characteristic, but has a true zero point.

reciprocal triadic causation The interplay between personal factors and environmental factors with behavior.

reinforcing factors External or internal rewards that shape continued acts of a given health behavior.

reinvention A user-centered application of the innovation which may not be compatible with the intended purpose.

relationship The connection between two or more people or things and the specific kind of interaction between network actors.

reliability The extent to which the scale or index consistently measures the same way each time it is used under the same condition with the same subjects.

resilient self-efficacy Enduring self-efficacy in spite of adverse conditions.

S

scientific innovation Any new knowledge, scientific advances, or technologies that may improve public health.

secondary prevention Second level of prevention that involves the use of health strategies, interventions, programs, or policies to diagnose and treat existing disease before it progresses and results in significant morbidity (e.g., screening programs to detect cervical cancer).

selective approach Public health interventions that target subgroups of the population who are at heightened risk of developing the disease by virtue of their membership in a particular segment of the population (e.g., men who have sex with men for HIV prevention).

self-efficacy One's confidence in one's ability to take action or to change a health-related behavior; a task-specific self-perception of one's personal ability.

self-liberation A process of change that is both the belief that one can change and the commitment and recommitment to act on that belief.

self-reevaluation A process of change that combines both cognitive and affective assessments of one's selfimage in conjunction with a given health behavior.

sick-role behavior Health behavior undertaken by individuals who perceive themselves to be ill and who seek relief or definition of the illness.

size The number of nodes/actors that constitute a network.

SMART objectives SMART objectives for evaluating a health promotion program include all of the following: the time period for expected changes, the specific direction of change that is expected, and how the change will be measured. In addition, objectives must be realistic and appropriate for the target population, precise in defining the behavior to be changed, and measurable in terms of health outcomes.

social etiology The underlying cause of the disease when it lies in the sociocultural environment.

social liberation A process of change that focuses on utilizing or increasing social opportunities that support health-promoting behavior change.

social marketing Applying commercial marketing strategies and techniques to achieve health-related behavioral goals that contribute to the wellbeing of society.

social norms Prevailing values, customs, and practices in a society.

split-half reliability A measure of consistency where the measure is split in two and the scores for each half are compared with one another. Stage-matched or stage-targeted intervention Interventions that use the transtheoretical model of change that are designed to be appropriate to the person's current stage of change.

staged A major premise of the transtheoretical model of change that suggests that people can be "staged," that is, they can be determined to be behavior. Staging is usually done with a staging algorithm.

stimulus control A process of change in which a person would remove cues for unhealthy behaviors and adds cues that support the adoption and maintenance of healthy behaviors.

strategy A strategy is the process employed to implement the program activity.

strong principle of progress As used in the transtheoretical model of change, it means that the pros of the health behavior change must increase by about 1 standard deviation from precontemplation to action.

structural barriers Social, cultural, economic, policy, regulation, or legal issues that preclude the easy adoption of a given health behavior.

subjective evaluation A personal favorable opinion of a given innovation.

subjective norm A primary construct in both the theory of reasoned action and the theory of planned behavior that is composed of a person's collective sense of what respected others would endorse as a "good" health behaviors.

successive-independent samples design A research strategy that incorporates multiple cross-sectional studies over successive time points using an independent sample for each time point.

summative evaluation Type of evaluation that is designed to produce data and information on the program's efficacy or effectiveness (its ability to do what it was designed to do) during its implementation phase.

superdiffuser A highly influential person who possesses the distinct traits of connectivity, persuasiveness, and mavenism to spread information within a social network.

T

task specific Because all health behaviors are different, it is important to think of each possible health behavior as a discrete task.

techniques (as used in transtheoretical model of change) Techniques are strategies, methods, or planned activities that are used to amplify a process of change.

temptation As used in the transtheoretical model of change, refers to the intensity of urges to engage in a specific behavior when confronted with challenging situations.

termination Sixth stage in the transtheoretical model of change that is generally omitted and represents zero temptation and 100% self-efficacy to cope without fear of relapse.

tertiary prevention Third level of prevention that involves health strategies, interventions, programs, or policies directed at assisting diseased and disabled people to reduce the impact of their disease. Medical care and rehabilitation are forms of tertiary prevention.

test–retest reliability Type of reliability of a measure that assesses the consistency of the measure across different time points.

theory of planned behavior An extension of the theory of reasoned action that involves the additional construct of perceived behavioral control.

threat appraisal A cognitive process involving an assessment of the rewards for engaging in an unhealthy behavior that may be offset or reduced by the seriousness of the health threat (i.e., the probability and severity of a negative outcome if no remedial action is taken).

traditional The physical contact and connections that occur in person.

translate Converting programs that have been deemed effective via rigorous research into a useable format and packaging the material for a large population of users.

transitivity The extent to which a relation that forms a tie between two actors is connected through another actor who serves as a link. If there is a tie between actor A and actor B, and a tie between actor B and actor C, then actor A will likely form a tie with actor C.

transtheoretical As used in the transtheoretical model of change. This model integrates processes and principles of individual-level behavior change from across major theories of psychotherapy, hence the name "transtheoretical."

triads The ties between three interconnected nodes.

U

universal approach Public health interventions that target the entire population versus specific risk groups.

V

validity The extent to which the scale or index measures what it is supposed to measure.

variable A measure that can take on more than one value.

verbal persuasion A primary method of building a person's selfefficacy, much like coaching.

vicarious experience A primary method of building a person's selfefficacy, based on learning by watching others and seeing their positive outcomes.

virtual Connections that occur online, particularly through social media websites.

volitionality A dimension of health behaviors that refers to the degree of personal control that somebody has over the performance of any given health behavior.

W

weak principle As used in the transtheoretical model of change, it means the cons of the health behavior change must decrease by 0.5 standard deviation from precontemplation to action.

whole network analysis Using a set of nodes as the study population to measure ties between selected nodes.

Index

Boxes, figures, and tables are indicated with *b*, *f*, and *t* following the page number.

"Goldilocks and the Three Bears" story as stage theory illustration, 95
Gonorrhea, 165
Granovetter, Mark, 182
Green, L., 42

H

Harmonic means, 268
Haythornthwaite, C., 186, 187
HBM. *See* Health belief model
Health and health behaviors, 3–23, 249
    attitude toward, 61
    barriers to change, 33, 37, 37*t*
    categories, 18, 18*t*
    causes of death, 4, 5*f*
    chronic diseases, 4, 6*t*
    complexity of health behavior, 9–11
    conceptualization of, 16–19, 16*t*, 18*t*
    defined, 4, 17
    dimensions of, 26–27, 28*f*
    diversity of, 26–27, 28*f*
    health promotion, 19–21, 20*f*
    individual and collective behaviors, 17
    multilevel causes and approaches, 33
    prevention, 8–16, 8*f*, 14*f*
    prioritization of, 16–19, 16*t*, 18*t*
    theory use in, 21–22, 22*f*, 31, 32*t*
Health belief model (HBM)
    perceived threat and fear appeals, 75, 77*f*, 79*f*, 82*f*
    SCT, relationship to, 125
    as value-expectancy model, 76–82
Health communication, 137–158
    applied examples, 155–158, 157*t*
    attributes of, 139, 140*t*
    central route processing, 144
    effects and dissemination, 138, 139*f*
    elaboration likelihood model, 144–147, 145*f*, 146*t*
    peripheral route processing, 147
    place, 151–152
    price, 150–151
    product, 148–149, 149*t*
    promotion, 152–153
    reception-yielding model, 141–143, 141*f*
    social marketing, 147–153, 149*t*
    tailored communications, 153–155, 154*f*
Health education, 49
Health effects, of social networks, 188–191

Health Program Planning: An Educational and Ecological Approach, 42
Health promotion, 250
    definition and background, 19–20, 19–21
    intervention, 296
    programs, 127*b*, 282–283
    in SCT, 58
    strategies, 20–21, 20*f*
    theoretical perspectives, 21–22
Health-protective behaviors, 241
Health-risk behaviors, 282
Health Utilities Index (HUI), 265
Healthy diet, TPB studies, 277*f*
Healthy People 2020 (Surgeon General's Report), 9–10, 26
Heart disease death rates, in U.S., 8
Helping relationships, 102
Hepatitis C, behavior change theories and, 32
Hereditary Genius (book), 256
Heuristics, 144–145
Hidden networks, 193
High-fidelity practitioner behavior, 237
HIV/AIDS
    applied examples, 155–158, 176–177
    EPPM and, 85
    PMT effectiveness and, 87
    social networking approaches for, 183
Homophily, 184, 188, 189*f*, 201–202
How-to knowledge, 203
HPV. *See* Human Papillomavirus
HUI. *See* Health Utilities Index
Human papillomavirus (HPV), 127*b*, 142, 145
    vaccination, 78–79, 79*f*
Hybrid corn adoption, 198, 199*f*
Hypothesized mediators
    determinant classification, 38
    identified factors and, 48
    as intervention targets, 33, 33*f*
    theory and, 34

I

IDU. *See* Injection drug use
Illness health behaviors, 18
IM. *See* Intervention Mapping
IMB model. *See* Information-motivation-behavioral skills model
Impact evaluations, 52, 52*b*, 287, 288–290

Implementation, 52*b*
    assessment, 236–237
    challenges, 237–238
    community participation importance, 45, 50–52, 51–52*b*
    core components, 234–236, 235*f*, 236*t*
    in DIT, 205
    drivers. *See* Core implementation components
    elements of, 233–234
    evaluation and, 50–52, 52*b*, 54
    factors affecting, 234
    funding requirements for, 274–275
    quality of, 219
    in SCT, 132–135
    as step in science to practice, 231–238, 232–233*f*, 233*b*
Importance, and changeability, 48
Impulsivity, 277–278
In-service training for implementation, 234–236
Indexes of constructs, 269, 270*f*
Indicated approach, as tertiary prevention, 14*f*, 15
Individual choice vs. environmental influence, 174
Individualized communications, 153, 154*f*
Induction, 188, 192*b*
Inductive approach to problem, 29–31
Infectious diseases, 4
Influenza vaccinations, HBM and, 77*f*
Information
    as assets of social network models, 186
    construct, 69–70
    flow, 186
    processing, 141, 141*f*
Information-motivation-behavioral skills (IMB) model, 68–71, 69*f*, 70*f*
Infrastructure, dissemination, 224–225*t*, 226
Inhibiting factors, 48, 65–68, 67*t*
Initial respondents, 191
"Injecting dyad level," 185*b*
Injection drug use (IDU), 184
Innovations and innovators
    adoption rates, 198, 199*f*
    in DIT, 199–200, 206–207
    innovation-decision process, 202–206
    innovation-evaluation information, 203
    use of term, 221–222